MIDWIFERY CONTINUITY OF CARE

2nd EDITION

MIDWIFERY CONTINUITY OF CARE

2ND EDITION

CAROLINE HOMER AO, PhD, MN, MScMed, RM

NICKY LEAP DMid, MSc, RM

PAT BRODIE AM, DMid, MN(Hons), RM

JANE SANDALL CBE, PhD, MSc, BSc(Hons), RM, HV

ELSEVIER

Elsevier Australia. ACN 001 002 357
(a division of Reed International Books Australia Pty Ltd)
Tower 1, 475 Victoria Avenue, Chatswood, NSW 2067

ISBN: 978-0-7295-4295-1

National Library of Australia Cataloguing-in-Publication Data

A catalogue record for this book is available from the National Library of Australia

Senior Content Strategist: Libby Houston
Content Project Manager: Fariha Nadeem
Edited by Christine Wyard
Proofread by Julie Ganner
Cover by Georgette Hall
Internal design: Standard
Index by Innodata Indexing
Typeset by Toppan Best-set Premedia Limited
Printed in China by 1010 Printing International Ltd.

Last digit is the print number: 9   8   7   6   5   4   3   2   1

CONTENTS

Foreword

Professor Lesley Page CBE
PhD, MSc, BA, RM, HFRCM, Honorary DSc
Visiting Professor, King's College London, United Kingdom
Adjunct Professor, University of Technology Sydney, NSW, Australia
Adjunct Professor, Griffith University, Queensland, Australia
Honorary Research Fellow, Oxford Brookes University, Oxford, United Kingdom

The development and evaluation of midwifery continuity of care ranks amongst one of the foremost developments in the progress of safe, high-quality and cost-effective maternity services, and the potential for a more satisfying role for those midwives who wish to practise in this way, over recent years. There is strong compelling evidence that midwifery continuity of care is associated with many benefits and no evidence of adverse effects. The benefits include a lower intervention rate, higher vaginal birth rate, lower assisted birth rate, lower pre-term birth rate and lower rate of fetal loss. In addition, women have found the care to be more satisfying, and feel better prepared for birth. There is evidence that women find the relationship with midwives satisfying. There are also benefits for the health system, including cost-effective care.

Through this research and development, we now have a deeper understanding of the problems of current maternity services in high-resource countries and the difficulties that many standard services face in providing responsive care. We now know of the problems with fragmented institution-focused services and complex systems of care, often operating to or beyond capacity. Fragmented services are littered with gaps and discontinuities—a risk to all, but particularly for vulnerable women and those with socially complex lives, or women living with other disadvantages. It is difficult to provide care responsive to the needs of individual women and their families, and to individual families and communities, through such fragmented and standardised services. There is also extensive variation in outcomes between different services, communities, places and countries. These outcomes include mortality and morbidity rates, and physiological birth and intervention rates. Inequalities in mortality and morbidity rates continue to prevail for those living in socioeconomic deprivation, between different ethnic groups, and for those women with mental health problems.

While services providing continuity of midwifery care have expanded, still far too few women have access to continuity of care, continuity of care of relationships, information and management. Scaling up and making services that support relationship-based continuity sustainable is now critical. Ensuring that continuity enables women and their midwives to get to know and trust each other over time is fundamental. This principle is key, but is often overlooked. Continuity of midwifery care should be embedded in health services that are woman centred and have a primary health or preventive orientation.

It is difficult to understand why midwifery continuity of care has taken so long to establish and scale up. But *Midwifery Continuity of Care* shows me we have in fact come a long way in understanding, and knowing what more needs to be explored and which questions need to be asked. Contained in the covers of this book is information that will give you the means to develop and practise in effective, sustainable and enjoyable models of care. I can't help thinking I wish we had known all this earlier—we could have avoided so many mistakes along the way!

I was also, as I read through the various chapters, reminded that the general advancement in understanding of implementation and improvement science, systems and cultures for the improvement of safety and quality, and knowledge of the socio-economic determinants of care, is now a great help to development.

From all sides—from high-quality international evidence, policy and surveys of quality of care and of midwife satisfaction—we are being shown that it is time to change. Although questions have been asked by many about the sustainability of midwifery continuity of care, it is becoming clear that it is the current mainstream systems of maternity care that are unsustainable. Many are working beyond capacity, with the dual problem of over- and under- intervention, and stretched resources as well as frustration and poor morale amongst midwives.

One of the difficulties, which so many of the chapters make clear, is that developing midwifery continuity is not just tinkering around the edges or running a pilot alongside the main service. Organising practice so that women and their midwives may work through a relationship of trust and respect is a transformative change. It is a change that depends not only on relationships between women and their midwives, professional autonomy, more flexibility and control over their practice arrangements, and a different culture of care, but also on collaborative and respectful work relationships. Collaboration is required within teams and between teams, between midwives doing continuity and core midwives, between midwives and doctors, midwives and managers, midwives and support staff, user representatives, and with the community served. Developing midwifery continuity of care requires a change of systems and culture. Given the tension of keeping stretched-at-the-seams services going, undertaking this transformation is highly challenging.

It would be remiss not to mention that developing relationship-based continuity of care sometimes creates antagonism and 'us and them' cultures, which must, if possible, be prevented or at least recognised. A bubbling resentment and fear of change often seems to boil over into a debate about on-call and overwork. This might of course be expected: it is a response to a fundamental change that alters power dynamics. The beautiful descriptions of different approaches help. Some of these are nationwide, for example in New Zealand, in the Netherlands and in Canada, as well as local developments in the UK, Australia and Ireland. The message is that, as long as continuity of relationship is provided, there are many ways of organising. This can include both pure forms of continuity and hybrid models that do not require on-call and are based around shift working.

You will have gathered by now that I really like this book! Above all, it is a really good read. It is well referenced and comprehensive. There are deeply reflective chapters that seem to race along. Whether you are a midwife in practice, an activist, a policy maker, a manager, a lobbyist or a parliamentarian seeking change, you will find chapters in this book that will inform, inspire to aspire, tell you the pitfalls and what works, and help you face 'the elephant in the room'.

It is a book that shows us there is still an important place for books—an important place particularly for books like this that gather together evidence, insights, advice and information. It is edited and written by people who have experience in practice, in planning and implementation, and in research and evaluation, who are deeply knowledgeable. *Midwifery Continuity of Care* will be the 'must have' resource to help in the thought, planning and ongoing support that is required to scale up and sustain midwifery continuity of care. Not only does it provide a wonderful synthesis of the plentiful evidence that makes such a compelling case for change, but also the chapters really make you think. At the same time, they give advice, describe theories, tell stories to illuminate, and analyse the development of midwifery continuity of care. There are boxes and vignettes and checklists too that help to focus. The contents will help those starting out and those more advanced in planning, implementation and practice. There are veins of wisdom throughout the book drawing on evidence and experience and relating to theory—for example, theories of sustainability. There are moments of bright illumination too, for example hearing about traditions and beliefs of Indigenous peoples, insight and experience. The likening of maternity care to a 'four-voice invention' (from Bach) is pure magic.

I have been involved in developing, implementing, evaluating and practising in midwifery continuity of care for many years. But nevertheless I found myself as I read being lifted by hope, inspired and better informed. There was a constant 'oh yes' and 'of course' or 'I never thought of that', or being moved by the ideals and rooted in its practical nature. Well I could go on but … .

Over to you now—read through, dip in, turn over page corners, make notes and take it to your colleagues and managers. Above all, enjoy. This is about a more positive future for women and their families, for midwives and for health services. We are here to help every woman and her baby and family get off to the best start. That one-to-one relationship between the woman and her midwife or midwives is crucial to the best start possible. Read so you can contribute, in one way or another, to this best start.

Lesley Page CBE
Oxford

ABOUT THE EDITORS

Pat Brodie AM is a well-known Australian midwifery leader with extensive experience in midwifery practice, management and policy reform over four decades. She has led and inspired the development of midwifery models of care to enable midwives to work to the full potential of their role and better meet the needs of pregnant women and new mothers.

Caroline Homer AO is an Australian midwifery leader with more than 25 years experience as a clinician, educator, researcher and advocate. She has studied, worked in, established and evaluated midwifery continuity of care for two decades and is a passionate believer that this type of care should be the norm for all women.

Nicky Leap has been involved in midwifery practice, education and research for over 40 years. She has been at the forefront of the development of midwifery continuity of care in mainstream maternity services in both the UK and Australia and has a wealth of practical experience in this area.

Jane Sandall CBE is a UK-based midwife academic and social scientist who has spent over 30 years as a clinician, educator and researcher. She has worked in, supported policy implementation and researched continuity of care in maternity care and for other groups. She is particularly interested in how continuity of care is at the heart of safe and high-quality care.

EDITORS

Pat Brodie
Adjunct Professor of Midwifery, Centre for Midwifery, Child and Family Health,
Faculty of Health, University of Technology Sydney, NSW, Australia

Caroline Homer
Co-Program Director, Maternal and Child Health, Burnet Institute, Melbourne, Australia;
Visiting Distinguished Professor of Midwifery, Centre for Midwifery, Child and Family
Health, University of Technology Sydney, NSW, Australia;
Visiting Professor, King's College London, United Kingdom;
Visiting Professor, Cardiff University, United Kingdom;
Adjunct Professor, School of Public Health and Preventative Medicine, Monash University,
Melbourne, Australia;
Honorary (Professorial Fellow), Melbourne School of Population and Global Health,
Faculty of Medicine, Dentistry and Health Sciences, University of Melbourne, Australia

Nicky Leap
Adjunct Professor of Midwifery, Centre for Midwifery, Child and Family Health,
Faculty of Health, University of Technology Sydney, NSW, Australia

Jane Sandall
Professor of Social Science and Women's Health, Department of Women and Children's
Health, School of Life Course Science, Faculty of Life Sciences and Medicine,
King's College London, United Kingdom;
Adjunct Professor, Centre for Midwifery, Child and Family Health, University of
Technology Sydney, NSW, Australia

CONTRIBUTORS

Jyai Allen
Senior Research Officer, Building On Our Strengths (BOOSt) project, Midwifery Research
Unit, Mater Research Institute, University of Queensland, Queensland, Australia

Andrew Bisits
Obstetrician and Gynaecologist, Royal Hospital for Women, Randwick, NSW, Australia;
Adjunct Professor, University of Technology Sydney, NSW, Australia;
Associate Professor, University of New South Wales, NSW, Australia

Helen Cheyne
Professor of Maternal and Child Health Research, RCM (Scotland);
Professor of Midwifery Research, NMAHP Research Unit, University of Stirling, Stirling, United Kingdom

Kirstie Coxon
Associate Professor (Research), Department of Midwifery, Faculty of Health, Social Care and Education, Kingston and St George's (a joint enterprise of Kingston University and St George's), University of London, United Kingdom

Susan Crowther
Professor of Midwifery, Faculty of Health and Social Care, Robert Gordon University, Aberdeen, United Kingdom

Lorna Davies
Associate Head of Midwifery and Principal Lecturer, School of Midwifery, Te Hoe Ora, Department of Nursing, Midwifery and Allied Health, Christchurch, New Zealand

Deborah Davis
Professor of Midwifery, University of Canberra and ACT Government, Health Directorate, Australia

Declan Devane
Professor of Midwifery, NUI Galway, Ireland;
Deputy Dean, College of Medicine, Nursing and Health Sciences;
Scientific Director, HRB-Trials Methodology Research Network;
Director, Evidence Synthesis Ireland;
Director, Cochrane Ireland

Roslyn Donnellan-Fernandez
Senior Lecturer in Midwifery, Director, Primary Maternity Care Programs, School of Nursing and Midwifery, Griffith University, Queensland, Australia

Natasha Donnolley
Project Officer, National Perinatal Epidemiology and Statistics Unit, Centre for Big Data Research in Health (CBDRH), NSW, Australia

Mandy Forrester
Head of Quality and Standards, The Royal College of Midwives, London, United Kingdom;
Visiting Fellow, Bournemouth University, Bournemouth, United Kingdom

Della Forster
Judith Lumley Centre, La Trobe University and Maternity Services, The Royal Women's Hospital, Melbourne, Australia

James Harris
Course Director, MSc Implementation and Improvement Science, King's Improvement Science Fellow, Lecturer in Midwifery, Florence Nightingale Faculty of Nursing and Midwifery, King's College London, United Kingdom

Andy Healy
Senior Health Economist, CLAHRC South London / King's Improvement Science and Kings Health Economics, Health Services and Population Research Department, Institute of Psychiatry, Psychology and Neuroscience, King's College London, United Kingdom

Billie Hunter
RCM Professor of Midwifery and Director, WHO Collaborating Centre for Midwifery Development, School of Healthcare Sciences, College of Biomedical and Life Sciences, Cardiff University, United Kingdom;
Adjunct Professor, University of Technology Sydney, NSW, Australia;
Honorary Professor, Nottingham University, Nottingham, United Kingdom;
Honorary Professor, University of Surrey, Guildford, United Kingdom

Holly Powell Kennedy
Helen Varney Professor of Midwifery, Yale School of Nursing, Connecticut, United States of America

Sue Kildea
Director, Midwifery Research Unit, Mater Research Institute University of Queensland (MRI-UQ), UQ School of Nursing, Midwifery and Social Work, Queensland, Australia; Mothers, Babies and Women's Services, Mater Health Service, Queensland, Australia; Affiliate Professor, Poche Centre for Indigenous Health, UQ, Queensland, Australia; Honorary Appointment, University of Nottingham, Nottingham, United Kingdom

Ann Kinnear
CEO, ACM Fellow, Paul Harris Fellow, Australian College of Midwives, Canberra, Australia

Christine McCourt
Professor of Maternal Health and Centre Lead, Centre for Maternal and Child Health Research, School of Health Sciences, City, University of London, London, United Kingdom

Helen McLachlan
Professor of Midwifery and Discipline Lead (Midwifery), Judith Lumley Centre, School of Nursing and Midwifery, La Trobe University, Melbourne, Australia

Michelle Newton
Director of Teaching and Learning, School of Nursing and Midwifery, College of Science, Health and Engineering, La Trobe University, Melbourne, Australia

Michael Nicholl
Clinical Director, Division Women's Children's and Family Health, North Shore Ryde Health Service;
Clinical Director, Maternal Neonatal and Women's Health Network, Northern Sydney Local Health District, NSW, Australia;
Clinical Professor, Northern Clinical School, Sydney Medical School, St Leonards, NSW, Australia

Jane Raymond
Manager, Maternity and Newborn Team, NSW Health, Australia

Mary Ross-Davie
Director for Scotland, The Royal College of Midwives, London, United Kingdom

Vanessa Scarf
Lecturer in Midwifery, Centre for Midwifery, Child and Family Health, Faculty of Health, University of Technology Sydney, NSW, Australia

Julie Simpson
Midwifery Manager, Industrial Relations and Workforce Management, Workplace Relations, NSW Ministry of Health, North Sydney, NSW, Australia

Suzanne Tyler
Executive Director for Services to Members, The Royal College of Midwives, London, United Kingdom

Cathy Warwick
Chair British Pregnancy Advisory Service, United Kingdom;
Non-executive Director, Kingston Hospital NHS Trust, London, United Kingdom;
Visiting Professor, King's College London, United Kingdom;
Visiting Professor, Chinese University, Hong Kong

Jan White
Clinical Manager, Women's Health, Neonatology and Paediatrics, Sydney Local Health District, NSW, Australia

REVIEWERS

Kerry Adams
Senior Lecturer, School of Midwifery, Otago Polytechnic, Dunedin, New Zealand;
Deputy Chair, Midwifery Council of NZ, New Zealand

Michelle Anderson
Research Midwife, Royal Free NHS Foundation Trust, London, United Kingdom

Cathy Ashwin
Head of MIDIRS;
Professional Editorial Advisor to RCM Midwives Magazine;
Honorary Assistant Professor, University of Nottingham, Nottingham, United Kingdom

Elaine Burns
Senior Lecturer, School of Nursing and Midwifery, Western Sydney University, Sydney, NSW, Australia

Lyn Francis
Lecturer, School of Nursing and Midwifery, Western Sydney University, NSW, Australia

Diane M. Fraser
Emeritus Professor of Midwifery, University of Nottingham, Nottingham, United Kingdom

Sadie Geraghty
Director of Clinical Education, Charles Darwin University, College of Nursing and Midwifery, Darwin, Australia

Michelle Gray
Lecturer in Nursing and Midwifery, School of Nursing, Midwifery and Paramedicine, University of the Sunshine Coast, Queensland, Australia

Lisa Johnson
Caseload Midwife, The Townsville Birth Centre, Queensland, Australia

Katrina Jones
Clinical Midwifery Manager, Western Australia Country Health Service, Bunbury, Australia

Susan McDonald
Professor of Midwifery at La Trobe University and Mercy Hospital for Women, Melbourne, Australia

Rachel Reed
Senior Lecturer in Midwifery, Discipline Leader: Midwifery, School of Nursing, Midwifery and Paramedicine, University of the Sunshine Coast, Queensland, Australia

Mary Sidebotham
Director, Primary Maternity Care Programs, School of Nursing & Midwifery, Griffith University, Queensland, Australia;
Program Lead, Education and Workforce, Transforming Maternity Care Collaborative (transformingmaternitycare.org)

FROM THE ROYAL COLLEGE OF MIDWIVES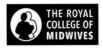

The Royal College of Midwives fully supports the aim that midwifery continuity of carer across the maternity journey should be the central model of maternity care for women. We know that the development of midwifery continuity of carer requires a very significant shift in the way our maternity services are delivered. In order to make the transition from our current models of care safely and sustainably, midwives, their managers and the wider teams need to be properly informed, prepared and supported. This latest edition of Midwifery Continuity of Care is an excellent addition to the resources and toolkits that help think through those knotty issues of flexibility and self-management, team working and mutual respect and safe levels of staffing.

By sharing the examples of those already on the journey this book provides confidence that, with commitment, resources and harnessing enthusiasm, midwifery continuity of care can work for women and midwives.

FROM THE AUSTRALIAN COLLEGE OF MIDWIVES

The Australian College of Midwives endorses this book — Midwifery Continuity of Care. We recognise that knowing your midwife — being cared for by, and able to build trust and rapport with, the same midwife or group of midwives during pregnancy, through labour and birth, and into the early weeks of mothering — has benefits for mothers, babies and society. It is known as the 'Gold standard' of maternity care and the Australian College of Midwives advocates for all women to have access to this model of care.

Prologue—Why Midwifery Continuity of Care Matters, for All Women in All Situations

We start our book with the voice of a woman who has generously written about her story of giving birth to her two children. This story highlights the importance of midwifery continuity to all women, regardless of possible complexities, planned mode of birth and context. We agreed to keep this woman's name confidential to protect her privacy. We hope you enjoy this story, which is unique but also familiar to many of us who work in or know maternity services.

Caroline, Nicky, Pat and Jane

'When I was pregnant with my first baby I was living in a city in the south-west of England and initially I was seeing the community midwife at my local GP surgery. So I did see one midwife briefly a few times at the surgery but, because the test for gestational diabetes was borderline positive, I had to see many different members of the hospital team for most of my antenatal care.

'I felt like I was pushed from pillar to post. I was in a system being told that I had to follow the rules and I felt like more of a number than a person. I had to do six blood tests every single day for months, recording my blood sugar level results as well as everything I was eating. The blood tests were, for the majority of the time, all in the normal range but no one seemed interested in discussing this with me and I had to keep telling my story to different people. I was told early on that I would have to be induced 2 weeks before my baby was due.

'I was seeing a different registrar and midwife at every visit. It was always just surface level conversations; there was never any in-depth discussion about my feelings or my thoughts about how the results were all normal. I constantly had to repeat to different people what had happened, why I was there, why I thought I wasn't really diabetic. No one seemed to listen and they were very busy.

'At 38 weeks I kept pushing the consultant team that I should go up to my due date and at that stage they did look at my book where they'd made me record all my blood sugar results and agreed that I could continue to my due date, at which stage they would then talk to me about induction. As it happened, I ended up developing pre-eclampsia—high blood pressure—just prior to my due date and so I ended up being admitted and induced anyway.

'I saw different teams of people throughout that induction and my labour. I think it wasn't helped by the fact that it fell over a weekend. I got to 8 cm over 36 hours but I ended up having an emergency caesarean as my baby was getting distressed.

'On the postnatal ward the staff were very busy. My baby was healthy and a normal weight for a baby born at 40 weeks. But because I'd been labelled with gestational diabetes—that's what it said in my pregnancy record—they kept pricking my baby's heel. He was "borderline low blood sugar" so they put down a tube through his nose and fed him formula. They then said he was jaundiced and so they took him away from me and put him in a special cot under lights. This made breastfeeding him very difficult and I had lots of different advice from a series of well-meaning staff.

'When we went home 4 days later I thought I would get on better in the calm of my own home but I was already having serious difficulties breastfeeding my baby. I had one home visit from the community midwifery team—someone who I hadn't met before. She came out to our home the day after I got back. She told me that for my subsequent postnatal visits I would have to go to a special clinic at the hospital. It was hard for me to do that; I couldn't drive after my caesarean and there was no direct bus route. We had to go in on a Sunday morning when my husband could drive me there to see somebody—another person who I hadn't seen before who knew nothing of my history. My baby and I continued to struggle with breastfeeding.

'When I was pregnant again a couple of years later, we had moved to a country area. I was lucky that a midwife attached to the small midwifery-led unit was the community midwife providing continuity of care for women in the area where I now live. I met Annie, my lovely midwife. She came to my house for our first visit and spent a couple of hours getting to know my husband and me. She took time taking a history and listening to how we both felt about my previous experience, what my thoughts were about this pregnancy, and what I wanted to happen this time. She said that from now on she would be my midwife and all my appointments would be with her, including after I'd had the baby. The relief was immense and immediately I felt a sense of calm, knowing that she would go on this journey with us.

'My husband too thought it was great being able to have one person to guide us. He was able to talk to her about how he felt last time—which was quite traumatised. He felt we were safe and was happy that I was being looked after, which eased the prospect of labour this time for him. Annie was able to get to know our two-and-a-half-year-old son too. At the antenatal visits she involved him in listening to the baby and took time to explain to him what she was doing when she was feeling the baby. It was lovely. For months his games involved him being "Annie the midwife" with a succession of soft toys.

'My pregnancy progressed well with no signs of gestational diabetes. Unfortunately, there was a rule that I could not have my baby in the little local midwifery-led unit because I'd had a previous caesarean and needed to be under consultant care. I was OK with going to the maternity unit in the nearest city but wanted to give birth in the midwifery-led birth centre attached to the labour ward there, an option not normally afforded to women who have had a previous caesarean. Annie spoke with the Head of Midwifery and together they made a special plan for me. I suspect that a lot of discussions took place on my behalf "behind the scenes". Annie organised for me to meet with the Head of Midwifery, who listened to me and reassured me that the plan stated that they would bend the rules so that I could labour and give birth in the alongside birth centre if all was well. She also constructed a written plan stating that if I needed to go to the labour ward and it wasn't an emergency situation I could still use the pool there to help me labour (not the policy for women with a previous caesarean). I felt that everyone was on my side and it was really comforting in the lead-up to labour.

'That feeling persisted during my labour. As it happened, I developed a fever from a flu infection and so was transferred to the labour ward soon after arriving in the birth centre. My temperature was high and the shared decision to have another caesarean felt appropriate and positive. I felt able to take that decision quickly and easily with no sense of disappointment. I knew it was for the best in the circumstances and felt completely fine about it. Because of the care I had had with Annie I was in a completely different head space compared with how I was when I faced labour and birth in my first pregnancy. I felt that all the staff knew about me; they understood my history, respected my wishes and were sensitive to my needs.

'The caesarean went well and my experience on the postnatal ward was completely different this time. Knowing that Annie would be visiting me at home to help me with breastfeeding was really comforting. By then she knew me so well. She understood how important it was to me that I would breastfeed successfully this time and she was really onto it. She visited me often in the first week after I went home and then less often up to 6 weeks. Had the breastfeeding not gone so well this time, I know she would have been there for me to help me get it right. But I felt so relaxed, possibly because of all the lead-up to giving birth, the care I had during that time. We all shared the joy of my milk flowing well and a peaceful baby putting on weight.

'The sense of calm that Annie brought to my experience of pregnancy, birth and breastfeeding is hard to explain. She listened to me and walked me through the build-up to labour, explaining all the steps and options, and discussing with my husband and me the implications of research evidence. She was also able to talk to the right people and ask them to bend the rules to get me what I wanted. That was amazing.

'Annie was a point of reference—someone I could turn to—throughout all the inevitable uncertainty of pregnancy, birth and new motherhood. This made me feel relaxed and grounded—just so much more in control of responding to everything that evolved than during my first pregnancy. I felt like somebody was looking out for me and that she had my best interests at heart. We became good friends. It was a brilliant system that enabled all of that and I feel really lucky to have moved to an area where I could have that continuity of care. I wish all women could have that. It should be available absolutely everywhere.'

Introduction

Caroline Homer, Pat Brodie, Nicky Leap, Jane Sandall

Contents

INTRODUCTION

Welcome to the Second Edition of *Midwifery Continuity of Care*. The initial idea for this book came about in response to an increasing number of requests from midwives, midwifery students, managers and policy makers for advice and direction on 'how to' establish midwifery continuity of care. Since our first edition was released in 2008 much progress has been made in many countries. The evidence base has strengthened with a number of new studies added to the Cochrane systematic review 'Midwife-led continuity models versus other models of care for childbearing women', further demonstrating the benefits of midwifery continuity of care for women and babies, especially in reducing pre-term birth and increasing safety (Sandall et al., 2016). More research has been published that shows benefits for midwives in terms of avoiding burnout and increasing job satisfaction (Newton et al., 2014, 2016) and cost benefits for health systems (Tracy et al., 2014). The most recent guidelines for antenatal care from the World Health Organization (WHO) recommend that:

> *Midwife-led continuity-of-care models, in which a known midwife or small group of known midwives supports a woman throughout the antenatal, intrapartum and postnatal continuum, are recommended for pregnant women in settings with well-functioning midwifery programmes.*
> **(World Health Organization, 2016, p. xv)**

In early 2018, the Health and Social Care Secretary in the United Kingdom announced that, by 2021, the majority of women will receive care from the same midwives throughout their pregnancy, labour and birth (Department of Health and Social Care, 2018).

Despite all the research and clear policy directions it is still a reality that too few women have access to midwifery continuity of care. The aim of this book therefore is to help in the establishment and sustainability of midwifery continuity of care within the mainstream public health systems of industrialised countries, especially in the United Kingdom (UK) and Australia. We hope that this book will also be of use to clinicians in all settings who are interested in the development of maternity services that respond to women's needs.

Midwifery Continuity of Care (2nd edition) begins with an analysis of the current evidence base for midwifery continuity of care and then proceeds to present a series of chapters that draw on research evidence and the experiences of a range of authors who have been involved in establishing and sustaining midwifery continuity of care in several countries. These experiences are used to 'bring to life' the everyday practices and challenges of introducing different ways of organising maternity services and the process of achieving sustainable change. We have also included some of the theory around the concepts related to midwifery continuity of care, quality and safety, sustainability and the organisation of mainstream maternity care, predominately in Australia and the UK.

This book is overtly about midwifery continuity of care across the spectrum of midwifery practice: antenatal, labour and birth, and postnatal. The focus is on the way that care is provided rather than the place in which it is provided, as many of the principles are the same. There is an emphasis throughout on 'how to' implement midwifery continuity of care. Some of the suggestions and experiences will be more relevant to you than others; some ideas may be really useful, whilst others may need to be adapted to assist you in making the case for and introducing midwifery continuity of care in your own settings.

OUR AUDIENCE

This book is written primarily for midwives, managers and policy makers engaged in the provision of publicly funded maternity services as well as for midwifery students. Our audience may include any of the following:

- midwives in practice, including midwives who already provide midwifery continuity of care and those who want to move towards working in this way
- managers of maternity units, especially those who want to expand their range of models of care but do not know 'how to' do it or where to begin
- commissioners and planners of health services who have responsibilities for the development, implementation and sustainability of maternity services budgets
- students and education providers, including undergraduate and postgraduate midwifery students as well as students from other disciplines, for example health services management or medicine
- policy makers and health service executives
- childbirth activists and organisations who advocate for better services for women
- health care workers such as maternity care assistants and doulas who provide support to women and families through their pregnancy, birth and postnatal experiences.

Essentially, this book will have relevance primarily for those who are engaged in the provision of midwifery continuity of care within publicly funded maternity services in high-income countries. In identifying our audience, we acknowledge the significant professional services that midwives in private practice also provide to women. Although this book is not specifically designed for them, they too may find many of the guiding principles and issues useful in their practice and in their negotiations with mainstream services. In addition, colleagues in low- to middle-income countries may find relevance in many of the strategies and examples in the book and these may be useful in maternity service development in such settings.

RATIONALE AND PHILOSOPHICAL PRINCIPLES

There is now strong evidence that models providing midwifery continuity of care should be established for all women. The evidence for this is discussed in detail in Chapter 1 and is woven throughout other sections of the book. Despite the evidence and subsequent policy developments in a number of industrialised countries, significant organisational change to enable midwifery continuity of care has been slow. In our view there are a number of reasons for this, including a lack of practical advice and information for midwives and managers on the processes of development and implementation. This book is a response to the need to provide information to support change in practice and policy. We have also addressed a number of organisational and political barriers and opposing views that we know exist in many contexts around the world.

The philosophical approaches for the book reflect primary health care principles and woman-centred care. Primary health care encompasses equity, access, the provision of services based on need, community participation, collaboration and community-based care. Primary health care involves using approaches that are affordable, appropriate to local needs and sustainable (WHO, 1978, 1997).

The book is also focused on woman-centred care as this is fundamental to all midwifery practice. Woman-centred care is a concept that implies that midwifery care:

- is focused on the woman's individual, unique needs, expectations and aspirations, rather than the needs of the institutions or professions involved
- recognises the woman's right to self-determination in terms of choice, control and continuity of care from a known or known caregivers
- encompasses the needs of the baby, the woman's family, her significant others and community, as identified and negotiated by the woman herself
- follows the woman across the interface between institutions and the community, through all phases of pregnancy, birth and the postnatal period, therefore involving collaboration with other health professionals when necessary
- is 'holistic' in terms of addressing the woman's social, emotional, physical, psychological, spiritual and cultural needs and expectations (Leap, 2009, p. 737).

A Cochrane review of midwifery-led care (Sandall et al., 2016) included a range of models, including team midwifery, suggesting that there are many ways to achieve the beneficial outcomes of continuity of care. Throughout this book, midwifery continuity of care means that care is provided by the same midwife or by a small group of midwives whom the woman is able to get to know throughout her pregnancy. The phrase 'continuity of carer' is used when referring to models where a primary midwife provides the majority of the woman's care through pregnancy, labour and birth and the postnatal period, is the first point of reference for her and is responsible for the coordination of her care. In different contexts, continuity of carer may be called 'one-to-one midwifery', 'caseload midwifery', 'midwifery caseload practice' and 'midwifery group practice' but definitions vary across and within countries. These terms are used throughout this book where relevant according to the context.

As editors we are committed to ensuring that midwifery continuity of care should be available and accessible to all women—not just those who are well informed about the benefits or who are deemed to be 'low risk'. Continuity of carer for women of 'any risk' has been shown to be beneficial for women and cost effective (Tracy et al., 2013). Rural and isolated women, Indigenous women, those living with poverty or lacking sufficient social support, women with mental health or drug and alcohol issues and adolescents are just some who stand to benefit most from midwifery continuity of care. We believe that systems need to change to benefit those women most in need of health gain. In primary health care terms this is called 'positive discrimination'. Models of care, particularly those that offer midwifery continuity of care and enable women to get to know their midwife, should prioritise women who have the poorest outcomes as we work towards access for all.

Throughout the book we use the feminine pronoun (she) when talking about a midwife, as more than 99% of midwives are women. This is not meant to discriminate in any way against men who are midwives.

HOW TO USE THIS BOOK

Each chapter addresses a different aspect of the process of introducing and sustaining midwifery continuity of care. The book is constructed in such a way that you may choose to start at the beginning and read each chapter in sequence. Alternatively, you may find it useful to go directly to the chapter that most meets your immediate needs. Each chapter has its own reference list.

Some chapters overlap a little and present similar information from slightly different perspectives. We recognise that this means there is sometimes a degree of repetition through the book but this is intentional. Some of the concepts are addressed in different ways by the various chapter authors. We feel this diversity of interpretation and writing style is useful, especially as we all learn and understand concepts in different ways.

Throughout the book we have also added stories from midwives who are involved in midwifery continuity of care. We do not propose that the examples you read in this book are the only ways that midwifery continuity of care might be designed and implemented. The stories bring to life the diversity of ways that midwifery continuity of care can be arranged, providing hints and ideas for others to consider.

We hope you will find *Midwifery Continuity of Care* (2nd edition) of use in your quest to plan, implement, evaluate and sustain midwifery continuity of care for the benefit of women, babies and communities.

REFERENCES

Department of Health and Social Care: *Women to have dedicated midwives throughout pregnancy and birth*, London, 2018, UK Government. Online: https://www.gov.uk/government/news/women-to-have-dedicated-midwives-throughout-pregnancy-and-birth.

Leap N: Woman-centred or women-centred care: does it matter?, *Br J Midwifery* 17(1):12–16, 2009.

Newton M, McLachlan H, Forster D, Willis K: Understanding the 'work' of caseload midwives: a mixed-methods exploration of two caseload midwifery models in Victoria, Australia, *Women Birth* 29(3):223–233, 2016.

Newton MS, McLachlan HL, Willis KF, Forster DA: Comparing satisfaction and burnout between caseload and standard care midwives: findings from two cross-sectional surveys conducted in Victoria, Australia, *BMC Pregnancy Childbirth* 14(1):1–16, 2014.

Sandall J, Soltani H, Gates S, Shennan A, Devane D: Midwife-led continuity models versus other models of care for childbearing women, *Cochrane Database Syst Rev* (4):CD004667, 2016. doi:10.1002/14651858.CD004667.pub4.

Tracy SK, Hartz DL, Tracy MB, Allen J, Forti A, Hall B, et al: Caseload midwifery care versus standard maternity care for women of any risk: m@NGO, a randomised controlled trial, *Lancet* 382(9906):1723–1732, 2013. doi:10.1016/S0140-6736(13)61406-3.

Tracy S, Welsh A, Hall B, Hartz D, Lainchbury A, Bisits A, et al: Caseload midwifery compared to standard or private obstetric care for first time mothers in a public teaching hospital in Australia: a cross sectional study of cost and birth outcomes, *BMC Pregnancy Childbirth* 14:46, 2014.

World Health Organization (WHO): *Primary health care: a report from the international conference on primary health care*, Geneva, 1978, WHO.

World Health Organization (WHO): *Declaration of Alma-ata*, Geneva, 1997, WHO. Online: http://www.euro.who.int/__data/assets/pdf_file/0009/113877/E93944.pdf.

World Health Organization (WHO): *WHO recommendations on antenatal care for a positive pregnancy experience*, Geneva, 2016, WHO.

CHAPTER 1

Is Midwifery Continuity of Care Better for Women and Babies? What Is the Evidence?

Helen McLachlan, Chris McCourt, Kirstie Coxon, Della Forster

Contents

INTRODUCTION

This chapter provides the rationale and discusses the evidence for midwifery continuity of care in relation to outcomes for women and babies. First, we discuss the evolution of continuity of care in the current context and policies that support midwifery continuity of care. Next, we summarise the evidence outlining the impact of midwifery continuity of care on pregnancy and childbirth clinical outcomes for women and babies, then its impact on women's satisfaction with care and childbirth experiences, and finally we look at issues associated with access for women who are in vulnerable or socially excluded groups.

THE EVOLUTION OF MIDWIFERY CONTINUITY OF CARE

Continuity of care has been a key aspect of maternity care policy since the 1990s in the United Kingdom (UK) (Expert Maternity Group, 1993; NHS England, 2016) and Australia (Department of Health (DOH), 1990; National Health and Medical Research Council (NHMRC), 1996) and there have been strong calls from consumers of maternity care that they want the opportunity to know their care provider

and to have greater access to continuity of care (Bryant, 2009). Although historically women were usually cared for by known midwives in their local communities,
women had increasingly limited access to continuity of midwife care as childbirth
moved into hospitals in the 20th century. By the 1970s and 1980s, women in
high-income countries were most often cared for by different clinicians across the
childbearing continuum; care was (and often still is in many instances) predominantly hospital based and fragmented, with little opportunity for women to get to
know their caregiver across the childbearing continuum. Today, pregnancy care is
provided mostly by doctors and midwives in either hospitals or community-based
antenatal clinics or by general practitioners (family doctors) in a shared care model.
Intrapartum care occurs mainly in the hospital setting, provided by midwives, junior
doctors, obstetric registrars and consultants. Postnatal care, likewise, is provided
mainly in hospital by midwives, and mostly overseen by the medical team. In the
UK and many parts of Australia, women return home after only a few days, and may
receive some visits at home from midwives or be invited to attend community-based
clinics.

Over the last few decades (since around 1990) there has been increased demand
for midwifery continuity of care from women, a plethora of evidence supporting
safety, efficacy and cost effectiveness, and subsequent policy reform in several countries including Australia, the UK and New Zealand. Many models of midwifery
continuity of care have been implemented within an evaluation framework, of
which a large proportion have been randomised controlled trials (RCTs): in the UK
(Flint et al., 1989; Hicks et al., 2003; MacVicar et al., 1993; North Staffordshire
Changing Childbirth Research Team, 2000; Turnbull et al., 1996), Ireland (Begley
et al., 2011), the Netherlands (The Royal Dutch Association of Midwives, 2017),
Australia (Biro et al., 2000; Homer et al., 2001; Kenny et al., 1994; McLachlan et al.,
2012; Rowley et al., 1995; Tracy et al., 2013) and Canada (Canadian Association
of Midwives, 2015; Harvey et al., 1996). In addition there have been a number of
retrospective and prospective studies regarding the evaluation of midwifery continuity of care (Benjamin et al., 2001; Brintworth & Sandall, 2013; Homer et al., 2017;
Lewis et al., 2016; Tracy et al., 2014). There has also been other important qualitative work on women's experiences of continuity of care (Allen et al., 2017; Boyle
et al., 2016; Jepsen et al., 2017a) and midwives' experiences of providing it (Dawson
et al., 2015; Jepsen et al., 2017b; Stevens & McCourt, 2002; Turnbull et al., 1995).
More recently, studies have mapped continuity models and women's access to them
(Dawson et al., 2014, 2016). This chapter summarises much of this evidence and is
also referred to in other chapters of this book.

RCTs of midwifery continuity of care models (including both team and caseload midwifery models) date back to the late 1980s (Flint, 1989). Along with other
research, this trial evidence, consolidated most recently in a Cochrane review on

midwife-led continuity (Sandall et al., 2016a), has consistently demonstrated the benefits of midwife-led continuity models for women and babies and for the midwives working in such models. Despite this evidence of benefit, as well as the policy documents recommending the introduction and expansion of continuity models (both discussed later in this chapter), the evidence suggests that most women in the UK and Australia *do not* have access to continuity of care (Care Quality Commission, 2018; Dawson et al., 2016; Redshaw & Henderson, 2014). A 2016 Australian study found that, although 31% of public services across the country have introduced midwifery continuity of care provided within a caseload model, only an estimated 8% of women can access the model, owing to the small scale of implementation (Dawson et al., 2016). The same study reported that 29% of providers have a team midwifery model and that approximately 12% of women across Australia in the public system had access to this care. In the UK, it is not known how many women have access to team or caseload midwifery care; however, a 2017 survey of 2500 women who gave birth in England and Wales found that the vast majority of women (88%) had never previously met any of the midwives who looked after them during labour and/or birth (Plotkin, 2017). The authors reported that 89% of the women saw between one and six midwives during the antenatal period, with those seeing fewer midwives (between one and four) reporting a better quality of antenatal care.

MIDWIFERY CONTINUITY OF CARE FOR WOMEN: POLICY SUPPORT

There is policy support for midwifery continuity of care models in a number of countries, including the UK, Australia and New Zealand, and this has been the case for many years. In the UK, the 'Changing Childbirth' report was an influential document informing maternity policy in the early 1990s, and emphasised women having 'choice, continuity and control' in pregnancy and childbirth (Expert Maternity Group, 1993). In 2016, the 'Better Births' report of the National Maternity Review in the UK also highlighted the importance of continuity of carer (NHS England, 2016), with implementation guidance published in 2017 (NHS England, 2017). Similarly, Scotland's new 'Best Start' policy, published in 2017, identified continuity of carer as a cornerstone of maternity services across Scotland to be implemented over the next 5 years (Scottish Government, 2017). The policy states (p. 6):

> *Continuity of Carer: all women will have continuity of carer from a primary midwife, and midwives and obstetric teams will be aligned with a caseload of women and co-located for the provision of community and hospital based services.*

Similar support for continuity of care is expressed in policies in Wales (Welsh Government, 2011) and Northern Ireland (Department of Health, Social Services and Public Safety, 2012).

In 1990 in New Zealand, the government passed the *Nurses' Amendment Act*, which gave midwives autonomy in their practice by restoring the professional and legal separation of midwifery from nursing (New Zealand College of Midwives (NZCOM), 2018). Following a series of reforms, a lead maternity carer (LMC) system was introduced in 1996 whereby pregnant women choose a LMC to coordinate and provide care. In New Zealand now, the majority of women (currently over 80%) choose a midwife as their LMC, with continuity of care provided by midwives working in small midwifery group practices (Midwifery Council of New Zealand (MCNZ), 2018).

In the Australian context, calls for the improvement of maternity services to facilitate midwifery continuity of care for women have been evident over the past 20 years, with reviews such as: 'Having a baby in Victoria' (DOH, 1990), 'Options for effective care in childbirth' (NHMRC, 1996), 'The NSW framework for maternity services' (NSW Department of Health, 2000), 'Future directions for Victoria's maternity services' (Department of Human Services, 2005) and 'Improving maternity services in Australia' (Bryant, 2009).

THE EFFECT OF MIDWIFERY CONTINUITY OF CARE ON CLINICAL OUTCOMES

There is significant evidence in high-income countries that midwifery continuity of care contributes to better outcomes for women and babies. A Cochrane review including 15 randomised trials and over 17,000 women, which compared midwifery continuity of care models (team or caseload midwifery) with medically led care or shared care models, found that midwifery-led care was associated with a range of improved maternal and infant outcomes (Sandall et al., 2016a). The review included eight trials with women identified as 'low' risk and six trials with women identified as 'low and high' and 'high' risk. All of the trials provided hospital birth care and none included birth at home, although four included intrapartum care in home-like hospital settings (Sandall et al., 2016a).

Women who received midwife-led continuity of care more often had a midwife whom they knew with them during their labour and birth. In terms of clinical outcomes, women were more likely to have a spontaneous vaginal birth and less likely to have an epidural, an episiotomy or an instrumental birth. Women were also less likely to have a baby born pre-term and their babies were at lower risk of death (including deaths before and after 24 weeks and neonatal deaths). For a range of other outcomes there were no differences between the groups; these included: fetal loss ≥24 weeks, neonatal death, low birth weight, Apgar score less than or equal to seven at 5 minutes, neonatal convulsions, admission to special or neonatal intensive care, labour induction, hospitalisation during pregnancy, antenatal haemorrhage,

Women who received models of midwife-led continuity of care

7 x more likely to be attended at birth by a known midwife	16% less likely to lose their baby	19% less likely to lose their baby before 24 weeks
15% less likely to have regional analgesia	24% less likely to experience pre-term birth	16% less likely to have an episiotomy

Figure 1.1 *Infographic:* Key outcomes for women from the Cochrane systematic review on midwife-led continuity of care *(Source: Sandall J, Mackintosh N, Rayment-Jones H, Locock L, Page L (writing on behalf of the Sheila Kitzinger symposium) 2016b. The infographics were created by Nisha Mattu, Alaur Rahman and Melanie Ward in the Technology & Information team at the Health Innovation Network, the Academic Health Science Network (AHSN) for South London for Jane Sandall, NIHR CLAHRC South London)*

labour augmentation, caesarean birth, opiate analgesia, perineal tears requiring suturing, postpartum haemorrhage, breastfeeding initiation and average neonatal hospital stay. The effects were the same across team and caseload models and also low- and mixed-risk models. The conclusion of the review was that 'most women should be offered midwife-led continuity models of care' (Sandall et al., 2016a, p. 3); however, the authors also stated that more research is needed to determine the most effective models of care for women with existing serious pregnancy or health complications. It should also be noted that all trials were conducted in high-income countries (Australia, Canada, Ireland and the UK). Fig. 1.1 provides an infographic that might be useful when explaining the findings of the systematic review.

The Cochrane review (Sandall et al., 2016a) was one of the reviews included in the development of a framework for quality maternal and newborn care in the *Lancet* midwifery series. In the series, continuity of care was emphasised as being central to quality care (Homer et al., 2014; Renfrew et al., 2014). The review was also cited in the report 'WHO recommendations on antenatal care for a positive pregnancy experience' published by the World Health Organization (WHO) in 2017.

The Cochrane review concluded that further research is needed to explore the association between midwife-led continuity of care models and fewer pre-term births, fewer fetal deaths less than 24 weeks, and fewer fetal losses / neonatal deaths overall (Sandall et al., 2016a). Another area that is lacking rigorous evidence in terms of midwife-led continuity of care models is the area of collaborative models providing care for at-risk women, and that is evident in the numbers of RCTs in the Cochrane review that included women at low risk of complications only (Sandall et al., 2016a). Of the 15 included trials, seven included women of 'all' or 'mixed' risk, and none included high-risk women only. There are no trials of women with complex social factors and vulnerability. It may be that some of the most vulnerable groups are the least likely to have access to midwife-led continuity of care models, and that is not surprising given the lack of available evidence. A study currently underway in the UK in an inner hospital in South London is the POPPIE pilot trial, which is investigating whether a model of midwifery continuity of care for women at increased risk of pre-term birth is feasible and whether it improves women's clinical outcomes and experiences and pregnancy outcomes (Ch. 5, Box 5.5 has more details about this trial).

In addition to randomised trials of continuity of midwifery care included in the Cochrane review (Sandall et al., 2016a), other randomised and non-randomised studies have reported similar findings (Page et al., 1999; Toohill et al., 2012; Turnbull et al., 2009) including some of the very early comparative studies such as the one-to-one study in the late 1990s, which found lower rates of epidural anaesthesia, episiotomy and perineal lacerations (Page et al., 1999) and, in the follow-up study performed 3 years post-implementation, a lower rate of assisted delivery or caesarean delivery and a shorter second stage of labour (Page et al., 2001).

IMPACT OF CONTINUITY OF MIDWIFERY CARE ON WOMEN'S SATISFACTION WITH CARE

Many studies of continuity of care, including both team and caseload models, have found higher levels of satisfaction with care for women receiving midwifery continuity of care compared with standard models of care (Biro et al., 2003; Forster et al., 2016; Kenny et al., 1994; MacVicar et al., 1993; Rowley et al., 1995; Shields et al., 1998; Waldenström et al., 2000). Measuring satisfaction can be complex, however, as there is a lack of consistent measures and ambiguity in the concepts. Given this, the Cochrane review of midwife-led versus other models of care for childbearing women was able to undertake only a narrative synthesis of the satisfaction data (Sandall et al., 2016a). It showed high ratings of satisfaction, although the authors concluded that it was difficult to conclude which aspects of care increased women's satisfaction with their care.

Three RCTs conducted in Melbourne, Australia, of team (Biro, 2000; Waldenström et al., 2000) and caseload (Forster et al., 2016) midwifery care respectively found increased satisfaction in a range of factors for women allocated to the midwife continuity model. Of particular note in the COmparing Standard Maternity care to One-to-one midwifery Support (COSMOS) caseload trial (Forster et al., 2016) was the impact on women's satisfaction with care *after* the birth, both in hospital and at home. Postnatal care is consistently rated by women as poor, and there have been almost no interventions that have increased women's satisfaction with postnatal care. Women allocated to caseload midwifery care in the COSMOS trial reported higher satisfaction with postnatal care overall, were more positive about a range of care factors and were more likely to report that they were given the advice they needed with breastfeeding, handling, settling and caring for the baby and about their own health and recovery after the birth (Forster et al., 2016). Women were three times more satisfied about overall care provision for themselves and their baby at home after the birth compared with women receiving usual care. This echoed the findings of an earlier caseload pilot evaluation, which found higher levels of satisfaction at all stages of care, including postnatal hospital and domiciliary care (Beake & Bick, 2006; McCourt et al., 1998).

A controlled prospective cohort study of caseload midwifery in England similarly found different rates of overall satisfaction with care in labour in a demographically and clinically similar sample: 62% of women in standard care compared with 89% of those receiving caseload care were 'very satisfied' with their care during labour (Page et al., 2001).

There has been significant discussion in the literature about continuity of carer versus continuity of care—i.e. seeing the same care provider (continuity of carer) versus continuity of philosophy and consistency of information and advice (continuity of care). In the Cochrane review, 10 trials were team midwifery models (continuity of care) and four were caseload models (continuity of carer) (Sandall et al., 2016a).

There have been conflicting findings regarding what women find most important. A critical review by Freeman (2006) did not find that continuity of carer was a clear predictor of women's satisfaction; similarly, a Swedish study of birth centre care concluded that, rather than continuity of carer being the most important factor, more important were care providers' attitudes, philosophy and the birthing environment (Waldenström, 1998). On the other hand, the COSMOS caseload midwifery trial found that women allocated to caseload were significantly more satisfied with their care (Forster et al., 2016), and there was also an association between increased satisfaction and increased numbers of visits, up to the point where a woman had met their midwife four times. After four visits, there did not seem to be an association with increased satisfaction.

Tilford (2015) undertook a qualitative synthesis of women's perspectives of midwife-led continuity of care models to further understand some of the mechanisms within the model that may contribute to improved outcomes. Key themes from the 27 included studies were that there were more positive outcomes when women felt care was tailored to their needs and when they felt supported, relaxed and comfortable (rather than worried) (Tilford, 2015). The positive views were facilitated by time spent with women, women's preferences, previous experiences of being understood, preparation, continuity of information, accessibility of midwives and the normalisation of birth in the context of women's lives. Included in this review, the study by Jenkins et al. (2015) of how women conceptualise continuity also identified that, as well as the benefit from relational continuity, women valued continuity across pregnancies, and across care locations (meaning that women received care at home and in facilities from a midwife or midwives they knew), adding further dimensions to how continuity of carer is experienced (Jenkins et al., 2015).

Other qualitative studies support Tilford's (2015) conclusions and provide additional evidence to extend understanding of how continuity impacts upon experiences of care. Jepsen et al. (2017a) explored experiences of caseload midwifery in Denmark and found that the relational benefits extended to partners as well as women (Jepsen et al., 2017a). The study by Kelly et al. (2014) of Australian Aboriginal and Torres Strait Islander women revealed how these women experienced continuity that was provided by midwifery students who shared their Aboriginal background. This type of continuity added to women's sense of feeling understood, as the continuity relationship drew on shared cultural understanding and cultural competency from the students, as well as enhancing the likelihood of women feeling able to ask questions and being comfortable attending for care (promoting cultural safety).

A qualitative analysis of the experiences of a sample of women from a caseload midwifery survey identified a set of themes that helped to explain women's increased satisfaction with this type of care: sense of control; confidence; person-centred care; social support; knowing and being known; reassurance, confidence and development; informed choice, control and autonomy and 'holistic care' (McCourt & Stevens, 2006, 2008). These themes were echoed in a qualitative study of women's experiences of caseload midwifery in a multiethnic area with a high proportion of women who were migrants or had low social support (McCourt & Pearce, 2000). The qualities of the relationship within these themes were illuminated further by an observational study of the interaction between women and midwives in caseload or standard maternity care models during the pregnancy booking visit (McCourt, 2006). This study was conducted to explore in more depth why women's survey and interview responses indicated greater satisfaction and sense of dialogue and control. The analysis identified different patterns of communication in the caseload model, in home- or hospital-based visits, with information provision characterised more by a learner-centred than by a didactic or disciplinary style compared with standard care midwives (McCourt, 2006).

Recent qualitative analysis of free text survey responses in the M@NGO RCT of caseload midwifery about factors women were particularly happy or unhappy with concluded that a key component of caseload was that it attracts midwives that go 'above and beyond', which in turn enables women to feel empowered, nurtured and safe during pregnancy, labour and birth (Allen et al., 2017).

IMPACT OF CONTINUITY OF MIDWIFERY CARE ON WOMEN'S EXPERIENCE OF BIRTH

A woman's *experience* of childbirth (as distinct from her satisfaction with care) has the potential to affect her future reproduction (Gottvall & Waldenström, 2002). Although, for most women, childbirth is a positive experience, those who have a negative experience of childbirth are less likely to have subsequent children or more likely to leave a longer time period before having another baby (McLachlan & Waldenström, 2005; Waldenström, 1999; Waldenström & Nilsson, 1994; Waldenström et al., 2000, 2004).

Although women's satisfaction with their care has often been measured in RCTs of continuity of care models, women's childbirth experience has received less attention.

It is possible that midwife-led continuity of care models can impact not only on women's satisfaction with care, but also on how they experience labour and birth. This is particularly likely given the evidence shows that in these models women have fewer interventions in labour and birth, use less pharmacological pain relief and have higher rates of spontaneous vaginal births compared with women in standard models of care (Sandall et al., 2016a). Three trials evaluating midwife-led continuity of care models, one conducted in a birth centre in Sweden (Waldenström & Nilsson, 1994) and two team midwifery trials in Australia (Biro et al., 2003; Waldenström et al., 2000), in which specific labour and birth questions were asked, did not find any differences in overall birth experience between the trial groups. However, the birth centre trial reported that women randomised to birth centre care felt freer to express their feelings during labour, and women having their first baby felt more involved in the birth process and were prouder of their own achievement (Waldenström & Nilsson, 1994). Similarly, a UK trial reported that team midwifery was associated with women feeling more prepared for labour, more in control and more likely to enjoy labour than women in standard care (Flint et al., 1989). A controlled prospective cohort study of caseload midwifery in England found women receiving caseload care were more likely to show strong personal expectations of control (60% vs 40% 'I should still be the one in control of the decision') and, reflecting back on the birth, were more likely to feel they had managed 'very well' (48% vs 33%) (Page et al., 2001). Women in caseload care reported seeing a median of two midwives in labour (including students) both of whom were known, whereas standard care group women reported seeing three midwives, none of whom they knew before. Caseload care women were also more likely to have a midwife who stayed with them all through the labour (92% vs 51%). The survey findings were illuminated further by open text responses and a set of qualitative interviews, where women spoke of the value of a known midwife in labour in terms of feeling supported, informed and encouraged and feeling a sense of confidence and control (McCourt, 2006; McCourt & Stevens, 2006b, 2008).

A large Australian caseload midwifery trial (COSMOS) found that caseload care was associated with more positive childbirth experiences for women (McLachlan et al., 2016). There were also fewer women in the caseload group who had a negative experience of childbirth—suggesting that caseload could potentially have a positive effect on future reproduction given the findings of the Swedish study that had shown a negative birth experience can impact future reproduction (Gottvall & Waldenström, 2002). Other key findings in the COSMOS trial were that women in the caseload arm of the trial were more likely to report that they 'coped better than expected', 'felt in control', rated their pain less negatively and were prouder of their childbirth achievements compared with women in standard care (McLachlan et al., 2016).

Key factors of the caseload model seem to be related to women's own management of their pain and their feeling of being in control. A number of studies have reported that feeling in control is a predictor of a woman's birth experience (Green et al., 2003; Waldenström, 1999). Feeling in control has also been associated with team midwife care and birth centre care (Green et al., 2003; Waldenström & Nilsson, 1994). A cohort study of women in a caseload model in England found that women in caseload care were less likely to use epidural pain relief (45% vs 69%) than women in usual care and were more likely to find other methods (pharmacological and 'natural') effective (Beake & Page, 2001). These findings appeared to be related to feeling informed (96% vs 82% felt staff explained things to them enough in labour), supported (87% vs 67% felt staff were 'very kind and understanding') and listened to during labour (97% vs 82% felt 'listened to enough by health professionals'). In the COSMOS randomised trial, women in caseload care were more likely to have said that they received support from midwives and that they could express themselves during labour; both of these factors may have strengthened women's self-confidence (McLachlan et al., 2016). Leap et al. (2010) have also reported that caseload midwives can help enhance a woman's sense of her ability to cope with the challenge of labour. The trust that develops between a woman and her midwife that starts during pregnancy is a key factor, as well as the encouragement to build a woman's confidence and ability to cope with the pain of labour.

Perhaps not surprisingly, existing qualitative evidence affirms these findings. Tilford's (2015) review of how women experience continuity also explored the impact of continuity of carer during labour, and found that knowing the midwife who provided care in labour was comforting and reassuring to them. Women talked about being 'known', as the midwife already knew what they wanted, understood their views on interventions or pain relief and were familiar with their feelings about previous births (Tilford, 2015). The opportunity to develop a relationship during pregnancy meant that women felt able to trust their midwives during labour. However, continuity models also generate a new challenge: women faced anxiety about what to do if a trusted midwife could not be there, or if their care was transferred to a different setting with new and unknown midwives.

Loss of continuity, or experiencing fragmented care during birth, is thought to be a factor in the development of postnatal morbidity for some women, especially if birth experiences are experienced as traumatic. Qualitative and case study evidence has shown that women who have previous traumatic births found the support of a known midwife invaluable during subsequent labours (Lyberg & Severinsson, 2010; Milan, 2003).

Despite such testimonies, there is currently little published evidence about the impact of continuity of midwifery care during pregnancy or labour on postnatal depression or other psychological sequelae. The Cochrane review of midwife-led continuity models (Sandall et al., 2016a) reported that only one included trial had postpartum depression as a measured outcome, and the results were therefore not included in the meta-analysis. A separate trial undertaken was with women who had pre-existing depressive disorders (Marks et al., 2003). In this study, women were randomised to either a continuity model or standard midwifery care. The trial found no difference in women's psychiatric outcomes, but reported that the continuity model was successful in engaging women in care, and that women in the continuity arm had a better experience of maternity care compared with those receiving standard midwifery care; however, the sample size was small and the study underpowered.

A qualitative evidence review that examined maternity care experiences of women with, or at risk of developing, mental health problems found that a lack of continuity was problematic, leading to feelings of isolation and difficulty disclosing symptoms, whilst having a single known carer, though uncommon, was experienced as beneficial (Megnin-Viggars et al., 2015).

CONTINUITY OF MIDWIFERY CARE FOR WOMEN WHO ARE FROM VULNERABLE GROUPS AND FOR MINORITY ETHNIC OR INDIGENOUS WOMEN

Quality of care for women who are vulnerable (for example owing to intimate partner violence or mental health problems) or socially disadvantaged or isolated, or from minority ethnic groups (particularly recent migrants and those who don't speak the majority language) is particularly important since successive reviews have identified they are more likely to receive suboptimal care and have higher rates of serious adverse outcomes, including mortality (Knight et al., 2017). In addition, subgroup analyses of national surveys in England show that women from minority ethnic groups are less likely to be satisfied with their maternity care experience (Henderson et al.,

2013), which is similar to Australian findings that women with more complex needs are less likely to be satisfied with their maternity care (Brown et al., 2014).

Few of the quantitative studies described above have reported on subanalyses relating to the experiences of women who are vulnerable or at higher social risk, so the main evidence in this area comes from qualitative studies. A systematic review of controlled (randomised and observational) studies of antenatal care models targeted for vulnerable women (Hollowell et al., 2011) did not include any studies of continuity of midwifery carer models, although other models studied (e.g. group antenatal care or additional home-visiting programs) may have increased the levels of continuity of care women received. The reviewers noted that the quality and extent of research was limited and that it was difficult to draw conclusions about models of care. A retrospective case note analysis of the outcomes of the Albany Midwifery Practice, which provides caseload care in an area with particularly high levels of social disadvantage, identified low intervention rates and lower than expected adverse neonatal outcomes when considering background rates for a comparable population (Homer et al., 2017).

A mixed methods study by Allen et al. (2016) examined possible explanations for the associations with reduced pre-term birth found in the Cochrane review of outcomes of continuity of midwife-led care (Sandall et al., 2016a), and in their own analysis of pre-term birth in young mothers (Allen et al., 2015). Using a cohort study of 1971 young women and babies and ethnographic interviews with 10 young women receiving caseload care, they hypothesised that promoting greater engagement with care, with subsequent impact on health behaviours, may be a key mechanism (Allen et al., 2015).

Qualitative studies provide evidence that illuminates how such beneficial outcomes might have been achieved. McCourt & Pearce (2000) conducted interviews with a subsample of women from minority ethnic groups and with teenage mothers who had not responded to a survey in a large evaluation of caseload midwifery. The subgroup analysis identified similar themes to those found in the larger survey and other qualitative analyses but identified that these issues were more important to women who lacked social support, or who traditionally reported poorer experiences of standard maternity care. For example, the women in standard care described experiences of lack of person-centred care, low levels of support, and discrimination, whereas those receiving caseload care emphasised the importance of the relationship with the midwife, of 'knowing and being known' and feeling that someone was 'there for you'. Consequently in the UK, following the 'Changing Childbirth' caseload midwifery pilot schemes, several services adopted caseload or small-team approaches for women identified as vulnerable. Few studies of these practices have been conducted. However, a retrospective observational study using case note analysis by Rayment-Jones et al. (2015) concluded that women receiving caseload care experienced lower rates of caesarean section, epidurals, and antenatal and neonatal admission, and shorter postnatal stay. Overall, they found that caseload midwifery care conveyed benefit and no harm. This was one of the few studies of a caseload practice established to provide continuity of care for women with complex social factors and it analysed findings for all women receiving this care over a 1-year period compared with a comparable control group of women receiving standard care. The authors recommended a full-scale trial be conducted to test these important findings further.

In the Australian context, a metasynthesis of qualitative studies that explored midwifery models of care for Aboriginal and Torres Strait Islander women and babies found that women had the most positive experiences when the services they accessed provided continuity of care, had strong community links and were controlled by Aboriginal communities (Corcoran et al., 2017). However, very few public maternity providers in Australia specifically prioritise Aboriginal women when allocating available caseload places each month (Dawson et al., 2018) and there are barriers to the provision of intrapartum midwifery care in remote areas (Corcoran et al., 2017). The authors of the metasynthesis concluded that expanding midwifery models of care for Aboriginal women would help improve cultural safety as well as women's clinical outcomes and birth experiences (Corcoran et al., 2017). There are several initiatives across Australia that aim to address this access issues, including two large partnership projects currently underway; in Victoria, four maternity service providers are aiming to offer caseload midwifery care to all Aboriginal women (or women having an Aboriginal baby) booking for pregnancy care at their services (McLachlan et al., 2017) (see Box 1.1, which illustrates the project), and in Queensland a similar project is underway (Kildea et al., 2018).

WHEN MIDWIFERY CONTINUITY OF CARE ACROSS THE CONTINUUM IS NOT POSSIBLE

The evidence presented in this chapter clearly supports the concept that, where at all possible, all women should have access to midwifery continuity of care throughout the pregnancy and birth continuum. In situations where continuity of care that starts in pregnancy and continues through labour and birth and the postnatal period is not an option, there are still potential benefits for women in receiving midwifery continuity of care during pregnancy and the postnatal period, as well as other factors that affect how women rate the care they receive. It is important to also understand the evidence in these instances, although high-level evidence is reasonably limited.

There are several areas that have been explored where there is continuity in some part of the pregnancy care continuum, and where there are improved outcomes for women who have had the continuity. A study in Australia compared levels of worry during pregnancy for women with risk-associated pregnancies (most commonly hypertension) with those in a concurrent RCT who had uncomplicated pregnancies and were

BOX 1.1 Partnerships and Collaboration

Implementing Continuity of Midwifery Care for Aboriginal Women in Four Maternity Services in Victoria, Australia

In Australia, maternity care outcomes such as pre-term birth, low birth weight, perinatal and maternal mortality are higher for Aboriginal and Torres Strait Islander mothers and babies. There have been many calls for strategies to address these inequities. One possible strategy that may improve outcomes is caseload midwifery; however, very few Aboriginal women have access to this model.

In Australia, a large project funded by the National Health and Medical Research Council[a] is exploring the implementation and sustainability of a caseload model specifically for Aboriginal women (and non-Aboriginal women having Aboriginal babies).

In 2017 and 2018, four health services located in the state of Victoria are proactively offering caseload midwifery to Aboriginal women. The project will measure the proportion of women that receive caseload care, key clinical outcomes (such as pre-term birth, low birth weight, infant admission to special care, birth type), costs and cost effectiveness as well as women's and midwives' views and experiences.

Prior to the project commencement, Aboriginal women were not proactively offered caseload midwifery care and non-Aboriginal women were substantially *more* likely to receive caseload care. At the time of writing (June 2018) the first site to implement the new caseload model has seen a more than tenfold increase in the number of women receiving caseload midwifery over the first 12 months of operation. Delays / challenges in implementation at two of the sites related to industrial agreements that required revision and staffing challenges across the health service generally.

Early findings show a major increase in update of caseload care at the first sites to proactively offer it to Aboriginal women with qualitative data to date showing high levels of satisfaction. Clinical outcome data are currently being collected. A crucial aspect of the success of the project to date has been engagement and collaboration with key stakeholders including the Victorian Aboriginal Community Controlled Health Organisation / s and the Aboriginal Advisory Committee. Models such as these can succeed only if they are based on the needs of women and their communities and ongoing consultation and engagement.

Footnote:

[a]Helen L McLachlan,[1] Della A Forster,[1] K Brintworth,[2] Sue Kildea,[3] Jane Freemantle,[4] Jennifer Browne,[5] Jeremy Oats,[6] Michelle Newton,[1] Marika Jackomos,[7] Jacqueline Watkins,[8] Simone Andy,[5] Sue Jacobs,[2] Ngaree Blow,[2] Karyn Ferguson,[4] Catherine Chamberlain,[9] Susan Donath,[10] Lisa Gold,[11] Helena Maher,[2] Jenny Ryan,[2] Belinda O'Connor,[1,2] Fiona McLardie-Hore,[1,2] Pam McCalman.[1,2]

1. La Trobe University, Melbourne. 2. The Royal Women's Hospital, Parkville. 3. University of Queensland, Brisbane. 4. University of Melbourne, Shepparton. 5. Victorian Aboriginal Community Controlled Health Organisation, Collingwood. 6. University of Melbourne, Parkville. 7. Mercy Hospital for Women, Heidelberg. 8. Western Health, St Albans. 9. Baker IDI Heart and Diabetes Institute, Melbourne. 10. Murdoch Children's Research Institute, Parkville. 11. Deakin University, Burwood.

(Reprinted from McLachlan H, Forster D, Kildea S, Freemantle J, Browne J, Oats J, et al. 2017 Partnerships and collaboration: implementing continuity of midwifery care for Aboriginal women in four Victorian maternity services. Women Birth *30: 38)*

receiving standard care or team midwifery care (Homer et al., 2002). The multidisciplinary team (including a small number of midwives, an obstetrician and a physician) provided predominantly antenatal continuity of care for the women with risk-associated pregnancies, with birth care only between 8 am and 8 pm from Monday to Friday. The study showed that, although the underlying level of anxiety was similar among all three groups, women cared for in the high-risk team reported a lower level of worry than women with uncomplicated pregnancies in either of the other models.

In Sweden, 'standard' care is usually separated into the different episodes of care. Most women receive continuity of midwife care in pregnancy, most commonly based in a community setting, and then have different hospital-based midwives providing intrapartum care. In this context the ratings of satisfaction with care are high (Waldenström, 1998) demonstrating that components of continuity of carer are also important.

Another consideration important for care providers (both in contexts where continuity is possible and also where it is not) is that other factors impact on women's satisfaction. Many studies have reported associations between positive ratings of satisfaction and different aspects of care, such as care being in a convenient location (Fellowes et al., 1999), safe care with skilled professionals (Fellowes et al., 1999; Goberna-Tricas et al., 2011), positive staff attitudes and behaviours (e.g. respectful, kind, empathetic) (Fellowes et al., 1999; Goberna-Tricas et al., 2011; Shafiei et al., 2012; Waldenström, 1998), being remembered between visits (Davey et al., 2005), having an active say in decision making (Bruinsma et al., 2003), having enough information (Bruinsma et al., 2003; Fellowes et al., 1999; Shafiei et al., 2012), perceiving care providers as helpful (Bruinsma et al., 2003) and a consistent philosophy of care (Waldenström, 1998).

CONCLUSION

This chapter has examined much of the evidence around midwifery continuity of care in terms of the effects for women and babies, and suggests that, wherever possible, midwife-led continuity of care models should be available for all women to access. In the parts of the world where it has been explored, the evidence suggests that midwifery continuity of care is associated with positive experiences for both women and midwives. It is also associated with a higher rate of normal birth and a lower rate of intervention.

Midwifery care has the capacity to impact on outcomes for women from marginalised and disadvantaged communities, yet the key evidence gap in the research on continuity of midwife-led care is the lack of rigorous research on midwife-led continuity of care for both medically and socially at-risk women. Less than half the trials in the Cochrane review of midwife-led care (Sandall et al., 2016a) include women with 'mixed' risk status, none included high-risk women only and there are no trials specifically targeting women with complex social factors and vulnerabilities.

When midwifery models of care such as caseload and team midwifery are implemented, it is essential to cater for the most disadvantaged, rather than the most advantaged, as these are the women already at most risk of poorer outcomes and where the greatest potential impact can be made. While the temptation is to provide services for those (predominantly middle-class) populations in our communities who are able to articulate a 'choice' agenda, this is unlikely to improve outcomes at a population level. In contrast, developing models that enable women from vulnerable and socially excluded communities to have access to midwifery continuity of care is more likely to demonstrate cost effectiveness and long-term health gain. Future work in this area should focus on these more vulnerable groups.

REFERENCES

Allen J, Gibbons M, Beckmann M, Tracy M, Stapleton H, Kildea S: Does model of maternity care make a difference to birth outcomes for young women? A retrospective cohort study, *Int J Nurs Stud* 52:1332–1342, 2015.

Allen J, Kildea S, Stapleton H: How optimal caseload midwifery can modify predictors for preterm birth in young women: integrated findings from a mixed methods study, *Midwifery* 41:30–38, 2016.

Allen J, Kildea S, Hartz DL, Tracy M, Tracy S: The motivation and capacity to go 'above and beyond': qualitative analysis of free-text survey responses in the M@NGO randomised controlled trial of caseload midwifery, *Midwifery* 50:148–156, 2017.

Beake SM, Bick D: Women's views of hospital and community-based postnatal care: the good, the bad and the indifferent, *Evid Based Midwifery* 3:80–86, 2006.

Beake SM, Page L, editors: *Evaluation of one-to-one midwifery. Second cohort study report*, London, 2001, Thames Valley University.

Begley C, Devane D, Clarke M, McCann C, Hughes P, Reilly M, et al: Comparison of midwife-led and consultant-led care of healthy women at low risk of childbirth complications in the republic of Ireland: a randomised trial, *BMC Pregnancy Childbirth* 11:85, 2011.

Benjamin Y, Walsh D, Taub N: A comparison of partnership caseload midwifery care with conventional team midwifery care: labour and birth outcomes, *Midwifery* 17:234–240, 2001.

Biro M: *The collaborative pregnancy care / team midwifery study: a randomised controlled trial*, Brisbane, 2000, Perinatal Society of Australia and New Zealand 4th Annual Congress.

Biro M, Waldenström U, Pannifex J: Team midwifery care in a tertiary level obstetric service: a randomized controlled trial, *Birth* 27:168–173, 2000.

Biro M, Waldenström U, Brown S, Pannifex J: Satisfaction with team midwifery care for low and high-risk women: a randomized controlled trial, *Birth* 30:1–9, 2003.

Boyle S, Thomas H, Brooks F: Women's views on partnership working with midwives during pregnancy and childbirth, *Midwifery* 32:21–29, 2016.

Brintworth K, Sandall J: What makes a successful home birth service: an examination of the influential elements by review of one service, *Midwifery* 29:713–721, 2013.

Brown S, Sutherland G, Gunn J, Yelland J: Changing models of public antenatal care in Australia: is current practice meeting the needs of vulnerable populations?, *Midwifery* 30:303–309, 2014.

Bruinsma F, Brown S, Darcy MA: Having a baby in Victoria 1989–2000: women's views of public and private models of care, *Aust N Z J Public Health* 27:20–26, 2003.

Bryant R: *Improving maternity services in Australia, the report of the maternity services review*, Canberra, 2009, Commonwealth of Australia.

Canadian Association of Midwives 2015 The Canadian midwifery model of care position statement. Online: https://canadianmidwives.org/wp-content/uploads/2016/06/CAM-MoCPSFINAL-OCT 2015-ENG-FINAL.pdf.

Care Quality Commission 2018 Maternity services survey 2017. Online: https://www.cqc.org.uk/ publications/surveys/maternity-services-survey-2017.

Corcoran PM, Catling C, Homer CS: Models of midwifery care for indigenous women and babies: a meta-synthesis, *Women Birth* 30:77–86, 2017.

Davey MA, Brown S, Bruinsma F: What is it about antenatal continuity of caregiver that matters to women?, *Birth* 32:262–271, 2005.

Dawson K, Newton M, Forster D, McLachlan H: *Exploring the introduction, expansion and sustainability of caseload midwifery in Australia*, Prague, Czech Republic, 2014, 30th Triennial Congress of the International Confederation of Midwives.

Dawson K, Newton M, Forster D, McLachlan H: Exploring midwifery students' views and experiences of caseload midwifery: a cross-sectional survey conducted in Victoria, Australia, *Midwifery* 31:e7–e15, 2015.

Dawson K, McLachlan H, Newton M, Forster D: Implementing caseload midwifery: exploring the views of maternity managers in Australia—a national cross-sectional survey, *Women Birth* 29:214–222, 2016.

Dawson K, Forster DA, McLachlan HL, Newton MS: Operationalising caseload midwifery in the Australian public maternity system: findings from a national cross-sectional survey of maternity managers, *Women Birth* 31(3):194–201, 2018. doi:10.1016/j.wombi.2017.08.132.

Department of Health (DOH): *Having a baby in Victoria: final report of the ministerial review of birthing services in Victoria*, Melbourne, 1990, Health Dept Victoria.

Department of Health Social Services and Public Safety 2012 A strategy for maternity care in Northern Ireland 2012–2018. Online: https://www.health-ni.gov.uk/publications/strategy-maternity-care -northern-ireland-2012-2018.

Department of Human Services: *Victorian maternity services performance indicators: complete set for 2003–2004*, Melbourne, 2005, Victoria State Government.

Expert Maternity Group: *Changing childbirth: the report of the expert maternity group (Cumberlege report)*, London, 1993, Department of Health.

Fellowes D, Horsley A, Rochefort J: Is continuity of care a top priority for all women?, *Br J Midwifery* 7:36–40, 1999.

Flint C, Poulengeris P, Grant A: The 'Know Your Midwife' scheme—a randomised trial of continuity of care by a team of midwives, *Midwifery* 5:11–16, 1989.

Forster DA, McLachlan HL, Davey MA, Biro MA, Farrell T, Gold L, et al: Continuity of care by a primary midwife (caseload midwifery) increases women's satisfaction with antenatal, intrapartum and postpartum care: results from the COSMOS randomised controlled trial, *BMC Pregnancy Childbirth* 16:28, 2016.

Freeman LM: Continuity of carer and partnership. A review of the literature, *Women Birth* 19:39–44, 2006.

Goberna-Tricas J, Banus-Gimenez M, Palacio-Tauste A, Linares-Sancho S: Satisfaction with pregnancy and birth services: the quality of maternity care services as experienced by women, *Midwifery* 27:e231–e237, 2011.

Gottvall K, Waldenström U: Does a traumatic birth experience have an impact on future reproduction?, *BJOG* 109:254–260, 2002.

Green J, Baston H, Easton S, McCormick F: *Greater expectations: interrelationship between women's expectations and experience of decision making, continuity, choice, control in labour and psychological outcomes*, Leeds, UK, 2003, Mother and Infant Research Unit.

Harvey S, Jarrell J, Brant R, Stainton C, Rach D: A randomized controlled trial of nurse-midwifery care, *Birth* 23:128–135, 1996.

Henderson J, Gao H, Redshaw M: Experiencing maternity care: the care received and perceptions of women from different ethnic groups, *BMC Pregnancy Childbirth* 13:196, 2013.

Hicks C, Spurgeon P, Barwell F: Changing childbirth: a pilot project, *J Adv Nurs* 42:617–628, 2003.

Hollowell J, Oakley L, Kurinczuk JJ, Brocklehurst P, Gray R: The effectiveness of antenatal care pro-
    grammes to reduce infant mortality and preterm birth in socially disadvantaged and vulnerable
    women in high-income countries: a systematic review, *BMC Pregnancy Childbirth* 11:13, 2011.

Homer CSE, Davis G, Brodie P, Sheehan A, Barclay LM, Wills J, et al: Collaboration in maternity
    care: a randomised controlled trial comparing community-based continuity of care with standard
    hospital care, *BJOG* 108(1):16–22, 2001.

Homer CSE, Farrell T, Brown M, Davis G: Women's worry and the risk-associated pregnancy team,
    Br J Midwifery 10:256–259, 2002.

Homer CSE, Friberg IK, Dias MA, ten Hoope-Bender P, Sandall J, Speciale AM, et al: The projected
    effect of scaling up midwifery, *Lancet* 384:1146–1157, 2014.

Homer CSE, Leap N, Edwards N, Sandall J: Midwifery continuity of carer in an area of high socio-
    economic disadvantage in London: a retrospective analysis of Albany midwifery practice outcomes
    using routine data (1997–2009), *Midwifery* 48:1–10, 2017.

Jenkins MG, Ford JB, Todd AL, Forsyth R, Morris JM, Roberts CL: Women's views about maternity
    care: how do women conceptualise the process of continuity?, *Midwifery* 31:25–30, 2015.

Jepsen I, Mark E, Foureur M, Nohr EA, Sorensen EE: A qualitative study of how caseload midwifery
    is experienced by couples in Denmark, *Women Birth* 30:e61–e69, 2017a.

Jepsen I, Juul S, Foureur M, Sorensen EE, Nohr EA: Is caseload midwifery a healthy work-form?—
    A survey of burnout among midwives in Denmark, *Sex Reprod Healthc* 11:102–106, 2017b.

Kelly J, West R, Gamble J, Sidebotham M, Carson V, Duffy E: 'She knows how we feel': Australian
    Aboriginal and Torres Strait Islander childbearing women's experience of continuity of care with
    an Australian Aboriginal and Torres Strait Islander midwifery student, *Women Birth* 27:157–162,
    2014.

Kenny P, Brodie P, Eckermann E, Hall J: *Westmead hospital team midwifery project evaluation*, Sydney,
    1994, final report, Westmead Hospital.

Kildea S, Hickey S, Nelson C, Currie J, Carson A, Reynolds M, et al: Birthing on country (in our
    community): a case study of engaging stakeholders and developing a best-practice Indigenous mater-
    nity service in an urban setting, *Aust Health Rev* 42(2):230–238, 2018. doi:10.1071/AH16218.

Knight M, Nair M, Tuffnell D, Shakespeare J, Kenyon S, Kurinczuk JJ, on behalf of MBRRACE-UK,
    editors: *Saving lives, improving mothers' care—lessons learned to inform maternity care from the UK and
    Ireland confidential enquiries into maternal deaths and morbidity 2013–15*, Oxford, 2017, National Perinatal
    Epidemiology Unit.

Leap N, Sandall J, Buckland S, Huber U: Journey to confidence: women's experiences of pain in labour
    and relational continuity of care, *J Midwifery Womens Health* 55:234–242, 2010.

Lewis L, Hauck YL, Crichton C, Pemberton A, Spence M, Kelly G: An overview of the first 'no exit'
    midwifery group practice in a tertiary maternity hospital in Western Australia: outcomes, satisfaction
    and perceptions of care, *Women Birth* 29:494–502, 2016.

Lyberg A, Severinsson E: Fear of childbirth: mothers' experiences of team-midwifery care—a follow-up
    study, *J Nurs Manag* 18:383–390, 2010.

McCourt C: Supporting choice and control? Communication and interaction between midwives and
    women at the antenatal booking visit, *Soc Sci Med* 62:1307–1318, 2006.

McCourt C, Pearce A: Does continuity of carer matter to women from minority ethnic groups?, *Mid-
    wifery* 16:145–154, 2000.

McCourt C, Stevens T: Continuity of carer—what does it mean and does it matter to midwives and
    birthing women?, *Can J Midwifery Res Pract* 4:10–20, 2006.

McCourt C, Stevens T: Relationship and reciprocity in caseload midwifery. In Hunter B, Deery R,
    editors: *Emotions in midwifery and reproduction*, Basingstoke, Hants, 2008, Palgrave Macmillan,
    pp 17–35.

McCourt C, Page L, Hewison J, Vail J: Evaluation of one-to-one midwifery: women's responses to
    care, *Birth* 25:73–80, 1998.

McLachlan H, Waldenström U: Childbirth experiences in Australia of women born in Turkey, Vietnam,
    and Australia, *Birth* 32:272–282, 2005.

McLachlan H, Forster D, Davey MA, Farrell T, Gold L, Biro MA, et al: Effects of continuity of care
    by a primary midwife (caseload midwifery) on caesarean section rates in women of low obstetric
    risk: the COSMOS randomised controlled trial, *BJOG* 119:1483–1492, 2012.

McLachlan H, Forster D, Davey MA, Farrell T, Flood M, Shafiei T, et al: The effect of primary midwife-led care on women's experience of childbirth: results from the COSMOS randomised controlled trial, *BJOG* 123:465–474, 2016.

McLachlan H, Forster D, Kildea S, Freemantle J, Browne J, Oats J, et al: Partnerships and collaboration: implementing continuity of midwifery care for Aboriginal women in four Victorian maternity services, *Women Birth* 30:38, 2017.

MacVicar J, Dobbie G, Owen-Johnstone L, Jagger C, Hopkins M, Kennedy J: Simulated home delivery in hospital: a randomised controlled trial, *BJOG* 100:316–323, 1993.

Marks MN, Siddle K, Warwick C: Can we prevent postnatal depression? A randomized controlled trial to assess the effect of continuity of midwifery care on rates of postnatal depression in high-risk women, *J Matern Fetal Neonatal Med* 13:119–127, 2003.

Megnin-Viggars O, Symington I, Howard LM, Pilling S: Experience of care for mental health problems in the antenatal or postnatal period for women in the UK: a systematic review and meta-synthesis of qualitative research, *Arch Womens Ment Health* 18(6):745–759, 2015.

Midwifery Council of New Zealand (MCNZ): *Professional standards*, Wellington, 2018, Midwifery Council of New Zealand.

Milan M: Childbirth as healing: three women's experience of independent midwife care, *Complement Ther Nurs Midwifery* 9:140–146, 2003.

National Health and Medical Research Council (NHMRC): *Options for effective care in childbirth*, Canberra, 1996, National Health and Medical Research Council.

NSW Department of Health: *The NSW framework for maternity services*, Sydney, 2000, NSW Government.

New Zealand College of Midwives (NZCOM): *Midwifery: an autonomous profession*, Christchurch, 2018, New Zealand College of Midwives.

NHS England: *Better Births: improving outcomes of maternity services in England. A five year forward view for maternity care. National maternity review*, London, 2016, NHS England. Online: https://www.england.nhs.uk/wp-content/uploads/2016/02/national-maternity-review-report.pdf.

NHS England: *Implementing Better Births: a resource pack for local maternity systems*, London, 2017, NHS England. Online: https://www.england.nhs.uk/mat-transformation/implementing-better-births.

North Staffordshire Changing Childbirth Research Team: A randomised study of midwifery caseload care and traditional 'shared care', *Midwifery* 16:295–302, 2000.

Page L, McCourt C, Beake S, Vail A, Hewison J: Clinical interventions and outcomes of one-to-one midwifery practice, *J Public Health Med* 21:243–248, 1999.

Page LA, Beake S, Vail A, McCourt C, Hewison J: Clinical outcomes of one-to-one midwifery practice, *Br J Midwifery* 9:700–706, 2001.

Plotkin L: *Support overdue: women's experiences of maternity services*, London, 2017, The National Federation of Women's Institutes and National Childbirth Trust.

Rayment-Jones H, Murrells T, Sandall J: An investigation of the relationship between the caseload model of midwifery for socially disadvantaged women and childbirth outcomes using routine data—a retrospective, observational study, *Midwifery* 31:409–417, 2015.

Redshaw M, Henderson J: *Safely delivered: a national survey of women's experience of maternity care*, Oxford, 2014, National Perinatal Epidemiology Unit.

Renfrew MJ, McFadden A, Bastos MH, Campbell J, Channon AA, Cheung NF, et al: Midwifery and quality care: findings from a new evidence-informed framework for maternal and newborn care, *Lancet* 384(9948):1129–1145, 2014. doi:10.1016/S0140-6736(14)60789-3.

Rowley MJ, Hensley MJ, Brinsmead MW, Wlodarczyk JH: Continuity of care by a midwife team versus routine care during pregnancy and birth: a randomised trial, *Med J Aust* 163:289–293, 1995.

Sandall J, Soltani H, Gates S, Shennan A, Devane D: Midwife-led continuity models versus other models of care for childbearing women, *Cochrane Database Syst Rev* (4):CD004667, 2016a. doi:10.1002/14651858.CD004667.pub5.

Sandall J, Mackintosh N, Rayment-Jones H, Locock L, Page L, writing on behalf of the Sheila Kitzinger symposium: *Relationships: the pathway to safe, high-quality maternity care*, Oxford, 2016b, Report from the Sheila Kitzinger symposium at Green Templeton College.

Scottish Government: *The best start: a five-year forward plan for maternity and neonatal care in Scotland*, Edinburgh, 2017, Scottish Government. Online: https://beta.gov.scot/publications/best-start-five-year-forward-plan-maternity-neonatal-care-scotland.

Shafiei T, Small R, McLachlan H: Women's views and experiences of maternity care: a study of immigrant Afghan women in Melbourne, Australia, *Midwifery* 28:198–203, 2012.

Shields N, Turnbull D, Reid M, Holmes A, McGinley M, Smith LN: Satisfaction with midwife-managed care in different time periods: a randomised controlled trial of 1299 women, *Midwifery* 14:85–93, 1998.

Stevens B, McCourt C: One-to-one midwifery practice. Part 3. Meaning for midwives, *Midwifery* 10:111–115, 2002.

The Royal Dutch Association of Midwives: *Midwifery in the Netherlands*, Utrecht, 2017, The Royal Dutch Association of Midwives.

Tilford R: *An exploration of women's perspectives of care in midwife led continuity models of care: a qualitative synthesis*, MPH thesis, London, 2015, King's College.

Toohill J, Turkstra E, Gamble J, Scuffham PA: A non-randomised trial investigating the cost-effectiveness of midwifery group practice compared with standard maternity care arrangements in one Australian hospital, *Midwifery* 28:e874–e879, 2012.

Tracy SK, Hartz DL, Tracy MB, Allen J, Forti A, Hall B, et al: Caseload midwifery care versus standard maternity care for women of any risk: M@NGO a randomised controlled trial, *Lancet* 382:1723–1732, 2013.

Tracy SK, Welsh A, Hall B, Hartz D, Lainchbury A, Bisits A, et al: Caseload midwifery compared to standard or private obstetric care for first time mothers in a public teaching hospital in Australia: a cross sectional study of cost and birth outcomes, *BMC Pregnancy Childbirth* 24:46, 2014.

Turnbull D, Reid M, McGinley M, Sheilds NR: Changes in midwives' attitudes to their professional role following the implementation of the midwifery development unit, *Midwifery* 11:110–119, 1995.

Turnbull D, Baghurst P, Collins C, Cornwell C, Nixon A, Donnelan-Fernandez R, et al: An evaluation of midwifery group practice. Part I. Clinical effectiveness, *Women Birth* 22:3–9, 2009.

Turnbull D, Holmes A, Schields N, Cheyne H, Twaddle S, Gilmour WH, et al: Randomised, controlled trial of efficacy of midwife-managed care, *Lancet* 348:213–218, 1996.

Waldenström U: Continuity of carer and satisfaction, *Midwifery* 14:207–213, 1998.

Waldenström U: Experience of labour and birth in 1111 women, *J Psychosom Res* 47:471–482, 1999.

Waldenström U, Nilsson C: Experience of childbirth in a birth centre. A randomised controlled study, *Acta Obstet Gynecol Scand* 73:547–553, 1994.

Waldenström U, Brown S, McLachlan H, Forster D, Brennecke S: Does team midwife care increase satisfaction with antenatal, intrapartum and postpartum care? A randomized controlled trial, *Birth* 27:156–167, 2000.

Waldenström U, Hildingsson I, Rubertsson C, Radestad I: A negative birth experience: prevalence and risk factors in a national sample, *Birth* 31:17–27, 2004.

Welsh Government: *A strategic vision for maternity services in Wales*, Cardiff, 2011, Government of Wales.

World Health Organization (WHO): *WHO recommendations on antenatal care for a positive pregnancy experience*, Geneva, 2017, World Health Organization.

CHAPTER 2

Introducing Midwifery Continuity of Care in Mainstream Maternity Services: The Foundations for Success

Cathy Warwick, Nicky Leap

Contents

INTRODUCTION

As outlined in Chapter 1, the evidence for developing maternity services based on midwifery continuity of care is now strong. If we are going to provide the highest quality of care for women and babies, we need to build services based on the important principles of care provided by small teams or groups of midwives, thereby enabling trusting relationships to develop over the antenatal, intrapartum and postnatal periods. Such care should be available to all women regardless of where they plan to give birth and whether or not they also need to receive care from obstetricians and other practitioners: 'Every woman needs a midwife and some women need a doctor too' (Sandall, 2012, p. 323). This is, however, a challenge given that in most middle- and high-income countries the dominant model of service delivery is based on a much more fragmented model of care—one which rarely enables a strong relationship to develop between the woman, her midwife and other caregivers. The questions are: 'How do midwives in a variety of roles who want to change this do so?', 'How do you get started?' and 'What considerations are necessary if successful change is to come about?' In this chapter we shall focus on addressing these questions. Some of our advice is based on evidence and some is based on our own experiences of working with others in setting up models of care based on the principles and practicalities associated with midwifery continuity of carer projects.

For the purposes of this chapter we shall focus on the setting up of projects that enable midwives to work in continuity of carer models: caseload practice within a midwifery group practice (MGP) or small team. Our rationale is the imperative to respond to policy directives (in countries such as the UK and Australia) that require continuity of carer models to be developed as the gold standard in mainstream maternity service provision. In England and Scotland, for example, the overarching policies 'Better Births' (National Health Service (NHS) England, 2016) and 'Best Start' (Scottish Government, 2017) respectively now specifically recommend that maternity services should be based on continuity of carer. At a national level, guidelines about processes of implementation are in place which should help innovative midwives to achieve these goals, for example: 'Implementing Better Births: continuity of carer' (NHS England, 2017). A resource provided by the Royal College of Midwives ((RCM) 'Can continuity work for us? A resource for midwives' (2017) is available to members of the RCM and helps midwives work through the issues and challenges associated with implementing continuity of care.

In Australia, the National Maternity Services Plan (Australian Government Department of Health, 2011; Australian Health Ministers Advisory Council (AHMAC), 2016) and various state and territory policy documents continue to include directives that midwifery continuity of carer for all women is an important goal. Various resources provide 'tool-kits' of how to go about setting up continuity of carer projects (Australian College of Midwives (ACM), 2016; New South Wales (NSW) Ministry of Health, 2012; Western Australian Department of Health, 2016).

Whether or not you have the advantage of being able to respond to policy imperatives, the principles and processes for planning to implement continuity of carer in mainstream maternity services will be similar. This chapter provides a road map to guide you through the initial stages of planning and implementation with sustainability in mind.

If you can establish your new service within your existing budget and staffing numbers, it is more likely to be sustainable. Implementation within an existing budget means the project will be embedded in the organisational structure from the outset; this makes it less vulnerable to discontinuation in times of budgetary constraint. Later in this chapter, however, we shall address the factors that need to be taken into consideration if you are applying for funding to set up a new midwifery continuity of carer service within the public health system.

WHERE TO START: INITIAL STEPS

Let us assume that the overall aim or vision is clear and that it is to improve the quality of your maternity service by ensuring that all of the women in your care can access a midwifery continuity of carer model. The next step is to plan and describe the building blocks that will enable you to get from where you are now to where you want to be. Whether you are the midwifery leader of a large maternity service or a midwife providing care to a small group of women, the initial three steps will be the same:

1. Audit what you are currently achieving.
2. Decide which women will access the new model.
3. Plan for scaling up.

Audit what you are currently achieving

The first step is an audit. As you make a coherent case for service development, sound information will be invaluable: firstly so you can benchmark future progress, secondly to enable you to work out the best place to start if you are planning to introduce continuity of carer incrementally, and finally to help ensure that any new developments cause minimum disruption to services already providing continuity of carer. If women are already receiving continuity, perhaps in a homebirth or birth centre service, you would not want to change that service unless there would be wider benefits of doing so.

You may be able to undertake an audit through a retrospective review of case notes, or you may want to design a short questionnaire describing what continuity of carer looks like and asking women to assess whether or not they received such a service. One caveat here: in many services, antenatal and postnatal continuity of carer are either already good or can be improved relatively easily. Although this is positive, it is vital that the evidence of improved outcomes relies on continuity of care from a known midwife or small team of midwives throughout the antenatal, labour and birth and postnatal periods.

The second aspect of audit will help a targeted approach. Have a look at the demographics of the women using your service and the outcomes experienced by women and their babies to find out, firstly, which women are most satisfied with their care and which are least satisfied and, secondly, which groups of women are experiencing the worst outcomes for themselves and their babies in terms of both mortality and morbidity. This information can usually be obtained from data that is already gathered in annual reports or statistics from your hospital, in local census documents or national reports on maternal and child health, or from a general review of the type of women who access your service. Demographic data might include the average age of women, parity, country of birth and language spoken at home. You can then analyse this data either against your own local statistics or by looking at national statistics and extrapolating from them how likely different groups of women in your service are to experience poor outcomes.

Decide which women will access the new model: a public health approach

Audits will enable you to decide which group or groups of women will have the first opportunity to access this model of care. It is important to justify your starting position using the data from your audit set against the improvements in outcomes that the evidence about continuity of carer shows. In health service provision, many take the position that if you cannot do something for everyone you should not do it at all. Continuity of carer is also often seen as a 'Rolls Royce' service—one that is assumed to be too expensive and so cannot be justified. In the UK the inequity of what is called a 'postcode lottery' in health care provision is often cited. You need to be able to address these arguments by clearly showing the logic for targeting a specific group of women. Of course if you are in the happy position of developing this model for all women immediately you can skip this step.

Essentially you are answering the question, 'Who in the population of women we serve is most likely to benefit from access to a continuity of carer model?' Undoubtedly, all women would prefer to receive care based on relationships but, initially, the main consideration may be which women and their babies are most likely to have improved outcomes. In Chapter 10, you can read about the primary health care principles that underpin a public health approach to addressing health inequalities when developing midwifery continuity of care for women in specific groups.

There is now evidence that the most dramatic impact of midwifery continuity of carer models is seen where midwives provide care to women in socially disadvantaged groups (Homer et al., 2017; Kelly et al., 2013; Rayment-Jones et al., 2015); yet these women are less likely than others to receive care in models where they are able to build a relationship with a midwife who understands the complex, interrelated issues that impact on their lives (Ebert et al., 2011; McCourt & Pearce, 2000). It thus makes perfect sense when introducing new models to prioritise continuity of carer for these women. Taking such an approach may also help to secure new funding.

Small groups of midwives practising caseloading have been part of the model of service delivery at St Mary's Hospital and Queen Charlotte's Hospital in London for some time. These maternity services are now amalgamated into the Imperial College Healthcare Trust. Vicki Cochrane was one of the caseload midwives from 2006. She had a number of leadership roles associated with the development of the models at Imperial College and in Box 2.1 she describes how caseload practice was able to improve outcomes for women in socially disadvantaged groups.

BOX 2.1 Midwifery Continuity of Carer for Women Living in Socially Complex Situations

Vicki Cochrane

Since it was impossible to provide all women across the new maternity service with a case-loading midwife, a decision was taken to focus on providing continuity of carer for women who are less likely to experience a good outcome. The women who can access caseload care live in the geographical area; they are in socially complex situations as defined by the National Insitute of Clinical Excellence (NICE, 2010) and the Centre for Maternal and Child Enquiries (CMACE, 2011). These definitions cover women in situations that include any of the following factors:

- domestic violence
- homelessness
- significant mental health issues
- substance or alcohol abuse
- asylum seekers or refugees
- learning difficulties
- teenagers under 20 years old
- members of the travelling community
- anyone with safeguarding (child protection) concerns.

Continued

BOX 2.1 Midwifery Continuity of Carer for Women Living in Socially Complex Situations—cont'd

There are now two caseloading groups of midwives: one on each hospital site. There are six midwives in each group, with a designated midwife as the coordinator. The midwife in this role takes responsibility for the day-to-day administrative tasks for her group. The midwives each have a caseload of 30 women a year, except for the coordinator, who has a caseload of 28 women a year.

The midwives work in pairs and share their on-call so that one of each pair is available 24/7. This means that 90% to 95% of the women are cared for by their named midwife or her buddy at the birth. The on-call hours might appear onerous on paper but experience has shown that being 'available' for a known group of women with flexible working arrangements is much less stressful than a traditional on-call rota.

The caseload midwives are all committed to providing continuity of carer. However, we identified early on that, if a caseloading model is to be sustainable for the midwives, the size of the caseload has to be lower than it might be for a less vulnerable group owing to the very complex care and extent of liaison required. It is also critical that the midwives are not expected to provide unit cover on a regular basis. Any request for caseload midwives to provide cover in the maternity unit has to go through the senior midwife for caseloading.

The midwives run a monthly Homebirth Information drop-in service and a Young Mums group. They attend all child protection conferences and obstetric appointments and have a joint hand over visits with the health visitor and the woman postnatally. Women can choose to have their care at home or in a community setting. They also have a choice around place of birth, which includes the option of giving birth at home if their pregnancy is healthy.

Interdisciplinary working, both within the maternity unit and in the community, is very important; for example, the midwives link with obstetricians, specialist midwives, social workers and staff in children's centres and housing services, to name just a few.

All midwives attend a weekly team meeting to discuss practice in relation to the women in their caseload and to support each other. On a monthly basis each group has a reflective session with the senior midwife for caseloading and the two groups also meet together monthly. Midwives who are core staff provide good support and respect the caseload midwives' autonomy.

There is a potential danger of midwives finding the needs of vulnerable women overwhelming if this is the bulk of their work. There are, therefore, ongoing discussions about whether it may be pragmatic to include some women who are low risk in the caseload—for example, multiparous women choosing homebirth.

A quantitative study within our maternity service compared birth outcomes for socially disadvantaged women who received care from a group of caseload midwives with outcomes for those receiving standard care.[a] The outcomes speak of the potential of caseload practice to improve outcomes for socially disadvantaged women and their babies; women receiving caseload care were more likely to experience:

- spontaneous vaginal birth (80% vs 55%)
- the use of water for pain management in labour (32% vs 10%)
- birth in the midwifery-led birth centre (26% vs 13%)

BOX 2.1 Midwifery Continuity of Carer for Women Living in Socially Complex Situations—cont'd

- assessment by 10 weeks gestation (24% vs 8%)
- a shorter postnatal stay in hospital (1 day vs 3 days)
- knowing their midwife (90% vs 8%)
- an intact perineum (46% vs 26%)
- referral to multidisciplinary support services: psychiatric services (56% vs 19%), domestic violence advocacy (42% vs 18%), other support services (56% vs 31%).
  Women receiving caseload care were less likely to experience:
- caesarean section (11% vs 34%)
- an epidural or spinal for pain management in labour (35% vs 56%)
- birth on the labour ward (70% vs 88%)
- antenatal admission (0.9% vs 1.1%)
- admission of their baby to the neonatal unit (4% vs 18%)
- extended postnatal stay in hospital.

[a]*Adapted from: Rayment-Jones H, Murrells T, Sandall J 2015 An investigation of the relationship between the case load model of midwifery for socially disadvantaged women and childbirth outcomes using routine data—a retrospective. observational study. Midwifery 31(4): 409-417.*

Plan for scaling up

You may decide that your starting point is to develop one or two models of service delivery based on a public health model but it is also important to think beyond the first step. Given the strength of the evidence that midwifery continuity of care improves outcomes, and certainly if there are local and national policies that all women should be able to access midwifery continuity of carer, the end point has to be exactly that. So, what is your plan for a further phase of development and for one after that? Which group of women would next access this service? How are midwives going to learn from the first phase of development? How will funding be accessed? Not only is this important so that all women receive the best possible service but also experience shows that one-off service developments are vulnerable when pressures and challenges emerge.

INVOLVING WOMEN AS USERS OF MATERNITY SERVICES

In any service development or change it is critical to involve service users. The days of professional paternalism (or maternalism) are now over. Partnership working and 'co-production' are very much advocated as the key to higher quality of services (Batalden et al., 2016) and it is especially important for health care providers to work in partnership with those affected by social inequities (Marmot et al., 2008).

The prime example of the value of working in partnership with women to develop maternity services occurred in New Zealand. In 1988, the New Zealand College of Midwives (NZCOM) was formed with a conscious decision to involve consumers as partners within the organisation (Donley, 1989; Guilliland & Pairman, 1995, 2010). Women and midwives worked together to bring about legislative and funding changes, which ultimately meant that each woman would be able to choose a publicly funded lead maternity carer (LMC) for her total care throughout pregnancy, labour and birth, and the postnatal period—a midwife, general practitioner or obstetrician. The majority of women choose midwives as their LMC and consistently value this service highly (Ministry of Health, 2017). The partnership relationship between midwives and women continues to underpin all processes involving the planning, implementation and evaluation of maternity service provision in New Zealnd (Grigg & Tracy, 2013) and has been shown to sustain the joy of practice for LMC midwives (McAra-Couper et al., 2014).

Identifying what local women want

On the face of it, making the case for midwifery continuity of care is relatively straightforward. If you are in the UK, you could argue that the overarching policy documents which recommend continuity of carer—Better Births in England and Best Start in Scotland—were based on very large surveys and extensive consultation processes, and that women were intricately involved in groups set up to determine the policy. Wherever you are, you could draw on Chapter 1 of this book and make the case that there is evidence that women appreciate midwifery continuity of carer and that it improves outcomes.

Despite all of this evidence, funders and others with influence may want specific local surveys. It is not at all uncommon to hear arguments based on, 'Our women are happy with the care they get'. The starting point always has to be related to improving services for *local* women with an emphasis on the advantages of midwifery as a public health strategy (Biro, 2011; Chief Nursing Officers of England, Northern Ireland, Scotland and Wales, 2010; Foureur, 2005) and so you may need to carry out local surveys.

The challenge is that surveys to identify women's satisfaction with maternity care often do not capture the complex mix of facets of women's experiences, both positive and negative, with women tending to uphold the status quo and not wanting to be critical of their care in retrospect (Redshaw, 2008; van Teijlingen et al., 2003). Finding out what women want from maternity services can be tricky if women have not had the opportunity to know what might be possible and have never experienced midwifery continuity of care. It is sometimes hard to imagine a type of care if you have never had it or even heard about it.

If another survey is needed to build your case, it is very important that women are fully informed about what a continuity of carer model offers that is different from the current model. Any consultation should also allow time for women to discuss the model and explore how it will impact on women and families in their communities. Sometimes, therefore, you need to develop an information leaflet describing options and addressing potential concerns.

Carrying out a SWOC analysis

As you are starting to gather your data and develop your plan with a few interested colleagues you may need to ask yourselves, 'How is our idea going to land?', 'How feasible is it going to be to implement our ideas?', 'Are they likely to get a good reception?' and 'How can we prepare the ground?' Your idea might fit very well with the direction of travel of both national and local policy makers—but are mid-wives in your maternity service keen or scared of the changes you want to propose? On the other hand, there might be a situation where the midwives are all keen but another group of professionals do not support midwifery continuity of care and they might be an influential voice in service planning. It is essential to get them on side by reviewing your own organisation and context in terms of what might be feasible or even possible and being clear about your strategy and tactics.

One way to review your situation is to do a SWOC analysis, which consists of working out the strengths, weaknesses, opportunities and challenges of your organisation. The **strengths** might include the fact that there are a large number of midwives who want to change to working in a continuity of carer project, a supportive manager and the presence of at least one obstetrician or general practitioner who believes it is a good idea. A **weakness** might be the fact that very few of your midwives are currently practising across the full scope of midwifery practice. An **opportunity** could include a recent review conducted in your country or area that recommended the implementation of midwifery continuity of carer. Working with local maternity service users can be included in your *opportunities*; the support of women in your community could also be an important *strength*. Your **challenges** might be a group of colleagues or managers whose actions have threatened previous changes, or the ongoing challenge of budgetary problems.

The SWOC analysis will not solve your problems but it may help you to be clear about where the difficulties lie ahead and may be useful when you start to develop your strategies for implementation. Knowing where the difficulties are before they arise may also help you plan a strategy to lessen the problems. In developing a plan to address the challenges and weaknesses you may find it useful to work out how you are going to learn from others, both those who have succeeded and those who have not. This might include setting up visits to other maternity units or inviting people to come to a meeting of your working group to talk about their experiences.

Forming a working group

Once it has been decided which population of women are going to access the new midwifery continuity of carer service, it is important to involve women who have used, currently use or potentially will use services in the detailed planning. We also recommend including women who may be accessing your service but who will not receive this model of care so that they understand the need for an incremental process and can help in designing subsequent phases. Beware of tokenism: having one or two service users amongst a group of professionals. A partnership or co-production process means equality of numbers, of voice and of weight given to each opinion (Batalden et al., 2016). In some situations it may be appropriate to have at least half of your steering group made up of local maternity service users.

You can approach local voluntary or non-government organisations for representatives, but advertising in the local paper or putting up notices in a community centre or health centre can be useful too. You may also want to think about approaching women who have recently given birth with your service and inviting them directly, particularly if you want to involve women from specific culturally and linguistically diverse (CALD) communities. The UK 'Maternity voices toolkit' website provides excellent resources about how to engage with maternity services user representatives, including the use of social media for networking and communicating with local women and families (Newburn & Fletcher, 2017).

You may choose to include in your working group some of the people who you decided in your SWOC analysis could potentially be *challenges*. Once people are involved in the process of design and implementation it is more difficult for them to be obstructive. Also, the experience of being exposed to evidence, enthusiasm and women's views may help change attitudes and beliefs. Box 2.2 lists considerations when setting up a working group.

Promoting positive working relationships

In the planning stages of your project it is important to involve all of the staff in your maternity service as well as staff in services based in the community. This might include those working in child health, allied health and community and social services as well as the emergency transport (ambulance) service. From a practical point of view, you might have to consolidate partnerships through developing service agreements or collaborative agreements but it is also more than just that—the reality is that communicating with potential stakeholders during the planning process about changes that might affect them directly or indirectly can be a useful way to maintain

BOX 2.2 Considerations When Setting Up a Working Group
Potential role of the working group:
- A forum for exchanging information and ideas regarding the implementation and integration of the new project
- An ongoing role addressing issues arising or resolving major problems
- Governance, once established

Include:
- those who might be affected in hospital and community services
- all who might be involved in consultation and referrals
- midwives who might be providing some care to to women despite their being cared for by caseload midwives
- general practitioners, particularly if they are providing some antenatal care for your maternity unit
- someone with a senior level role in your organisation who can provide guidance about strategies and available resources, keep the development of the model on the agenda at relevant meetings, and convince others to be champions of your project (Shaw et al., 2012).

Practicalities:
- Establish a regular meeting pattern with dates well in advance.
- Draw up terms of reference to include leadership of the group and an outline of who is responsible for arranging dates, finding a venue, minute taking and circulation of minutes to the group and staff in the unit.
- Identify decision-making processes and who will carry decisions to the next stage.
- Identify clear lines of communication from the working group to other groups or leaders within the organisation.

or promote positive working relationships down the track. This might be in the form of an email bulletin or circulation of minutes, or through arranging face-to-face meetings to explain and discuss the plans. (You will find more ideas about promoting positive working relationships in Chapter 5, which discusses ways of building alliances.)

PREPARING THE ORGANISATION: TEACHING AND LEARNING INITIATIVES TO SUPPORT CONTINUITY OF CARE

Increasingly, universities are organising modules or courses that focus on addressing the continuing professional development (CPD) needs of midwives and managers in light of changes to enable midwifery continuity of care. Within maternity units, midwifery educators or consultant midwives are also developing courses to support

> ## BOX 2.3 Preparing the Organisation: a Graduate Certificate in Midwifery Continuity of Care for All Staff
> *Ali Teate*
>
> During the years leading up to the implementation of the MGPs, the Graduate Certificate in Midwifery Continuity of Care set the scene, provided theoretical background and explored the practicalities for midwives wishing to work in midwifery continuity of carer or support others working in this way. The course was accessed by a number of core staff, who identified that it enabled them to understand the context and support the development and implementation of the MGPs.
>
> The Graduate Certificate brought together midwives with diverse clinical experiences and philosophical beliefs about midwifery. The group was a dynamic mix of midwives who came together to study: from delivery suites, antenatal clinics and birth centres. The participants included managers, new graduates, old graduates and dedicated caseload junkies. This mix of midwives enabled the concept of continuity of midwifery carer to be disseminated throughout the Women's and Children's Hospital. In particular, core staff came to understand continuity of carer and this assisted with the general acceptance of the model when it was implemented eventually in 2002.

such changes. An early example is a course that was established at the Women's and Children's Hospital in Adelaide in partnership with Flinders University of South Australia. Drawing on texts from the UK identifying the importance of developing continuing education programs for midwives moving into continuity of carer roles (Page, 1995; Turnbull et al., 1995; Warwick, 1995), the course paved the way for the establishment of 4 MGPs comprising 24 full-time equivalent (FTE) midwife positions and 2 unit head positions that were to provide a caseload model of care to approximately 1000 women and babies per annum across all risk categories (see Chapter 11 where the sustainability of this project is discussed). Ali Teate, one of the original MGP midwives, reflects in Box 2.3 on the role the course played in paving the way for the initiative.

DESIGNING AND PLANNING MIDWIFERY CONTINUITY OF CARE

When designing midwifery continuity of care programs the starting point is identifying your overall vision, which ideally should be compatible or even the same as the overall vision for your whole maternity service. If this is not the case then it may be harder to resolve difficulties as time goes by.

The planning phase is an opportunity for discussion, negotiation, information sharing and collaboration—all of which are essential to the success of new projects. It may take a number of meetings and discussions to agree on the project you hope to develop; it would not be unusual to take at least 6 months or longer to get to the point where the group can actually write a clear proposal about the project. Challenges will always need to be faced, even when you have been meticulous in your planning; just when you think you have anticipated everything, the unanticipated happens.

Flexibility in enabling the project to evolve and change over time is important. Midwifery continuity of carer projects are often 'works in progress' that may change quite considerably as midwives find their way and grow in confidence over the first couple of years. In light of this, it may be necessary to delay your initial evaluation or ensure that you re-evaluate once the project is settled. Any major evaluation or research on the outcomes should be delayed until the project is well established. (Chapter 8 on monitoring and evaluation will provide you with more information about how to set up appropriate systems.)

Deciding the type of continuity of care model

The Cochrane review of midwifery-led care (Sandall et al., 2016) included a range of models, suggesting that there are many ways to achieve the beneficial outcomes of continuity of care. As identified in Chapter 1, though, a growing body of evidence about midwifery continuity of carer or caseload practice enables us to identify the specific elements of a continuity of carer model. These are that:

- each woman has a primary or named midwife who takes responsibility for overseeing her care and who is the first point of contact for her
- continuity of care is provided by the primary midwife throughout the antenatal, labour and birth and postnatal periods, with backup from another midwife or small group of midwives working together in a team, often referred to as a midwifery group practice.

Other than these elements, the model needs to be built according to local considerations as discussed fully in Chapter 3.

In Box 2.4, Annie Lester, who currently works in a rural free-standing midwifery-led unit (MLU) in the UK, discusses her experience of working in different models aiming to provide continuity of care and carer. She highlights several important issues: the support that is needed for midwives, the fulfilment that continuity of carer brings, a way of facilitating continuity of friendships and social support for women, and the need to make sure that we do not disrupt care that is already of a high quality as we develop new models.

Working out the detail when designing your project

You will find information in other chapters in this book that will help you to consider a range of important issues when designing and planning your project. We shall discuss some of these in turn briefly.

BOX 2.4 Experiences of Providing Continuity of Care in Different Ways

Annie Lester

As a relatively newly qualified midwife I was lucky enough to get a job in a caseload practice in inner London looking after a multirisk, vulnerable population. This felt like a proper apprenticeship into the world of autonomous midwifery practice, where midwives enabled situations where women felt empowered to make evidenced-based choices and were supported in these choices. I was on-call 24/7, I attended more than 90% of the births of the women I was midwife to and 50% had a homebirth. The breastfeeding rates were high and birth outcomes were positive. I had amazing support from the other midwives in the practice through, among other things, weekly team meetings, great job satisfaction and flexible working hours. I am very passionate about this model of midwifery care; however, due to the on-call burden it does not suit everyone at all points in their midwifery career.

When I left London I found work in a rural free-standing midwifery-led unit (MLU). I was an 'integrated midwife'. I was attached to a GP surgery and provided the antenatal and postnatal care to the women there. I also, along with all the other community midwives, worked shifts in the MLU and once a week was on-call for the unit and homebirths. However, this role gave me the flexibility to go on-call if I wanted to for women in my caseload who planned to give birth at home or in the MLU. I tried to continue the ethos of caseload practice, but this time as an individual as not all the other team members worked this way and the team support in relation to weekly team meetings and named second midwives at the birth etc. was absent. I could not sustain that level of on-call without the support and soon burnt out. Shortly afterwards the integrated role was eroded by new management and I retreated into the less fulfilling, but comfortable, role of a traditional community midwife with the odd shift in the MLU. I found my job satisfaction still through the relationships I developed with women, but at a personal level I compensated for the lack of births I attended through obtaining a secondment as a midwifery lecturer and developing other projects such as piloting group pregnancy care.

Group pregnancy care is a model where women whose babies are all due in the same month receive their antenatal care together in a 2-hour group session; this includes facilitated discussions on topics relevant to the women's pregnancies, lives and interests. Importantly, group pregnancy care also creates community. The women develop relationships with the other women in the group and these endure into the postnatal period and beyond once the midwives have discharged them. Suddenly the concept of continuity means more than continuity of named midwife, and encompasses a more profound element—that of continuity of peer support. As a midwife working in this model I enjoyed getting to know women well as they interacted with each other in the group; many of the discussions were profound. I also greatly appreciated working alongside another midwife—each session is run by two midwives—as it is sadly a rare luxury to work together and to learn from and support one another in this way.

Now, with the call of Better Births to increase levels of continuity through possibly working in teams of four to six midwives, it will be interesting to see whether the national emphasis on intrapartum continuity will in fact impact on the levels of continuity during pregnancy and the early postnatal weeks as some midwives fear. I am eagerly waiting to see how our Trust responds to the challenge of Better Births and what part our free-standing rural MLU will play in it.

Addressing midwives' potential concerns

The concerns of some midwives may already have become obvious during your SWOC analysis. Addressing these is of critical importance. It may not be possible to overcome concerns fully before you start to design your project, but if you can address some major concerns at an early stage then other planning may become easier. Time should be spent on having detailed discussions with midwives including managers of services and taking their concerns seriously. Midwives may or may not be keen on the concept of continuity of carer—but what do they understand by that? Does their interest extend to working in the model and are there limitations to that? How might the model work for midwives who are employed on a part-time basis? What might the new model of care mean for midwives who will need to support the changes but who work in core services, such as antenatal, labour and birth or postnatal services? (You will find useful information in Chapter 4, which addresses how to make continuity of care work for midwives and managers.)

Addressing women's expectations

One important point to remember as you think through these issues is that women using the service will need to have a very clear understanding of how the model will work so that they know exactly what to expect; for example, how strong is the possibility that they will be looked after by their primary midwife or her buddy? Always remember that what you are trying to do is improve care and that increasing the number of women who get a known midwife looking after them in labour from a very low percentage to even 50% would be a brilliant improvement.

Addressing the size of caseload

The number of women per year for whom each midwife will be the primary or named midwife needs to be decided. We do know that it is important to make sure the caseloads are not too big, as the risk is that midwives will get tired and be unable to work to their full potential. Of course the opposite also holds true: it is important to have the midwives working to their full capacity to ensure that the models of care are cost effective. In working through these issues it is important to consider the particular service the model will provide:

- Which women will be cared for—do they have high physical, social or emotional needs?
- What is the ratio of primiparous to multiparous women?
- Will antenatal care be provided in the woman's home or from a central location?
- What is the geographical area—will the midwives need to travel considerable distances to provide care in women's homes?
- What is the length of postnatal care that will be provided?
- Will recently qualified midwives have a reduced caseload?

The detail behind discussing these issues is very important—for example, if a woman is lost from a midwife's caseload, is that woman replaced? Or, if a woman has an induction of labour, how much of her care during the induction process will be managed by the MGP midwife / midwives? If women are not home within 24 hours after giving birth, will the midwives be visiting them on the postnatal ward?

Guidelines for consultation and referral

You will need to consider systems to promote timely and effective consultation and referral. In some instances the women's general practitioner will be the first point of call or there may be a consultant obstetrician who is the lead obstetrician for the MGP; for non-urgent consultations during a woman's pregnancy the midwives would refer to that particular obstetrician or their team. This would also apply if the midwives wished to discuss an area of uncertainty or concern regarding anything that might necessitate obstetric opinion. The Australian College of Midwives' *National Midwifery Guidelines for Consultation and Referral* (ACM, 2014, reprinted 2017) is a resource that is being used and adapted in countries outside of Australia. (See Chapter 6, which explores safety and quality issues.)

Identifying the cost of your new project

One of the big challenges when you are arguing for the development of midwifery continuity of care models is to show how they are value for money. You can, however, draw on the evidence presented in Chapter 7 showing that cost benefits can be associated with setting up MGPs based on a caseload model in mainstream maternity services.

In both Australia and the UK, Birthrate Plus (2015), a well-respected workforce-planning tool for maternity services, is continuing to develop a methodology to calculate the different staffing levels that will be needed for different maternity services if they encompass continuity of carer models. This is important because it will be the number of midwives needed that will largely drive service costs. (See Chapter 9 for more details about Birthrate Plus.)

In considering the potential costs of your project the following factors will need to be addressed:

- the size of caseload per midwife and the number of women whom the continuity of care midwives will be expected to attend in labour
- the expectations about the work that will be undertaken by the continuity of care midwives and the amount that will be undertaken by core staff (ultimately the number of core staff should reduce as continuity of carer models develop)
- the potential improvements in outcomes and associated cost savings
- any increased salary costs—for example, any additional payments that may be expected for additional on-call arrangements

- the degree to which midwifery costs can be reduced by including other staff in the model; depending on your context this might include, for example, clerical workers, maternity support workers, Aboriginal health workers or midwifery care assistants
- the impact of introducing new models of care on recruitment and retention or on reducing agency staffing costs.

Addressing issues around terms and conditions of working

The midwifery continuity of carer model that you ultimately design will be influenced by industrial relations issues in your context. In the UK all midwives working as NHS employees work under 'Agenda for Change' terms and conditions. In most instances, midwives are paid hourly rates with clearly defined rules around hours of work, hours off between shifts, on-call arrangements and days off. There is often more potential for flexibility within national pay agreements than people realise and it should be possible with good local negotiation to develop a salary agreement that is acceptable to midwives and suitable to the model of care, but is still compliant.

In many parts of Australia, managers of midwives working in caseload projects have successfully negotiated an annualised salary agreement. These agreements are negotiated between the health service or provider and the industrial union. Midwives are paid an annualised salary with an extra loading (usually 30%–35%) on top of their usual award rates. The loading compensates midwives for not receiving 'penalty rates' (allowances normally paid to shift workers, such as overtime and working outside of office hours).

When you start designing your model and working out the logistical arrangements of how it will work, it is worth having a meeting with a representative from your industrial organisation / trade union (if there is such a group in your country). You will need to have a clear proposal and idea about what you hope to achieve and how you would like the project to work before this meeting. It is also helpful if the midwives who are going to work in the new project are also included in the meeting. This is an important part of ensuring that a transparent process exists in the development of the project and that choosing to work in this way does not disadvantage the midwives. (Chapters 5 and 9 elaborate further on these matters.)

Plans for ensuring the sustainability of the project

Designing a project that will be sustainable starts with designing the foundations of your project and having a clear understanding of factors in your organisation that might promote or challenge implementation (Forster et al., 2011). Chapter 11 provides you with an opportunity to consider some of these issues.

Overall, there are three overarching factors that will enhance the sustainability of midwifery continuity of care projects; first described by Jane Sandall in 1997, midwives working in successful continuity of care projects enjoy the following:

- **meaningful relationships with women**—enough continuity through pregnancy, labour and birth and the postnatal period for a two-way, meaningful relationship to evolve
- **occupational autonomy**—the opportunity for midwives to have flexible arrangements regarding how they organise their working lives, including working out on-call arrangements with colleagues in their MGP or team
- **social support at home and at work**—this means that midwives meet at least once a week with other midwives in their team or MGP for collegial support: to plan work and discuss pressing issues, but also to support each other around any potential uncertainty, overload of work or emotional difficulties that may be affecting their working lives.

WRITING A PROPOSAL

As you start to become clear about how your new midwifery continuity of care model will operate, writing a short proposal with members of your working group can help you develop your ideas and become clear about the new project and what it will involve. The process of writing the proposal and then sharing it with others is also a good way to inform others and gather support for the idea and for the implementation process.

The proposal does not need to be very long; two to three pages is often enough. As shown in Box 2.5, a series of headings can help you structure the document.

Writing the proposal takes time, as does refining and making your ideas clearer, accessible to all parties and more succinct. Be prepared to go through a significant number of drafts, during which time you might show your proposal to others in your maternity unit, talking them through your plans and considering their feedback carefully. Remember to take into account what are likely to be key concerns of different groups.

IMPLEMENTING YOUR NEW PROJECT

The question is often asked: 'What sort of midwife can provide continuity of carer?' Essentially, all midwives educated in high-income countries are qualified to provide continuity of carer. They may, however, need help to ensure their skills and competencies are up to date, they will need adequate support, and they will need to be enthusiastic about practising according to the full potential of their role (Forster et al., 2011).

Including recently qualified midwives

Including recently qualified midwives in continuity of carer models can be seen as an important strategy for workforce capacity building and sustainability (Hartz et al.,

BOX 2.5 Suggested Template When Writing a Proposal for a Continuity of Care Project

- **Aim** (What do you hope to achieve?)—e.g.: To establish a new midwifery continuity of care project that will provide women with a known midwife through pregnancy, labour and birth, and the postnatal period.
- **Background** (What has informed this new project?)—Briefly describe the evidence around continuity of care and why it has been shown to be beneficial (see Chapter 1).
- **Proposed project** (What are the project that you want to implement and the proposed processes?)—Describe your project and how it will operate: the group of women you hope to cater for and the percentage of women who will receive continuity of carer, the proposed caseload size, the number of midwives and the way in which they will work including their working arrangements, and clinical outcomes measures.
- **Implementation** (How will the project be put into practice?)—Describe the timeframe and process, how you propose to recruit midwives and arrangements for support, upskilling and continuing professional development.
- **Evaluation** (How will you know that you have met your aims?)—Describe how you will evaluate the success of your new project. (Chapter 8 has some useful strategies and approaches to guide your evaluation.)

2012). Having many years of experience as a midwife is not necessarily the only criterion to use when selecting or inviting midwives to work in continuity of carer models. Recently qualified midwives have advantages. For example they have had less socialisation into an institutionalised style of care and are usually enthusiastic and keen, with up-to-date knowledge—all of which makes them ideally placed to provide continuity of carer (Cummins et al., 2015, 2016; Passant et al., 2003).

In many instances, recently qualified midwives have had some experience in providing continuity of carer (or learning about continuity of carer) during their preregistration education. This may have included being placed with midwives providing continuity of care, having their own caseload of women in their final year, or working through the 'continuity of care' experiences that are a regulatory requirement of Australian midwifery education programs (Gray et al., 2016). In many cases this means that new graduates feel ready to provide continuity of care and are keen to work in this way (Cummins, 2013; Cummins et al., 2015; Gray et al., 2012, 2016). However, visionary leadership is often required, particularly in managing the myths and fears that abound about the inadvisability of placing new graduates in such roles (Cummins et al., 2016). Initial and ongoing supportive measures from managers are crucial; this might include a prolonged period of orientation and reduced caseload while recently qualified midwives build their confidence about providing care across the full midwifery scope of practice (Cummins et al., 2016).

Including experienced midwives

Clearly, experienced midwives are also important to include in your new project. These midwives will provide invaluable support, role modelling, education and expertise to less experienced midwives. However, midwives who have worked in only one area of maternity care for a long time may need additional support.

Including students

Including midwifery students in midwifery continuity of carer projects is essential. This is one effective way that students understand continuity and can prepare to work in this way once qualified. It may be difficult for students to have a complete understanding of continuity of carer until they are placed with a caseload midwife from an MGP.

Medical students also benefit from exposure to midwifery continuity of carer. Opportunities can be explored to ensure that the obstetricians and general practitioners of the future have an understanding of the role of the midwife and the importance of midwifery continuity of carer.

The selection process

A general principle around selecting midwives, particularly in the beginning, is to let midwives select themselves (McCourt et al., 2006). Calling for 'expressions of interest' for the new model within your unit may be a good place to start. Before you distribute this you may need to do some education within the unit about what midwifery continuity of carer is all about and how it might work, including being very clear about the model you have designed and the expectations of midwives working in the scheme.

Another issue you will need to decide is whether or not to have a lead midwife in the team. This is a decision that will need to be made locally: in some models it is considered important, whereas in others it is felt that shared leadership is better for high-quality team working.

Working closely with a small group of midwives means that a certain level of trust and camaraderie will need to exist or develop, and midwives may ask for some control over the people with whom they choose to work. It is important to adhere to the usual fair processes of recruitment. This could, however, include a group discussion attended by existing midwives in the group practices. This process mirrors the ways that midwives work together in a group practice, where midwives need to respect one another's similarities and differences as well as to be able to discuss issues, share uncertainty, manage conflict, negotiate solutions and embrace compromise. Having a group interview process where these skills and attitudes are demonstrated can be very useful for applicants and interviewers.

Preparing midwives to work in continuity of care models

Once you have selected the midwives who will work in the new model, the next step is to ensure that they are well prepared to fulfil their role. A self-assessment process has been used to help midwives determine which practice-based skills need further development. This started out as a skills inventory and was adapted with permission from research at the Midwifery Development Unit in Scotland (McGinley et al., 1995). The Australian College of Midwives subsequently developed the inventory into a 'Practice development resource: a self-assessment tool for midwives', which enables midwives to assess their own professional development needs in terms of skills, knowledge and experience. The resource is available from the College (ACM, 2018a).

Team-building workshops

In preparing for working in a group practice we have already outlined how it is important to involve the midwives in deciding how they will work. It is also important to remember that most midwives will not have had experience of working in a small autonomous team and it is generally agreed that, if continuity of carer models are to be successful, teams will need both initial and ongoing support. We have found great benefit in the provision of a number of team-building days or workshops. Topics that might be covered during the set-up phase are 'reaching consensus', 'conflict resolution' and 'negotiation skills'. Support may be ongoing—for example, a weekly supervision session or ad hoc meetings to address issues or reflect on a difficult situation. Such sessions will ideally be facilitated by someone who does not have a 'stake' in the group.

MANAGING MIDWIVES IN CONTINUITY OF CARE PROJECTS

A major challenge in some contexts is the issue of how midwives working in continuity of carer schemes will be 'managed'. In many countries, midwifery management is quite hierarchical and rule bound. Close attention is paid to detail such as when midwives come on duty and who is in charge. If continuity of carer schemes are to flourish it is important that midwives are left to self-manage and to negotiate how they work within their team. The organisation should be focusing on whether or not the midwives are meeting the agreed outcomes rather than on day-to-day working. As self-management develops a process of clinical governance becomes essential. Midwives in these models of care must expect to submit data on process outcomes—for example, the percentage of women who are attended by their named midwife in labour, and on clinical outcomes in a timely manner. These issues are discussed further in Chapters 4 and 6.

CONTRACTING ARRANGEMENTS IN PUBLIC HEALTH SYSTEMS

In Australia and the UK there are examples of midwives forming their own contracts with publicly funded maternity services / the NHS in order to provide women with continuity of carer.

Contracting arrangements for midwives in Australia

Since November 2010, after meeting certain criteria and being endorsed by the Nursing and Midwifery Board of Australia (NMBA), privately practising midwives can apply for a Medicare provider number; this means that women can claim Medicare rebates from the national government for the care they receive from their midwife. The intrapartum care rebate only applies if the woman gives birth in a hospital or birth centre facility.

Once endorsed, a midwife can purchase professional indemnity insurance through the Midwives Practice Insurance Scheme (MPIS), a national government-subsidised scheme which covers pregnancy and postnatal care in any setting and labour and birth care in a hospital or birth unit.

As identified on the website of the Australian College of Midwives (ACM, 2018b), in order to provide Medicare rebatable services, endorsed midwives have to have '… a collaborative arrangement with either a doctor who provides obstetric services; a hospital that has credentialed the midwife; or a health service / organisation that employs or engages at least one obstetric specified medical practitioner'. A growing number of endorsed midwives with collaborative arrangements, some of them in group practices, have negotiated agreements with maternity units for access or 'visiting' rights so that they can provide rebated continuity of carer for women who wish or need to give birth in hospital.

Contracting arrangements for midwives in the UK

In the UK the *National Health Service Act* of 2006 allowed clinical commissioning groups to contract with approved independent providers to deliver NHS services. To date very few midwives have taken advantage of this but two organisations—'One to One Midwives' and 'Neighbourhood Midwives'—have contracted into the NHS and are helping maternity services to understand how this can best be achieved.

One issue that concerns UK midwives is the question of how they can work if they are not covered by the vicarious liability that comes from employment within the NHS. This is a real issue as individual independent midwives have found it impossible to purchase insurance which is deemed adequate by the Nursing and Midwifery Council to cover the whole episode of maternity care. Both Neighbourhood Midwives and One to One Midwives originally overcame this problem by forming an organisation which could be insured as the 'employer' of the midwives. In other words, they became the body responsible for governance of their model. However, if an MGP is contracting into the NHS it can ask for insurance cover from the NHS scheme Clinical Negligence Scheme for Trusts (CNST).

Neighbourhood Midwives (NM) is an employee-owned social enterprise organisation that was incorporated as a company under the *Companies Act* in March 2012. This organisation has always aimed to become a service commissioned by the NHS and thereby free to women at the point of access. In order to establish a track record, it provided private midwifery services until 2016 when it got its first NHS contract with Waltham Forest Clinical Commissioning Group (CCG) in North London. In the first year of the contract, NM booked 190 women with straightforward pregnancies; each midwife had an annual caseload of 35 women (fewer if there were complex social needs). The midwives work from a children's centre where there is also a weekly ultrasound scanning service. The group has links to named NHS consultants. The midwives are making arrangements to work clinically in local hospitals so that they can give direct care to all their women, not just those giving birth at home.

Midwife and NHS commissioner Kate Brintworth was instrumental in the process that led to NM contracting with Waltham Forest CCG. In Box 2.6, she describes what midwives need to consider if they are preparing to negotiate with NHS CCGs.

BOX 2.6 Negotiating With NHS Clinical Commission Groups for Continuity of Carer Funding

Kate Brintworth

NHS commissioning is a structured, bureaucratic process. Each Clinical Commissioning Group (CCG) assesses the needs of its local population and procures services to meet those needs. Commissioners are motivated to improve the health of their population, so your service needs to be able to show what you can offer to meet the need. This means demonstrating improvement in a measurable way, such as increasing breastfeeding rates or homebirth rates, not just describing how well your service is structured and claiming how much women will like it. Commissioners need to be clear that your service represents value for money and will improve outcomes, particularly for the more vulnerable women.

Prepare for more paperwork than you ever imagined. Commissioners must assure themselves that you are a safe, sustainable service that is on a sound financial footing and that involves you engaging with multiple assurance processes.

Questions you may want to ask yourself to make sure you will succeed might include:

- How do I get registered with the UK regulatory body—the Care Quality Commission (CQC)—and what will I have to do to maintain registration and respond to the request for inspection (this may occur within a few months of starting)?
- How do I get registered with the UK health service insurance scheme—the Clinical Negligence Scheme for Trusts (CNST)?

Continued

BOX 2.6 Negotiating With NHS Clinical Commission Groups for Continuity of Carer Funding—cont'd

- Do I fully understand tariff, how money moves around the system and the determinants of how payment is managed?
- What financial backing do I have? You should not assume that because you have a contract you will have income to match your outgoings.
- Do I understand my outgoings fully? You have to think about premises, accountants, IT, administration, equipment, subcontracts you may require (for bloods, scans, etc.), CNST, national insurance, mobile phones, tax, disposables and drugs to name a few.
- How will I capture and report on data? You will need to report to a variety of organisations such as the Maternity Services Data Set, the antenatal and newborn screening committee, NHS England and your local maternity system, as well as reporting activity to be paid and your commissioner's request as part of the NHS standard contract including a dashboard and ad hoc requests.
- Do I have the right policies? You will need to have good policies for everything including safeguarding, information governance, managing staff, escalation, etc. as well as clinical issues.
- How am I managing governance? You will need to identify, manage and report on all of the above, including maintaining a risk register, and keep clear records of all of this work. But it is possible. What you can see is that you need support and some professional help to succeed.

Top tips
- Use the knowledge and skills of those who have already done this.
- Consider sharing backroom services with another organisation to reduce costs.
- Do your research! There is lots of information about CCGs and local authority populations on their websites.
- Understand your local maternity system. What position are current providers in? Do they have concerns about your service? Working through their issues together will support your relationship establishing positively.

In Box 2.7, Annie Francis describes what it has meant being commissioned by Waltham Forest CCG from the point of view of NM.

Another example of a midwifery service which contracts into the NHS is One to One Midwives. The founder of the organisation, Jo Parkington, explains how the project was developed in Box 2.8.

BOX 2.7 Contracting Into the NHS: the Experience of Neighbourhood Midwives

Annie Francis

The first question is, why do you want to do this? This is an important place to start because the answer will need to sustain you throughout the long, challenging process ahead.

For us, the search for affordable indemnity insurance for independent midwives was a key driver. This was combined with our passionate belief that the future for midwifery lies in the development and scalability of an holistic, social model of midwifery care delivered through small, self-managing, caseloading teams.

We felt that the social model of midwifery care was probably most sustainable if delivered not from within the traditional NHS structures but from an employee-owned social enterprise—'Neighbourhood Midwives' was our vehicle, working alongside and in partnership with the wider system and regulatory framework, but in charge of our own destiny and with the freedom and flexibility to make our own 'rules'.

An important key ingredient for success is timing. You need some luck and a few planets to align in your favour. For us the recommendations of the Better Births report in 2016—specifically around welcoming independent providers into the NHS to increase choice—supplied the required impetus to our early talks with an interested and engaged CCG. You need to know what it is you can offer that is different from what is already available and then demonstrate how you plan to deliver it.

Our route to a 'track record' was through the launch of a small private service in the first instance, which enabled us to put all the required governance structures in place, including registering with the CQC. We put in years of groundwork in developing the policies, guidelines and processes needed—and we are still working on them. We feel strongly though that these should be 'open source' and are happy to support other groups wanting to explore this route—there is absolutely no point in everyone re-inventing the wheel!

For our pilot in north-east London, we created a project plan, based on the long list of 'to-do's' outlined in Kate's vignette above, and had a countdown to launch day (which was set back at least three times). A cornerstone of the project was the recruitment and 'onboarding' of our first midwives. As for every other provider, it is a challenging and time-consuming task to find midwives who want to work in this way, especially in the current climate, when so many feel anxious about what 24/7 on-call means and how it might affect them and their work–life balance.

The more control midwives have over this key aspect of caseloading though, the more they can weave this way of working into their own personal circumstances. We are a Teal organisation (go to Teal organisation wiki to get an idea of what that means) in which 'self-management' means so much more than just planning your own diary. It is a concept that we believe fits perfectly with autonomous midwifery practice—but is at odds with how midwives currently work in the wider system. It has been a steep learning curve for all of us to adopt and then adapt to a very different set of principles and values underpinning everything we do—but the supportive culture and positive working environment it creates is definitely worth the effort.

Continued

BOX 2.7 Contracting Into the NHS: the Experience of Neighbourhood Midwives—cont'd

So, almost 5 years since we first launched, and just over 1 year into our first NHS service delivery, we currently have 6 F/T midwives in our NHS practice, 10 in our private service and we plan to start a second NHS team soon. Our outcomes are fabulous—very similar to other caseloading models—and the feedback and evaluation of our service from women and their families is hugely positive. We still face daily challenges though and, although immensely rewarding, it does require total commitment, resilience in bucket loads and I would have to say it is not an option for the faint hearted.

BOX 2.8 Contracting Into the NHS: the Experience of One to One Midwives

Jo Parkington

The One to One Midwives model is based on one midwife providing continuity of care for 32 women at any one time. Since 2010, One to One has been commissioned by the NHS and has grown from 2 midwives to 60 midwives today working across 8 teams. We have provided care for over 11,000 women with a normal birth rate of 78% and a homebirth rate of 30% against a national average of 2.4%. Women of all risk categories can be accepted into the service.

One of our major challenges has been retention of our workforce. In a country where there is a recognised national shortage of midwives and where midwives receive very little training or exposure to continuity of carer models, it has been a major challenge to retain midwives to work in a model that requires 24/7 on-call commitment. We also recognised that the midwives of today hail from the millennial culture—it is well researched that this generation has little interest in traditional hierarchical structures and does not expect to remain in the same job for a long period of time.

So here at One to One we have focused on giving our workforce maximum autonomy, not just in their clinical decision making but also in how they work. We wanted to create an environment that decentralised leadership and have created a non-hierarchical structure where everyone is recognised as a leader. We have devolved our decision-making process to individuals and into self-managed teams supported by a governance framework that provides clear boundaries and robust processes to ensure that all decisions remain compliant with our contractual and regulatory requirements.

An example of this is that different teams have established their own working patterns. We have set parameters that each midwife has to achieve a continuity of carer rate of 85% or above for the whole pathway of care: antenatal, birth and postnatal. Within this framework the teams have evolved their way of working to meet this parameter but provide themselves with the work–life balance that is so important to them. One team is working with buddy teams rotating 2 months on and then 2 months off; another team works within a 'protected time' model where each midwife within the team is allocated protected time each week. The continuity rates have actually increased across all teams, achieving rates for antenatal care of 88% and postnatal care of 95%, with birth continuity up to 70% across the buddy team. We believe that this is due to midwives feeling in control and empowered and we tap into the concept that everyone wants to be the best that they can be; we trust them to do just that.

WHEN WIDESCALE CHANGE IS POSSIBLE: SEIZING THE MOMENT

Occasionally, opportunities present that enable you to make widescale changes to your service. This enables you to ensure that midwifery caseload practice is the chosen model of care that is developed. In Box 2.9, Professor of Midwifery Sally Tracy describes two such experiences, both of which highlight many of the issues that we have discussed in this chapter.

BOX 2.9 Implementing Caseload Practice in a New Midwifery-Led Unit and a Large Tertiary Hospital

Sally Tracy

When planning for change, never underestimate the serendipitous opportunities that arise around you. Let me describe the way we used local factors to lever change to set up a stand-alone midwifery-led primary birth unit (Tracy et al., 2005), and a few years later a reorganisation of the midwifery workforce at a large teaching hospital in Sydney (Hartz et al., 2012). Both changes were based on being able to respond to local challenges when the time was right; and the success of both changes relied on implementing caseload midwifery care.

The primary level midwifery-led unit (PMU) was established at a peripheral metropolitan hospital in 2003. The area health service was going through a stringent cost-cutting exercise and decided it was unprofitable to continue providing anaesthetic registrars when there were only about 500 births a year. The management solution was to close the maternity section of the hospital and encourage women to travel to the large tertiary maternity hospital about 15 kilometres away. The most obvious fallout from this move was the loss of jobs for 23 full-time midwives who were employed by the unit and who mainly spoke Chinese languages, and the disadvantage caused to the mainly immigrant Asian community of women who often did not have any other means of transport other than the bus—but the bus route didn't extend to the tertiary hospital 15 km away.

The solution was to propose a PMU that did not require anaesthetics or a caesarean section capability and would employ the very capable 23 full-time midwives who had clocked up years of experience working at the unit. There were no precedents in New South Wales at the time for this type of unit or caseload midwifery care.

The resistance was huge. The anaesthetists clamoured about the unsafety of a low-risk birth unit and said that women would die on the road in the night having to travel urgently for a caesarean section. The local and major daily papers ran stories about the deaths and devastation that would ensue. The doctors' union, the Australian Medical Association, ran an editorial condemning such a move and demanded to visit the unit with the state health minister. Specialists of all creeds, obstetricians, paediatricians and anaesthetists, joined forces to resist such a mad-cap idea.

To combat all these barriers we had to be very patient and inclusive and carefully plan the change using the positive factors we had on the balance sheet against the risks or challenges that we also faced. Along with identifying key management level people to support

Continued

BOX 2.9 Implementing Caseload Practice in a New Midwifery-Led Unit and a Large Tertiary Hospital—cont'd

our plan, the one safety card up our sleeve was the plan to offer continuity of care—based on the fact that we had an experienced and capable group of midwives. This is the most important way of ensuring that problems do not suddenly arise, or that women are left to worry or even transfer to more specialist medical care on their own. A midwife who has got to know a woman during the 6 months of her pregnancy is able to recognise early signs of change well within time to make decisions that will affect the safety of that woman and her infant. Not only was our plan to set up a free-standing unit; the non-negotiable element was the ability for midwives to work in the caseload model. We knew this was the one way we could guarantee the safety of the mothers and the midwives.

We identified key supporters amongst the senior management and obstetric personnel and held weekly meetings for 6 months to identify all the 'dangers' in such a plan; we prepared an evidence-based proposal outlining our vision to the area health clinical council, and in it we noted all the risks, benefits and challenges of such an idea; we responded to the media and we provided updates for question time in state parliament; we audited and noted just how often an obstetrician and an anaesthetist had to be called between the hours of midnight and 6 am for an urgent caesarean section (zero times in the two preceding years); we ran workshops with the midwives on how to manage caseload and how to survive in a PMU, and the midwives achieved a level of competency and confidence through using a self-assessment skills audit; we planned a call system for the ambulance service; we provided a 24-hour telephone mentoring system for senior midwives to support those on-call; and we sat with the Nurses Union to redraft a wage agreement so that the midwives could work within an annualised salary agreement to follow women through the service.

The old stables at the hospital came in handy, and several families held 'working bees' to revamp those spaces to make way for women to attend antenatal visits with the midwives; we prepared a set of midwifery guidelines that had to appease the anaesthetists and act as a signpost for women and midwives about when it was appropriate to transfer or go straight to the tertiary unit to give birth. And finally we helped to mobilise the local women to write to the CEO of the area health service and request to keep the unit open.

The midwives organised themselves into working partnerships and where midwives could only manage a part-time caseload they partnered up with another midwife who would also work part time. The group was an organic whole of about eight midwives consisting of closer partnership pairs. All major system-based decisions were made at the weekly peer review meeting held at the unit.

The first-year audit of caseload midwifery care within the PMU was tabled in the NSW parliament and it was noted that caseload midwifery group practice supported the provision of maternity care within a community hospital as a safe alternative to tertiary hospital-based obstetric care. No adverse outcome was reported. A quality audit based on focus groups with the women found that having a known midwife for pregnancy, birth and postnatally enhanced the experience of birth for the women. Having a caseload midwife lowered the need for obstetric intervention and pharmacological pain relief in the birth process and it increased the perception of control and comfort for women. The screening procedures, guidelines and

BOX 2.9 Implementing Caseload Practice in a New Midwifery-Led Unit and a Large Tertiary Hospital—cont'd

protocols established were well adhered to. The PMU placed much greater emphasis on primary level health services with an enhanced risk management structure to refer and safely obtain tertiary medical assistance as the need arose. In doing so it offered midwives the opportunity to provide midwifery care based on following the woman's needs rather than on primarily addressing the staffing needs of a maternity hospital (Tracy & Hartz, 2006).

Ten years on, the PMU is still providing a safe, cost-effective service (Monk et al., 2014). It has won several government awards for safety and innovation.

Similar opportunities were identified and grasped in favour of setting up caseload care for women of all risk categories at a major teaching hospital. The Area Health Service in this case was very keen to cut costs by 'lopping off' funding to the alongside birth centre (which was one of the first established in Australia in the 1970s). Managers pointed out that many of the rostered birth centre staff were only fully utilised when there were busy times, and that because they sat outside the staffing quota for the delivery suite it would be economical to close the birth centre and fund birth services in one cost centre. The midwives had been working very effectively in a team structure for at least 5 years, and were extremely unhappy at the thought of losing the alongside birth centre.

This was a golden opportunity. It is often very difficult to effect a smooth transition from a rostered staff situation to having midwives on an annualised salary being able to follow a caseload of women. But in this situation we were faced with losing the birth centre or being imaginative and brave! The other magical ingredient here was our having received funding to undertake a randomised controlled trial (RCT) of caseload midwifery. After many meetings and workshops with senior managers and staff in the unit, including birth centre midwives and midwives interested in working in caseload practice, eight MGPs were established, made up of 32 FTE midwives.

A couple of supportive obstetricians were identified to attach themselves to the different caseload groups to ensure women who had health problems would appropriately receive both medical and midwifery care as needed. The RCT was set up and women who began booking at the hospital were offered caseload care—they could give birth in the birth centre space or the routine delivery ward and if they had no special preference they were ran-domised to routine care or caseload. When caseload midwives left on maternity leave they often returned to work part time and work in the rostered ward, populating the 'core' staff with a deeper understanding of how to support caseload midwifery in a busy teaching hos-pital. Again, offering continuity of midwifery care ensured the health problems that emerged were attended to in good time and again the birth outcomes for mothers and infants were excellent (Tracy et al., 2013).

The dream of course, is to have caseload care for all women—and this is the next major challenge. I suspect again it will be managed when the time is right to move to a national government-funded bundled price for maternity care (similar to that in New Zealand). The important thing is to be ready to act when the time is right!

MAPPING THE DEVELOPMENT OF YOUR PROJECT

Our final suggestion in this chapter is that you keep a diary record of the journey you take during the process of planning and implementation. This serves as an important source of data when you are writing the evaluation of your project. You will forget where the trials and tribulations were along the way and how these were tackled. These are usually the most useful tips to pass on to others embarking on a similar exercise. It is also beneficial to have your story recorded, particularly on the 'bad days'. It can be very heartening and encouraging to read over where you have come from, and remember how much has really been achieved.

CONCLUSION

In conclusion, when implementing midwifery continuity of carer in mainstream services, it is essential to join forces with users of services in the planning, implementation and ongoing evaluation of services. It is also important to make sure that, at every stage, processes are enacted to involve, inform and consult with all staff in hospital and community settings who may be affected by the changes you are planning. These overarching factors form the foundations for success and sustainability.

REFERENCES

Australian College of Midwives (ACM): *National midwifery guidelines for consultation and referral*, ed 3, issue 2, Canberra, 2014, (reprinted May 2017 with amendments), ACM. Online: https://issuu.com/austcollegemidwives/docs/consultation_and_referral_guideline.

Australian College of Midwives (ACM): *ACM continuity of care handbook*, Canberra, 2016, ACM. Online: https://www.midwives.org.au/resources/continuity-care-handbook-electronic.

Australian College of Midwives (ACM): *MidPLUS practice development resource: a self-assessment tool for midwives*, Canberra, 2018a, ACM. Online: https://www.midwives.org.au/resources/midplus-practice-development-resource-self-assessment-tool-midwives.

Australian College of Midwives (ACM): Endorsement & Medicare, Canberra, 2018b, ACM. Online: https://www.midwives.org.au/endorsement-medicare.

Australian Government Department of Health: National Maternity Services Plan, Canberra, 2011. Online: http://www.health.gov.au/internet/publications/publishing.nsf/Content/pacd-maternityservices plan-toc.

Australian Health Ministers Advisory Council (AHMAC): National Maternity Services Plan: 2014–15 annual report, Canberra, 2011, AHMAC. Online: https://health.gov.au/internet/main/publishing.nsf/content/8985FF7FE467D0AACA257D330080BCD2/$File/NSMP%20Annual%20Report-FINAL%20ENDORSED%20(D16-524081).PDF.

Batalden M, Batalden P, Margolis P, Seid M, Armstrong G, Opipari-Arrigan L, et al: Coproduction of healthcare services, *BMJ Qual Saf* 25:509–517, 2016.

Biro MA: What has public health got to do with midwifery? Midwives' role in securing better health outcomes for mothers and babies, *Women Birth* 24:17–23, 2011.

Birthrate Plus: Birthrateplus: safe staffing for maternity services, 2015. Online: https://www.birthrateplus.co.uk.

Centre for Maternal and Child Enquiries (CMACE): *Saving mothers' lives: reviewing maternal deaths to make motherhood safer: 2006–08*. The eighth report on confidential enquiries into maternal deaths in the United Kingdom, *BJOG* 118:1–203, 2011.

Chief Nursing Officers of England, Northern Ireland, Scotland and Wales: *Midwifery 2020: delivering expectations*, London, 2010, Department of Health. Online: https://www.gov.uk/government/publications/midwifery-2020-delivering-expectations.

Cummins AM: Facilitation of new graduate midwives into midwifery continuity of care models, *Women Birth* 26:S25–S25, 2013.

Cummins AM, Denney-Wilson E, Homer CSE: The experiences of new graduate midwives working in midwifery continuity of care models in Australia, *Midwifery* 31(4):438–444, 2015.

Cummins AM, Denney-Wilson E, Homer CSE: The challenge of employing and managing new graduate midwives in midwifery group practices in hospitals, *J Nurs Manag* 24:614–623, 2016.

Donley J: The importance of consumer control over childbirth, *NZCOM J* 1:6–7, 1989.

Ebert L, Ferguson A, Bellchambers H: Working for socially disadvanted women, *Women Birth* 24:85–91, 2011.

Forster DA, Newton M, McLachlan HL, Willis K: Exploring implementation and sustainability of models of care: can theory help?, *BMC Public Health* 11(Suppl 5):S8, 2011.

Foureur M: Next steps: public health in midwifery practice. In Luanaigh PO, Carlson C, editors: *Midwifery and public health: future directions and new opportunities*, London, 2005, Elsevier, pp 221–237.

Gray JE, Leap N, Sheehy A, Homer CSE: The 'follow-through' experience in three-year bachelor of midwifery programs in Australia: a survey of students, *J Nurs Educ Pract* 12:258–263, 2012.

Gray JE, Taylor J, Newton M: Embedding continuity of care experiences: an innovation in midwifery education, *Midwifery* 33:40–42, 2016.

Grigg CP, Tracy SK: New Zealand's unique maternity system, *Women Birth* 26(1):e59–e64, 2013.

Guilliland K, Pairman S: *The midwifery partnership: a model for practice*. Department of Nursing and Midwifery monograph series, Wellington, 1995, Victoria University.

Guilliland K, Pairman S: *Women's business: the story of the New Zealand College of Midwives 1986–2010*, Christchurch, 2010, New Zealand College of Midwives.

Hartz D, White J, Lainchbury KA, Gunn H, Jarman H, Welsh A, et al: Australian maternity reform through clinical redesign, *Aust Health Rev* 36(2):169–175, 2012.

Homer CSE, Leap N, Edwards N, Sandall J: Midwifery continuity of carer in an area of high socio-economic disadvantage in London: a retrospective analysis of Albany midwifery practice outcomes using routine data (1997–2009), *Midwifery* 48:1–10, 2017.

Kelly C, Alderdice F, Lohan M, Spence D: 'Every pregnant woman needs a midwife'—the experiences of HIV affected women in maternity care, *Midwifery* 29:132–138, 2013.

McAra-Couper J, Gilkison A, Crowther S, Hunter M, Hotchin C, Gunn J: Partnership and reciprocity with women sustain lead maternity carer midwives in practice, *NZCOM J* 49:23–33, 2014.

McCourt C, Pearce A: Does continuity of carer matter to women from minority ethnic groups?, *Midwifery* 16:145–154, 2000.

McCourt C, Stevens T, Sandall J, Brodie P: Working with women: developing continuity of care in practice. In Page LA, McCandlish R, editors: *The new midwifery: science and sensitivity in practice*, ed 2, Philadelphia, 2006, Churchill Livingstone Elsevier, pp 141–166.

McGinley M, Turnbull D, Fyvie H, Johnstone I, MacLennan B: Midwifery development unit at Glasgow Royal Maternity Hospital, *Br J Midwifery* 3(7):362–371, 1995.

Marmot M, Friel S, Bell R, Houweling TA, Taylor S: Closing the gap in a generation: health equity through action on the social determinants of health, *Lancet* 372:1661–1669, 2008.

Ministry of Health (MOH): *Report on maternity 2015*, Wellington, 2017, MOH.

Monk A, Tracy M, Foureur M, Grigg C, Tracy SK: Evaluating midwifery units (EMU): a prospective cohort study of freestanding midwifery units in New South Wales, Australia, *BMJ Open Access* 4: e006252, 2014.

National Health Service (NHS) England: *National maternity review. Better Births: improving outcomes of maternity services in England. A five year forward view for maternity care*, London, 2016, NHS England. Online: https://www.england.nhs.uk/wp-content/uploads/2016/02/national-maternity-review-report.pdf.

National Health Service (NHS) England: *Implementing Better Births: a resource pack for local maternity systems*, London, 2017, NHS England. Online: https://www.england.nhs.uk/wp-content/uploads/2017/03/nhs-guidance-maternity-services-v1.pdf.

National Insitute of Clinical Excellence (NICE): *Pregnancy and complex social factors: a model for service provision for pregnant women with complex social factors*, London, 2010, NICE.

New South Wales (NSW) Ministry of Health: *Midwifery continuity of carer model tool-kit*, Sydney, 2012, NSW Ministry of Health.

Newburn M, Fletcher G (co-production editors / section authors): *Maternity voices partnerships toolkit. Developed in collaboration with Kath Evans*, London, 2017, NHS England. Online: http://national maternityvoices.org.uk/wp-content/uploads/2017/03/Using-social-media-How-to-get-started -Maternity-Voices-Partnership-Toolkit-0617v.1.pdf.

Page LA: *Effective group practice in midwifery: working with women*, Oxford, 1995, Blackwell Science.

Passant L, Homer C, Wills J: From student to midwife: the experiences of newly graduated midwives working in an innovative model of midwifery care, *Aust J Midwifery* 16(4):18–21, 2003.

Rayment-Jones H, Murrells T, Sandall J: An investigation of the relationship between the case load model of midwifery for socially disadvantaged women and childbirth outcomes using routine data— a retrospective. Observational study, *Midwifery* 31(4):409–417, 2015.

Redshaw M: Women as consumers of maternity care: measuring "satisfaction" or "dissatisfaction"?, *Birth* 35:73–76, 2008.

Royal College of Midwives (RCM): Can continuity work for us? A resource for midwives. London, 2017, RCM. Online: https://www.rcm.org.uk/can-continuity-work-for-us.

Sandall J: Midwives' burnout and continuity of care, *Br J Midwifery* 5(2):106–111, 1997.

Sandall J: Every woman needs a midwife and some women need a doctor too, *Birth* 39(4):323–326, 2012.

Sandall J, Soltani H, Gates S, Shennan A, Devane D: Midwife-led continuity models versus other models of care for childbearing women, *Cochrane Database Syst Rev* (4):CD004667, 2016. doi:10.1002/14651858. CD004667.pub5.

Scottish Government: *The best start: a five-year forward plan for maternity and neonatal care in Scotland*, Edinburgh, 2017, Scottish Government. Online: https://beta.gov.scot/publications/best-start-five -year-forward-plan-maternity-neonatal-care-scotland/.

Shaw EK, Howard J, West DR, Crabtree BF, Nease DE Jr, Tutt B, et al: The role of the champion in primary care change efforts: from the state networks of Colorado ambulatory practices and partners (SNOCAP), *J Am Board Fam Med* 25(5):676–685, 2012.

Tracy SK, Hartz D: *The quality review of Ryde Midwifery Group Practice. September 2004 to October 2005. Final report*. Northern Sydney and Central Coast Health, Sydney, 2006, University of Technology. Online: https://www.uts.edu.au/sites/default/files/ryde-midwifery-caseload-practice.pdf.

Tracy SK, Hartz D, Nicholl M, McCann Y, Latta D: An integrated service network in maternity—the implementation of a midwifery-led unit, *Aust Health Rev* 29(3):332–339, 2005.

Tracy SK, Hartz DL, Tracy MB, Allen J, Forti A, Hall B, et al: Caseload midwifery care versus standard maternity care for women of any risk: M@NGO, a randomised controlled trial, *Lancet* 382(9906): 1723–1732, 2013. doi:10.1016/S0140-6736(13)61406-3.

Turnbull D, Reid M, McGinley M, Shields NR: Changes in midwives' attitudes to their professional role following implementation of the midwifery development unit, *Midwifery* 11(3):110–119, 1995.

van Teijlingen ER, Hundley V, Rennie A-M, Graham W, Fitzmaurice A: Maternity satisfaction studies and their limitations: "what is, must still be best", *Birth* 30(2):75–78, 2003.

Warwick C: Small group practices. Part 1, *Mod Midwife* 22–23, 1995.

Western Australian Department of Health: *Midwifery continuity of carer model toolkit*, Perth, 2016, Health Networks Directorate, Western Australian Department of Health. Online: https://ww2.health.wa.gov. au/~/media/Files/Corporate/general%20documents/Health%20Networks/Womens%20and%20 Newborns/Maternity-Continuity-of-Carer-Toolkit.pdf.

CHAPTER 3

Ways of Providing Midwifery Continuity of Care

Susan Crowther, Mary Ross-Davie, Deborah Davis, Natasha Donnolley

Contents

INTRODUCTION

It is now well established that midwifery continuity of care is evidence based, safe and desirable with benefits for women, babies, midwives and health systems. Nevertheless the setting up, scaling up and sustainability of midwifery continuity of care require significant thought, planning and ongoing support. One size does not fit all and it is vital that contextual considerations are fully appreciated in any planning and implementation. Failure to acknowledge contextual differences between settings can lead to unsustainable working practices and negative effects on the wellbeing and morale of midwives.

The purpose of this chapter is to explore the different ways that midwifery continuity of care can be provided in different contexts and settings. Previous chapters have examined the various definitions of midwifery continuity of care and carer. In this chapter, we unpack these definitions further, introducing some recent detailed work on characterising different models of midwifery continuity of care provision using terminology from the Australian Maternity Care Classification System (MaCCS).

The key to our discussion is an emphasis on the diversity of practice arrangements and the similarities and differences between the definitions and models of care that exist across and within different countries and regions. Our purpose is to showcase the degree of flexibility, innovation and creativity that midwives have fostered to make midwifery continuity of care work for them.

This chapter will illustrate different practice arrangements through examples taken from published practice-based evidence and includes two vignettes, one written by a practitioner working in a model that provides continuity of carer and one by a senior midwife working in a trade union / professional body. All our examples are taken from actual practice experiences which highlight the principles of successful midwifery continuity of care models.

We are acutely aware that often the 'elephant in the room' of any discussion of setting up midwifery continuity of care is the issue of the on-call arrangements (Royal College of Midwives (RCM), 2017). This chapter therefore dedicates a whole section to this 'elephant' and attempts to defuse many of the misconceptions around this concern—one that is often at the heart of resistance to changing to this way of practising (Crowther, 2017).

It is also vital that midwives' voices are heard and that they are protected from feeling vulnerable as practice arrangements change. Therefore, we include a short exploration of the potential role of professional bodies in supporting midwives and managers to successfully approach implementation in ways that are inclusive and supportive of midwives. The chapter will conclude with some exploration of sustainability of working this way with a focus on the significance of collegial relationships and avoiding burnout.

DEFINITIONS AND CHARACTERISTICS

As models of care have evolved over the years and around the globe, so too has the terminology we use to describe them. At the time of writing this chapter there continues to be diversity in the terminology used to describe the various practice arrangements for midwifery continuity of care. Although an expansion in the choice of models of care available to women is likely to be a positive outcome, it has led to confusion—both for women and for those providing maternity care—especially in understanding what the name of a model of care means and what it provides. For example, what is the difference between continuity of *care* and continuity of *carer?* What is *midwifery group practice* and what is *midwifery caseload care?* Is midwifery-led care the same thing as team midwifery care? The answers to these questions can differ both between and within countries, and until recently there was no standardised way to describe and define models of maternity care.

Previous chapters have referred to the difference between continuity of *care* and continuity of *carer*, the latter often being referred to as 'caseload practice'. Notwithstanding these differences in terminology, there are still variations in how models offering continuity of care / carer are organised and named that need to be explored further. The name of a model of care can be misleading if the details of what it involves are not properly understood. What one person calls 'midwifery group practice' may mean something else entirely in a different location or context, and there are a multitude of different models of care covered by the term 'midwifery-led continuity of care' (Sandall et al., 2016).

So how do we know to what we are referring when speaking about midwifery continuity of care(r)? The newly developed Australian Maternity Care Classification System was developed to do just that. The MaCCS classifies models of care based on the characteristics of the women for whom the model is intended, the carers working in the model and aspects of how the care is provided (Donnolley et al., 2016). By using the characteristics of the models, the classification system adds granularity that enables similar models of care to be grouped together regardless of their name. Names are an important feature in terms of communicating to women and within 'the system' but when these are applied inconsistently, even within a single jurisdiction let alone globally, understanding breaks down. It is hoped that removing the reliance on the model name reduces some of the confusion.

One of the more important characteristics captured by the MaCCS is the *extent of continuity of carer*. Within the MaCCS, this is defined as:

> *The extent to which continuity of carer is provided across the continuum of maternity care within a model of maternity care …*
>
> *This data element measures 'continuity of carer' which is a measure of whether relational continuity or 'one-to-one care' is provided by the same named caregiver being involved throughout the period of care even when other caregivers are required. A defining requirement of 'continuity of carer' is that the care is provided or lead over the full length of the episode of care by the same named carer in a model of care.*
>
> **(Source: Australian Institute of Health and Welfare. n.d. National Health Data Dictionary:**
> **http://meteor.aihw.gov.au/content/index.phtml/itemId/562423)**

This definition allows us to distinguish between models of care that provide differing degrees of continuity, thereby identifying those that provide continuity of *carer* across the continuum of pregnancy, birth and the postnatal period. This is not only continuity of *care*, but also of *carer*.

Recognising that providing full continuity of carer across the whole continuum of maternity care is not always possible, some models of care attempt to provide continuity of carer to women in the antenatal and postnatal periods only. This is still defined as women having a single named midwife as responsible for her care during those periods, but intrapartum care would be provided by a different health care professional. Midwives working in these models may be allocated a 'caseload' of women for antenatal and postnatal care, but the midwives are not on-call for intrapartum care, which is provided by 'core' midwives rostered at the hospital. Rather than have a blanket yes/no for continuity of carer, values for this characteristic in the MaCCS cover the different periods of maternity care: antenatal, intrapartum and postpartum and combinations of these periods. In this way, models of care offering some level of continuity of carer can be identified, even if they do not meet the definition of a full caseload model.

In addition to the extent of continuity, there are a range of characteristics that may vary between models that offer continuity of midwifery carer (regardless of the model's name). Some of these are captured in the MaCCS, and some are reflective of differences between countries in their funding models and health systems. Identifying these characteristics can assist in understanding how a model of care is constructed and being able to identify and compare similar models of care (Table 3.1).

WAYS OF WORKING THIS WAY: PRINCIPLES OF EACH MODEL

Despite the difficulties in standardising the naming of models of care, having agreed terminology is still important. In addition to classifying models of care based on their characteristics, the MaCCS allocates each model of care to one of 11 major model categories (MMCs) representing the main types of models of care found in Australia.

Although developed for the Australian context, the MaCCS terminology can be applied to other maternity care contexts and could be adapted for use in other countries. Box 3.1 details the descriptions of the MMCs relevant to models of care that could provide midwifery continuity of carer, although to different extents. What varies across these different model types is the extent of continuity of carer, where care is provided and the relationship between the midwife providing care and other health care providers involved. It also highlights the variation that is possible in how models offering midwifery continuity of carer can be structured and named. Some of these variations are influenced by funding models and legal frameworks, and will not necessarily apply to all countries or jurisdictions, but many of these permutations are seen around the world, albeit called different things.

Box 3.1 provides a summary of the different ways that midwives can work in continuity of carer models. We have chosen to use the model names used in the MaCCS for simplicity, while acknowledging that they may be referred to differently in your own country or facility. Examples are provided from different contexts and countries; however, these are by no means exhaustive. One of the wonderful things about providing continuity of midwifery care is the innovative ways in which it can be done.

Variations in model structures

Under the Better Births program recently implemented in the UK, two models of care were identified as providing continuity of carer by a known midwife—these

Table 3.1 Characteristics that differ between types of midwifery continuity of care models

Model characteristic	Examples/detail
Target group of women in the model (equivalent to risk status)	All women; low-risk/normal pregnancy; young mothers; breech births; high-risk/complex pregnancy; geographic area; specific ethnic group
Extent of continuity of carer	Antenatal period only; antenatal and intrapartum periods; antenatal and postpartum periods; whole duration of maternity period—antenatal, intrapartum and postpartum
Midwifery caseload and size	Caseload yes/no; number of women per FTE caseload
Routine relocation for intrapartum care	All women are relocated from their local areas for intrapartum care as birthing services are not provided in their local area
Setting for antenatal/intrapartum/postnatal care	Home; hospital clinic; birth centre; community facility
Compulsory planned medical visits	All women have a minimum number of planned visits with a medical practitioner (obstetrician or GP) as well as their routine care with a known midwife
Length of time for planned postnatal care	How many weeks planned postnatal care is provided for in the model
Planned collaborative carers	Are other healthcare providers included routinely in the model for all women—e.g. obstetrician, Aboriginal health practitioner, perinatal mental health worker, endocrinologist, etc.?
Ongoing involvement after transfer[a]	Whether the primary midwife continues to provide care for women in the model even after they have been referred for secondary/tertiary care
Funding source[a]	Public (government); private health insurance; private out of pocket; contract bundle; individual items
Employment/remuneration type[a]	Employed under annualised salary; employed on rostered hourly wage; self-employed
Employment status[a]	Contracted; hospital employee; self-employed

[a]Characteristics not included in the MaCCS and added here for information.
FTE=full-time equivalent.

were known as 'team continuity (midwifery group practice)' and 'full caseloading' (NHS England, 2017). Based on the MaCCS classifications, however, they would both be categorised as *midwifery group practice caseload care*. Both of these models provide continuity of carer across the full continuum of care, with each midwife being allocated a 'caseload' of women for whom they provide primary care. The main difference is how backup care is provided when a midwife is unavailable for her primary caseload—such as when she is already providing care to another woman in labour, when she is sick or on leave, etc. In the team model, midwives organise themselves into small teams (suggested to be four to eight in number), each having their own

BOX 3.1 Ways of Providing Midwifery Continuity of Care Based on the MaCCS Definitions

Private midwifery care

Antenatal, intrapartum and postnatal care is provided by a private midwife or group of midwives in collaboration with doctors in the event of identified risk factors. Antenatal, intrapartum and postnatal care could be provided in a range of locations including the home.

Shared care

Antenatal care is provided by a community maternity service provider (doctor and / or midwife) in collaboration with hospital medical and / or midwifery staff under an established agreement, and can occur both in the community and in hospital outpatient clinics. Intrapartum and early postnatal care usually takes place in the hospital by hospital midwives and doctors, often in conjunction with the community doctor or midwife (particularly in rural settings).

Combined care

Antenatal care is provided by a private maternity service provider (doctor and / or midwife) in the community. Intrapartum and early postnatal care is provided in the public hospital by hospital midwives and doctors. Postnatal care may continue in the home or community by hospital midwives.

Team midwifery care

Antenatal, intrapartum and postnatal care is provided by a small team of rostered midwives (no more than eight) in collaboration with doctors in the event of identified risk factors. Intrapartum care is usually provided in a hospital or birth centre. Postnatal care may continue in the home or community by the team midwives.

Midwifery group practice caseload care

Antenatal, intrapartum and postnatal care is provided within a publicly funded caseload model by a known primary midwife with secondary backup midwife / midwives providing cover and assistance in collaboration with doctors in the event of identified risk factors. Antenatal care and postnatal care is usually provided in the hospital, community or home with intrapartum care in a hospital, birth centre or home.

Private obstetrician and privately practising midwife joint care

Antenatal, intrapartum and postnatal care is provided by a privately practising obstetrician and midwife from the same collaborative private practice. Intrapartum care is usually provided in either a private or public hospital by the privately practising midwife and / or private specialist obstetrician in collaboration with hospital midwifery staff. Postnatal care is usually provided in the hospital and may continue in the home, hotel or hostel by the privately practising midwife.

(Source: Donnolley et al., 2016)

primary caseload and providing backup to each other, with the intention that women get to meet the other midwives at some point in their pregnancy in case their primary midwife is unavailable. The on-call component may be shared in various ways in this model, with midwives 'buddying up' in pairs or sharing it across the team. The aim is to still provide women with continuity of carer across the whole continuum, but for the midwives to better manage 'protected time'.

The alternative model relies on 'core midwives' rostered on at the hospital to provide backup care when a caseload midwife is unavailable for one of the women in her caseload. The caseload midwife arranges her time according to her caseload, including being on-call for all the women in her care. Relying on 'core midwives' for backup means that women may be cared for by midwives they have not met previously if their own midwife is unavailable. Both models are intended to provide women with relational continuity across the whole spectrum of their care by a known midwife but can have different impacts on the midwives involved. The differences between these two models are subtle, and not really identified by their different names.

To illustrate the difference a name can make, in Australia 'team midwifery' has a different meaning entirely, with midwives in a team sharing a caseload of women and often being rostered to provide antenatal, intrapartum and postnatal care for all the women in the caseload, without the women having relational continuity with a single primary midwife. The midwives' caseload is not 'self-managed' in the same way that a caseload or MGP model is, and women could see any one of the midwives in the team during her pregnancy and birth. In this model of care, there is no planned continuity of *carer;* however, there may be continuity of *care* as the team midwives share a philosophy and information. In terms of the industrial arrangement, midwives employed in a team midwifery model like this would usually be paid on an hourly rostered basis as opposed to an annualised salary with a self-managed workload.

Some large hospitals in Australia have implemented a version of team midwifery in an effort to have a model that is sustainable for the midwives (see Box 3.2).

This 'team midwifery' approach is very similar to the types of arrangements set up shortly after publication of *Changing Childbirth* (Department of Health, 1993) in the UK where centres like the Chelsea and Westminster Hospital NHS trust had several. These were named 'group practices' and functioned with six to eight midwives (depending on part-time and job share needs within a team) in much the same way as team midwifery is described in the MaCCS. It is clear why there has been so much confusion over the names of these arrangements!

In addition to the models suggested in the UK's Better Births implementation, there are many other examples of models offering continuity of midwifery carer that are based either within a hospital service or independently. In New Zealand, midwives working as a lead maternity carer (LMC) can be hospital based but are more

BOX 3.2 Team Midwifery at the Royal Women's Hospital (RWH) in Melbourne

Della Forster, RWH and La Trobe University, Melbourne, Australia.

The Royal Women's Hospital in Melbourne (RWH) has two midwife-led continuity of care models in operation—caseload midwifery and team midwifery. The evidence supports both these models, so it has been a deliberate management strategy to have both options operating, to enable more women to have access to continuity of midwife care across the continuum.

How it works

The RWH team midwifery model is known as MIST—midwives in a small team. There are four MIST teams across the main RWH campus, and each team is made up of eight midwives maximum, regardless of FTE (full-time equivalent), as continuity becomes compromised over this number. The midwives work from 0.6 to 1 FTE, but the most common is 0.8. On average, this means there are 6.5–7 FTE of midwives per team. MIST teams take approximately 45 women per year per midwife FTE in any one team, which works out to about 300 women per year per MIST team (25 women due per month). The MIST teams are set up to care for women with a variety of complexity to ensure that not only those women considered at low risk of complications can access the model. To moderate this and to avoid 'overloading' the team, the allocation of women is 10 primiparous women, 10 multiparous women and 5 more complex women each month.

Women are not allocated to any one midwife—it is a team approach to care. Each MIST team operates slightly differently, but generally each covers all MIST antenatal clinics, and aims to have one MIST midwife on per shift across birth suite, and postnatal care in hospital and at home, with the coverage of home-based postnatal care posing the biggest challenge. The MIST midwives work on rostered shifts—so there is no on-call component for midwives, but there is some flexibility for the midwives in that as long as the scheduled shift is covered they can swap among themselves.

Monitoring outcomes

Electronic clinical outcome data are provided monthly by the MIST team and as a total to enable regular review of outcomes and of how the MIST team outcomes compare with the overall outcomes at the RWH, as well as with previously generated evidence. Regular audits also explore continuity; while the percentage of MIST women who have a MIST midwife for labour and birth is a little lower than when the team midwifery randomised controlled trial (Waldenström et al., 2001) was conducted at the RWH, there is increased postnatal continuity—with at least half of the women receiving some of their home-based postnatal care from a MIST midwife.

Sustainability issues

The team midwifery model is one that is sustainable over time; it provides an alternative for midwives who want to work in a continuity model but cannot commit to the on-call requirement of the caseload model. Midwives can move in and out of the two models as their life circumstances and needs change. In either case, the ability of the models to be fluid enough to ensure the midwives have autonomy in how they work is a key issue for sustainability.

usually self-employed and based in the community, contracting their services to the NZ Ministry of Health (Grigg & Tracy, 2013). They provide one-to-one maternity care to women across the full spectrum of pregnancy, birth and the postnatal period with backup provided by other midwives in a group practice setting (see Box 3.3, a vignette from New Zealand, as an example). The midwives may work in conjunction with other care providers in the hospital.

A similar system exists in the Netherlands where midwives are autonomous primary maternity care providers and offer continuity of care across the continuum for women without complications in pregnancy, and refer women for secondary and tertiary hospital-based care when necessary. However, in the New Zealand midwifery system a self-employed continuity of carer midwife can work across institutions following the woman's needs and choices. The interface between primary and secondary services in New Zealand is based on the need and requirement for continuity of carer midwives to work across sites to facilitate this partnership smoothly. Each midwife in the New Zealand model needs to apply for access agreements to hospital and birth centre facilties and to have these updated annually to ensure required skills and orientation to the various sites are contemporary. This is easier and more practicable for urban and semirural continuity of carer New Zealand midwives but can be signifianctly more challenging the further away a midwife works from a hospital.

The Rodney Coast Midwives example from New Zealand in Box 3.3 illustrates how a rural and semirural practice can facilitate this interface for the majority of the women in their care across all risk catogories. However, this may not be feasible for all rural and remote continuity of carer midwives who need to prioritise staying in their region to ensure adequate and safe 24-hour coverage for their remaining caseload; an aspect of remote practising continuity of carer midwives is that they can find themselves without consistent local support and backup from other midwives.

Not all midwives want to, or are able to, work in a full continuity of carer model. This can be due to lifestyle, family or health reasons or because they just do not enjoy the on-call component (see section below for more about these issues). Sometimes health services struggle to implement MGP caseload models and look for alternatives. There are, however, some 'hybrid' models of care that have appeared to bridge the gap between full continuity and completely fragmented models of care. In these models, midwives provide continuity of care to an individual caseload of women during the antenatal and postnatal periods but are not on-call for women for birth. Intrapartum care is either shared amongst the team based on a roster or provided by 'core midwives' in the hospital. Models such as this are often seen in remote and regional locations in Australia, including models of care specifically for Aboriginal women, when birthing services are not available locally and women must be relocated for labour and birth care in the weeks prior to birth. These models do

BOX 3.3 Midwifery Group Practice Caseload Care Example From New Zealand

Kathy Carter-Lee, Rodney Coast Midwives, New Zealand

Rodney Coast Midwives are a collegial group of midwives committed to support each other in their work as lead maternity carer (LMC) midwives. Our area is a mix of rural and remote rural locations, but two are based in the urban south. Each of us has our own caseload and is self-employed. Women choose who they book with, but none of us can work without a break sometimes, so we try to ensure women are birthing with someone they know. Two midwives in our group partner to cover each other regularly, have similar size caseloads and work in the same area so can tell their women from the start of pregnancy they have one backup. In this pair, if one midwife has been up in the night or has a family emergency and they are both working, the other can fill in and cover a day or half day of clinic, as they do clinics at different times. Others have a less structured approach, and ask women to choose a backup midwife and meet them if they wish. Women are told then that we try to have their backup available if their LMC is not on-call when they go into labour. This backup midwife will be called as second midwife in the second stage of labour if the woman is birthing at home or at one of the two local birth units. Some choose a backup, and others say 'whoever is available', or reflect the partnership we have with women, saying 'whoever you trust'.

Women also choose where they give birth. Local primary options are home, Wellsford Birth Unit, or Warkworth Birth Centre. LMC midwives will have more or less influence, especially for primigravidae, but women are encouraged to choose for themselves. Often the small number of uncomplicated women who choose hospital birth will have changed to the primary unit by the time they have been to classes. Also if they arrive at the unit for an assessment in labour and realise that they are doing well or realise there is a car journey to hospital, they stay at the primary unit.

The Ministry of Health currently pays us in modules of care. From this we have worked out a system of payments within the group. Some of us who work together a lot will 'washup' after 6 months. Others will invoice each other as needed. To encourage midwives to take time off regularly, if another midwife from the group births one of my clients while I am off-call for the weekend, she will get two-thirds of the birth fee and the off-call midwife will retain one-third.

We try to have at least four midwives on-call in the weekends, in addition to the midwife manager at the WWBC (Warkworth Birth Centre). Because we attend women at their chosen birthplace, these four midwives could theoretically all be with birthing women in four different places at the same time. In this environment the commitment to and support of colleagues is important to make it work, and flexibility is a key. Occasionally an early return to work is needed if there are stretched midwife reserves. The phrase 'swings and roundabouts' describes the give and take that is the culture of support here. We support each other, and we support the women we care for. It is important to us that we meet as a group on Thursday mornings for an hour or so. We discuss issues, share stories and give and receive support. This gives us cohesion, gives us strength and builds a sisterhood that has and will keep us going.

provide the benefit of continuity of carer for much of pregnancy (prior to relocation) and then after the women return home with their babies.

Where publicly funded midwifery continuity models are not available, another option for some women is accessing a privately practising midwife. Privately practising midwives may work on their own, with an obstetrician or in group practices, and provide care in the woman's home, community facilities and the clinician's rooms in a birth centre or in hospital. Depending on the country and health system, women may have to pay the full cost of these services or they may be funded through their health insurance (government or private). In some countries, care by privately practising midwives may be restricted to women with uncomplicated pregnancies, whereas in others the care may be co-managed with an obstetrician or hospital maternity service.

The major principle behind all these models is to maximise the relational continuity of a single named midwife to coordinate (and where possible provide) the care for a defined group of women. The next section explores the often thorny issue of on-call arrangements that accompany continuity of carer models of care.

ON-CALL ARRANGEMENTS: ENGAGING WITH UNPREDICTABILITY

Providing continuity of carer over 24 hours for 7 days a week requires different ways of working if a known midwife is to provide intrapartum care. Unlike antenatal and postnatal care, which, for the most part, can be provided within allocated and prebooked schedules, intrapartum care (other than elective caesarean sections and induction of labours) is unpredictable. Therefore to embrace relational continuity of care requires engagement with some degree of unpredictability and on-call arrangements. This is not to imply that all continuity of carer models require a named midwife to be on-call 24/7, but rather that some 24-hour cover is required, within either a team or a group practice arrangement as explored above.

Paradoxically, though being at the birth of a baby for a woman and family known to the midwife brings much joy to practice and is welcomed by mothers, being on-call can for many midwives also bring fear and create resistance to working in continuity of carer models owing to the unpredictability of being called out for labour and birth. Many midwives (some authors of this chapter included) find that being on-call for our 'own women' (women we have booked and continue to see through the childbirth year) is fundamentally different to being on-call for a whole team midwifery caseload. Being called in by someone with whom a relationship has been formed over time is different to being called at 2 am by someone you have never previously met.

Let us unpack this further. In continuity of carer models where the named midwife is called out to the women in their caseload only (e.g. in a group practice arrangement or private practice), and occasionally for backup support to their practice partner, is very different in terms of being called out when sharing the on-call in a team approach, when on-calls are rostered (e.g. team midwifery care or an MGP sharing the on-call). In team midwifery models, the on-call midwife is rostered to be on-call for all the women in the team practice, not only her own women. In other words, there is a real difference between

- being on-call more often, but called out for fewer women and more of them 'known women' (such as in the Better Births 'full caseloading' model), and
- being on-call less often, yet called out more when on-call for women who you do not know with rostered times for on-calls (the 'team continuity group practice caseloading' model).

Whichever way the on-calls are arranged, and it could also be a hybrid of models as suggested above, it is crucial that it is sensitive to the needs of midwives. This means that women and families have realistic expectations of the on-call arrangements, and it is made explicit to women the reasons for using the on-call service and that it should not be abused. For example, using the on-call facility to change non-urgent appointments or calling to ask advice about travel is unacceptable and could place unnecessary burden on the on-call system. Most on-call midwives have found it important to provide women in their care with information about the appropriate times to call outside of scheduled appointments (Gilkison et al., 2015). This is a skill that continuity of carer midwives learn and often struggle with at the start, as they may feel they have to be available for all things to all 'their' women—however, that is not what continuity of carer means or needs to be. Women are generally grateful for the guidance about when to use the on-call facility and respect the personal time of their midwife knowing they will be available when needed. It is about working *in partnership* with women and not working *for* them (McAra-Couper et al., 2014).

Obviously, some women have more complex needs. For this reason, it is vital that midwives working within communities of high social deprivation with multiple public health concerns have smaller caseload numbers. For example, in Scotland it has been suggested that midwives working with this type of client base have no more than 18 compared with the recommended 35 (Scottish Government, 2017).

Inappropriate use or misuse of the on-call system can also come from the institutions that employ midwives working in these models. For example, being pulled in to 'help out' the core hospital rostered midwives when the midwife is not 'actually out' on a call creates tensions. The perception is that the midwife is on-call yet not actually working, so can be 'used'—yet she may have been busy the night before and may become busy again within a short period of time. Servicing the institution as well as a caseload of women (whatever the model) is simply unsustainable when the hospital, particularly the hospital intrapartum area, remains the priority. The unsustainability of having two 'pulls' on the continuity of carer midwife is a common story, and is reminiscent of the experiences of many midwives in the UK following the sporadic implementation of the Changing Childbirth (Department of Health, 1993) recommendations, in which provision of relational continuity was often seen (or interpreted) as a luxury by many and therefore not a priority.

Of equal importance is where to be based whilst on-call (e.g. home, clinic, hospital, community hub). This needs to be decided according to circumstance, context and local self-directed practice arrangements. For many midwives, working in the group practice way is about being on-call wherever they are—at home, doing a clinic or on the labour ward. For others, who perhaps work in challenging geographical locations, staying at a local birth centre within the community is better when taking the rostered on-call in the team approach, as discussed above. Likewise, part-time and job share positions need to be available to midwives who are unable to work a full-time caseload (e.g. if they have young children) but wish to work within a continuity of carer model. There are various solutions to this.

One solution which can work well is job sharing in group practice arrangements. A job share between two midwives who hold a full caseload between them is feasible—they can share the workload and on-call commitments across any division of time that suits them as a partnership (e.g. 40%–60%, not necessarily 50/50). In a team approach, part-time and job share midwives are both workable options, although the concern would be if there are too many part-time/job share midwives. If there are more than eight such midwives this reduces the degree of continuity provided to women (and midwives).

Whatever the arrangements, maintenance of personal and professional boundaries is vital and is found to be a major aspect of sustaining on-calls over time (Gilkison et al., 2015). For an example of what a month of on-call 'call outs' looks like by one of the authors (Susan), whilst managing a personal caseload of 40–60 women within a group practice, refer to a detailed description taken from her practice diary (Crowther, 2016—online blog). The vignette from New Zealand in Box 3.3 provides a further example of how midwifery group practice caseload care and on-calls can work well and not burn out the midwives. As you read through, see what key advice is given that you feel would work in your own practice environment, within either a current continuity of carer model or one that you want to set up.

There are key points in the vignette in Box 3.3 that can be used in different settings to support being on-call:

- flexibility
- mutual support to take time off (come off-call) when needed
- commitment to ensuring everyone gets time off being on-call on a regular basis
- shared philosophy—e.g. the group practice meets regularly and discusses issues and shares stories
- supporting each other—which is vital and makes it all work

- each midwife carrying her own caseload yet feeling collegially supported by the practice of midwives
- tailored and flexible care that is congruent with provision of choice
- choice in ways midwives work, and ensuring choice for women—both core values
- women being in partnership with the midwives—this reciprocity engenders trust
- midwives educating and informing women of the system of care provided
- financial arrangements that have been mutually agreed within the practice (unique to the New Zealand self-employed arrangements); other arrangements could include mutually agreed off duty, rostered on-call scheduling, clinic re-stocking, etc.
- cohesive group practice of midwives, meeting both individual and group needs.

The example in Box 3.3 is taken from a rural practice based at a rural free-standing birthing centre in New Zealand, yet the constituent qualities that appear to make it all work smoothly could be applicable in any locality. It is important to re-emphasise that the notion of midwifery continuity of care is essentially about providing quality primary care with acute episodes across sites (home, birth centres and hospitals).

The bottom line is that these models of care are about staffing women 'as needed', not about staffing organisations / institutions. Any continuity of carer model can be enabled only through some sort of dedicated team or practice in which mutually agreed local on-call arrangements have been established and when local hospitals and employing bodies of midwives respect and appreciate the work and commitment involved in providing on-call arrangements.

It is imperative that, whatever model is adopted, midwives are given guidance and support to ensure they are not treated unfairly within any system of care provision that does not listen to their individual context-dependent concerns. The next section explores the role of professional bodies in providing support and guidance to midwives as they move to a different way of working, or to midwives who seek advice on how to sustain or upscale a practice that already provides relational continuity.

PROFESSIONAL BODIES: SUPPORT AND GUIDANCE

The International Confederation of Midwives states that there are three key pillars for a strong midwifery profession: education, regulation and association (International Confederation of Midwives (ICM), 2016). Professional associations for midwives have a significant role to play when models of midwifery continuity of care are being proposed and implemented. The roles of the association in this context are several:

1. **Lobbying**—a professional association should lobby governments and funding bodies to ensure that any change in the model of care is appropriately funded. Any significant organisational change or change in the ways that midwives work will require investment to ensure that there is adequate project planning,

leadership and management and that midwives receive appropriate training, time and support to adapt to working in different areas and in different ways. Planning should include adequate workload and workforce scoping activities. Where significant shortfalls in midwifery staffing are identified, the professional association has a responsibility to lobby clearly and consistently that these shortfalls are addressed in order to ensure any model of care is safe and sustainable.

2. **Support and education for midwives**—a professional association will have a role in promoting evidence-based service change and in advocating for high-quality maternity services. The strong evidence base for midwifery continuity means that professional associations have a responsibility not only to represent the interests of their members, but also to advocate for the implementation of continuity models. This role is likely to involve professional associations in helping to provide their midwife members with information about the benefits of continuity for women, families and midwives; to provide examples of successful models and to provide support to midwifery leaders and managers in implementing and managing change successfully.

3. **Representation of members' needs and rights**—professional associations, whether or not they are also trade unions, have a role in representing the needs of their members. Working in a midwifery continuity of care model may not be possible for all midwives, and professional associations should offer a strong voice to support the continued existence of a variety of midwifery roles and ways of working for midwives. The development of continuity models should not lead to a removal of opportunities for midwives to specialise in particular areas of care and will not remove the need for a cohort of midwives who provide core hospital-based care. For example, in New Zealand over 50% of the midwifery workforce are hospital or core staff on shift-work basis (Grigg & Tracy, 2013). Despite this, most of the New Zealand population have access to a continuity of carer midwife who provides care across primary and acute settings. There is room in the profession and maternity services for both cadres of midwife; indeed it is vital that these different midwifery roles exist to ensure that all types of services for women are available in the primary and acute sectors. Professional associations should provide expert guidance and representation to ensure that midwives' workloads and working lives enable them to have adequate rest and time off, to have a good work–life balance and to have adequate support from the wider team where they are not able to cover the care of their own caseload. The vignette in Box 3.4 describes the role of a professional body and trade union (in this case the Royal College of Midwives, UK) in implementation of a midwifery continuity of care.

There is a need to have realistic expectations of what is doable. It is crucial that any implementation is sensitive and proactive to the contextual realities when forming communities of continuity of carer midwives. In addition, the importance of support

BOX 3.4 The Role of a Professional Organisation in Supporting Midwifery Continuity of Care

A review of maternity and neonatal services in Scotland was undertaken during 2015 and 2016. The professional body and trade union for the great majority of midwives in Scotland is the Royal College of Midwives (RCM). The RCM was represented on the review board and each of the three working groups and contributed actively to discussions, development of the recommendations and the review of current evidence. It was active in ensuring that the voices of midwives were heard by the review team at local engagement and listening events across Scotland during the review process.

The review findings and recommendations were published in January 2017—'The Best Start: a five-year forward plan for maternity and neonatal care in Scotland'. The Best Start review places continuity of carer as the central model of maternity care for Scotland.

Since publication, the RCM team in Scotland have been proactive in ensuring that members across Scotland are aware of the review recommendations and how they might be successfully implemented. This has been done through a series of six regional workshops. These workshops have shared the review recommendations and then provided detailed exploration of the evidence for continuity of carer, how continuity of carer models work and interactive sessions to help midwives and student midwives understand how their working lives might look and feel in a continuity model of care.

The RCM has continued to be strongly represented at the national implementation board level and on the working groups, representing its members' interests and concerns, and providing a strong professional voice for high-quality maternity services. The RCM has lobbied the Scottish Government to ensure that the implementation of the Best Start recommendations is adequately funded through submission of a detailed, costed proposal that covers the need for adequate training, equipment and working environments for midwives working in a continuity model of carer.

At a local level, RCM workplace representatives have received training from the RCM team to ensure that they are aware of the implications of a continuity model of care and the parameters provided by employment regulations to support members and ensure that organisational change does not lead to detriment for midwives.

As part of the wider RCM UK organisation, the RCM is continuing to develop a range of learning resources for midwives, managers and support workers to help them to understand continuity of carer and how it may best be implemented. These include an online interactive workbook 'Can continuity work for us?' (RCM, 2017) and an online learning module, available for members.

The RCM continues to lobby strongly to ensure that midwife vacancies are addressed as a matter of urgency at both a national and local level. For any model of maternity care to provide high-quality care, there needs to be a safe number of midwives and support staff.

and guidance from professional organisations illustrates how midwives need to be heard and not silenced. In this final section we turn briefly to an exploration of the principal qualities that can help make this model of care sustainable.

MAKING IT SUSTAINABLE

The theoretical and conceptual frameworks of the notion of sustainability is addressed in more depth in Chapter 11. What we highlight here is the significance and importance of relationships between midwives and with others in different models that promote midwifery continuity of carer. At the same time, we focus on the importance of finding ways that enable midwives to work in self-directed ways so that it is fit for any context in which they practise. In exploring the literature, it is apparent that sustainability of this model depends, unsurprisingly, on partnership, collegiality, flexibility, collaborations and professional autonomy.

Professional autonomy

The word 'autonomous' has its origins in Ancient Greek, meaning 'self-governing'. In contemporary times and in relation to the professions, autonomy refers to the profession's ability to determine its own standards for education, regulation and the freedom of professionals to make clinical decisions in accordance with their own professional knowledge base (ICM, 2011; Skar, 2010). Autonomy in practice can also refer to the ability of professionals to have control over their work schedule. Professional autonomy is positively associated with wellbeing, productivity and job satisfaction (Daniel, 2017; Tyssen et al., 2013). Although some may think that providing continuity of carer with on-call commitments is a recipe for burnout, evidence suggests otherwise. Studies in Australia and New Zealand have shown that midwives working in continuity models of care demonstrate less burnout and greater wellbeing than their counterparts not working in continuity models. This may be related to autonomy, as the midwives working in continuity also rated themselves more highly on autonomy than those not working in continuity (Dixon et al., 2017; Fenwick et al., 2018).

In midwifery continuity of carer models, the ability to organise, structure and control work practices and flow positively contributes to midwifery sustainability (Crowther et al., 2016). The previous sections and the New Zealand vignette in Box 3.3 have born this truth out. Wherever possible, midwives should be enabled to determine their own ways of working—for example, with whom they partner, where and when they visit women, how they structure their day, how they work with colleagues, and how they plan for time off and structure on-call commitments. This approach recognises that one size does not fit all and that there are many ways to successfully 'do continuity'. Autonomy over these aspects of midwifery work may also enable midwives to care better for themselves and achieve greater work–life balance—factors identified as essential to successful continuity of carer practices (Crowther et al., 2016).

Although the 'auto' in autonomy refers to the 'self', midwives and other health professionals never operate in isolation from others, regardless of the model of care in which they work or their employment status (self-employed or employed). Beyond the partnership midwives have with the women for whom they care, these professional collaborative relationships include (but are not limited to) those with midwifery, medical and allied health colleagues and health service managers. These relationships are crucial to successful midwifery (Crowther et al., 2016). We must establish strong collaborative relationships with others to ensure that women and their babies receive the best possible care and to ensure that we as midwives are provided with the support and care we need to do the work of midwifery well. More broadly, midwives should consider their relationships with relevant professional associations and colleges as these organisations can be excellent sources of information and support for midwives.

Collaborative relationships

While the concept of professional collaboration has several dimensions (including organisational), the relational dimension is paramount. As discussed in Chapter 5, this dimension includes effective communication, trust, reciprocity, synergy and respect (Smith, 2015). The foundation to any successful collaboration is trust and respect (National Health and Medical Research Council (NHMRC), 2010). Midwives know well from working with diverse groups of childbearing women that respect can be afforded to one another, despite differences in backgrounds, beliefs, opinions or philosophy.

Collaborating well with others (whether a medical colleague or another midwife, for example) requires that each individual understands and values the knowledge, expertise and skills of the other (NHMRC, 2010). Synergy acknowledges the common goal of health professionals and the recognition that more can be achieved with health professionals working together towards a common goal than independently (Smith, 2015).

In professional collaborations, our common ground is in wanting what is best for the women in our care. It can be helpful to come back to this point as a first principle in any difficult collaborative negotiation, because it is rare that this is not the case. Reciprocity refers to the need for health professionals to rely on each other to be responsible and accountable for their practice. Whatever the midwife's role in a woman's care, whether as lead carer, backup midwife or support in an obstetric-led situation, the midwife (as are other professionals) is wholly accountable and responsible for her own practice. In health care in general, effective communication amongst health professionals is key to patient safety (NHMRC, 2010). This includes reciprocal sharing of accurate and appropriate information in a timely way to best inform decision making in relation to a woman's care.

Midwives should consider the importance of this relational dimension of collaboration not only for direct clinical care (e.g. transfer of clinical information, advocacy) but also for enhancing midwifery professionalism and the midwife's personal well-being (and hence her effectiveness and longevity as a midwife). Midwives who have developed strong collaborative relationships will be more likely to achieve excellent outcomes for the women in their care, be able to more clearly articulate and assert their own professional knowledge (which informs their decision making), help others to understand their expectations, perspectives and needs, and negotiate successful outcomes for themselves and the women in their care.

Although midwives often need to collaborate with individuals with whom they may not have developed a relationship, it is important to consider strategies that can enhance the development of collaborative relationships over time. Research has shown that spending time talking with others can enhance relationships (Schofield et al., 2009). Creating regular opportunities for talking, especially in the interprofessional context, is important. These may include shared learning opportunities, structured meetings or social events.

Additional strategies could include 'talking circles'—a practice originating with Native Americans that aims to reach creative solutions to problems while fostering group cohesion and collective responsibility for the welfare of those within the group (Lombard, 2016). Although the evidence for this approach still needs to be established in midwifery the emphasis on finding co-creative or co-designed ways of working on midwifery practice issues through building cohesive relationships is worthy of further examination.

Relationships between continuity of midwifery team members is most important because it is this group with whom the continuity midwife will be working most closely and will gain most support. The New Zealand vignette in Box 3.3 highlights the importance of the weekly meeting of the caseload midwives in the group practice.

Much of the research about what makes caseloading practice sustainable comes from New Zealand, where nearly half of all midwives work in this way (New Zealand College of Midwives, 2016). Studies from New Zealand (Crowther et al., 2016; Gilkison et al., 2015; Hunter et al., 2016) highlight the importance of open and honest communication, shared philosophy, clear expectations and boundaries, and generosity of spirit. Open and honest communication in an atmosphere of generosity ensures that midwives are able to 'clear the air' with each other and also to critique practice (their own and that of others) in a way that is constructive and leads to learning and growth.

Shared philosophy means that midwives in the practice are on the same page and that they can take time off, safe in the knowledge that the women in their care are in good (similar) hands. Time off and work–life balance is critical to midwifery sustainability. Clear expectations and boundaries similarly ensure that midwives are also on the same page in relation to the role, and generosity of spirit means that midwives can ask for and rely on their partner or team members for emotional or practical support and assistance when it is needed.

As in interprofessional relationships, structuring time to talk and build these important professional relationships is important. A successful and long-lasting continuity of carer practice in New Zealand privileges 'time and talking' by building this into the working week (Thorpe, 2005). This group holds a meeting each week and there is an expectation that all team members will attend (except if they are attending a birth). They bring nice food and sometimes flowers and they give over a good amount of time to talk. Talking focuses not only on operational issues but on critique of their practice and any issues with which they might be struggling. The team are then able to arrange their working week (the operational issues), learn from constructive debate focusing on their practice and offer practical and emotional support to their colleagues. This kind of support enables midwives to do the work of caseload midwifery well.

CONCLUSION

This chapter has shown that there are many approaches to realising relational continuity of midwifery care and each approach provides further support and guidance to those seeking to implement, sustain and upscale such an approach of care provision in different settings. Meaningful relationships, autonomy, self-determined ways of working, self-management and support have all been shown to be central to the sustainability of these models of care. It is crucial that midwives within a practice, professional advisors and managers all seek ways to ensure wellbeing across the workforce. There is room in the profession to work in myriad ways either within a variety of continuity of carer arrangements or in a core / hospital position that supports and contributes to the safe delivery of relational continuity. This chapter has clearly shown that one size does not fit all; context and the voices of individual midwives must be heard, supported by strong professional midwifery associations. Finally, yet so important, the outcome of working in this way often brings a joy to midwifery practice which often sustains midwives.

REFERENCES

Australian Institute of Health and Welfare: Maternity model of care—extent of continuity of carer, code N[N]. National Health Data Dictionary, n.d. Online: http://meteor.aihw.gov.au/content/index. phtml/itemId/562423.
Crowther S: Caseload midwifery is sustainable: personal example. Blog, 2016. Online: https://drsusan crowther.com/2016/05/14/caseload-midwifery-is-sustainable-personal-example/.

Crowther S: Who's afraid of working as a continuity of carer midwife?, *Practis Midwife* 20(6):2017. ePub 1.

Crowther SB, Hunter J, McAra-Couper L, Warren A, Gilkison M, Hunter A, et al: Sustainability and resilience in midwifery: a discussion paper, *Midwifery* 40:40–48, 2016.

Daniel W: Autonomy in paid work and employee subjective well-being, *Work Occup* 44:296–328, 2017.

Department of Health: *Changing childbirth*, London, 1993, HMSO.

Dixon L, Pallant J, Sidebotham M, Fenwick J, McAra-Couper J, Gilkison A: The emotional wellbeing of New Zealand midwives: comparing responses for midwives in caseloading and shift work settings, *NZCOM J* 53:5–14, 2017.

Donnolley N, Butler-Henderson K, Chapman M, Sullivan E: The development of a classification system for maternity models of care, *Health Inf Manag* 45:64–70, 2016.

Fenwick J, Sidebotham M, Gamble J, Creedy DK: The emotional and professional wellbeing of Australian midwives: a comparison between those providing continuity of midwifery care and those not providing continuity, *Women Birth* 31:38–43, 2018.

Gilkison A, McAra-Couper J, Gunn J, Crowther S, Hunter M, Macgregor D, et al: Midwifery practice arrangements which sustain caseloading lead maternity carer midwives in New Zealand, *NZCOM J* 51:11–16, 2015.

Grigg CP, Tracy SK: New Zealand's unique maternity system, *Women Birth* 26:e59–e64, 2013.

Hunter M, Crowther S, McAra-Couper J, Gilkison A, MacGregor D, Gunn J: Generosity of spirit sustains caseloading lead maternity carer midwives in New Zealand, *NZCOM J* 52:50–55, 2016.

International Confederation of Midwives (ICM): *Midwifery: an autonomous profession. Position statement*, The Hague, 2011, ICM.

International Confederation of Midwives (ICM): *Education, regulation and association*, The Hague, 2016, ICM.

Lombard K: The circle way to authentic leadership, *Nurs Manag* 47(5):13–16, 2016.

McAra-Couper J, Gilkison A, Crowther S, Hunter M, Hotchin C, Gunn J: Partnership and reciprocity with women sustain lead maternity carer midwives in practice, *NZCOM J* 49:27–31, 2014.

National Health and Medical Research Council (NHMRC): *National guidance on collaborative maternity care*, Canberra, 2010, NHMRC.

New Zealand College of Midwives (NZCOM): *Media kit*, Christchurch, 2016, NZCOM.

NHS England: *Implementing Better Births: a resource pack for Local Maternity Systems*. London, 2017, NHS England. Online: https://www.england.nhs.uk/wp-content/uploads/2017/03/nhs-guidance-maternity-services-v1.pdf.

Royal College of Midwives (RCM): *Can continuity work for us?—a resource for midwives*, London, 2017, RCM.

Sandall J, Soltani H, Gates S, Shennan A, Devane D: Midwife-led continuity models versus other models of care for childbearing women, *Cochrane Database Syst Rev* (4):CD004667, 2016. doi:10.1002/14651858. CD004667.pub4.

Schofield D, Fuller J, Wagner S, Friis L, Tyrell B: Multidisciplinary management of complex care, *Aust J Rural Health* 17:45–48, 2009.

Scottish Government: *The best start: a five-year forward plan for maternity and neonatal care in Scotland*. Edinburgh, 2017, Government of Scotland. Online: https://beta.gov.scot/publications/best-start-five-year-forward-plan-maternity-neonatal-care-scotland/.

Skar R: The meaning of autonomy in nursing practice, *J Clin Nurs* 19:2226–2234, 2010.

Smith DC: Midwife–physician collaboration: a conceptual framework for interprofessional collaborative practice, *J Midwifery Womens Health* 60:128–139, 2015.

Thorpe J: A feminist case study of the collegial relationships within a home birth midwifery practice in New Zealand. MMid thesis, Otago, 2005, Otago Polytechnic.

Tyssen R, Palmer KS, Solberg IB, Voltmer E, Frank E: Physicians' perceptions of quality of care, professional autonomy, and job satisfaction in Canada, Norway, and the United States, *BMC Health Serv Res* 13:516, 2013.

Waldenström U, McLachlan H, Forster D, Brennecke S, Brown S: Team midwife care: maternal and infant outcomes, *Aust N Z J Obstet Gynaecol* 41:257–264, 2001.

CHAPTER 4

How Can Managers Make Midwifery Continuity of Care Work?

Michelle Newton, Jan White, Pat Brodie

Contents

INTRODUCTION

In this chapter, we share our experiences as managers and researchers involved in leading the establishment, implementation and evaluation of midwifery continuity of care models. The reorganisation of maternity services to include midwifery continuity of care models is possible and generally acceptable to most stakeholders, although this is not without challenges. From the outset, it is important to recognise that one size does not fit all; any model needs to take account of women's needs, midwives' needs and what is the right organisational fit. A growing body of evidence is now available to assist managers and midwives to better understand the enablers and facilitators, as well as the barriers that need to be overcome, in order to support midwifery continuity of care within the health care system. There are also particular attributes of effective leadership and innovative ways of working that can make this more readily achievable. This chapter discusses how to make midwifery continuity of care work for all midwives and managers. We explore how midwifery leaders can become agents for change, conveying their belief in the importance of midwifery continuity of care using the transformational language of 'why', 'how' and 'what' in order to inspire and convince others (Sinek, 2010, 2011).

The implementation and sustainability of continuity models is not a concrete or finite outcome; it is more evolutionary. Our ways of working to ensure long-term viability are continuously changing as we learn, adjust and integrate new understandings about how to act to achieve the best from the models for women, midwives and managers. Of equal importance is the need for midwives, and those charged with managing midwives, to develop an appreciation, understanding and ability to articulate the wider challenges of health service innovation. This includes consideration of health policy, workforce sustainability, resource management and the various industrial relations and other regulatory frameworks that influence maternity service provision (Shaw et al., 2016).

Many successful midwifery continuity of care models have been the result of starting out on a positive note with a shared vision, bringing interested others together to share ideas, building relationships and making good decisions early on in the development and implementation phases of the new model. Sometimes these opportunities are serendipitous or unexpected, but it is always important to make the most of the opportunities when they present themselves. Supporting midwives and managers as they evolve into new ways of leading and managing the many and varied challenges and demands encountered professionally is a shared responsibility.

PRIORITISING CONTINUITY MODELS—MANOEUVRING, NEGOTIATING AND INFLUENCING FOR CHANGE

At a time when health services face political, financial and organisational challenges, responding to emerging catalysts or stimuli for change may present managers of midwifery services with unexpected opportunities. For example, the prioritisation of midwifery continuity of care models can become part of the broader solution. This is highlighted by Shaw et al. (2016) who identify that, in high-income countries, a focus on normalising birth for most women and improving quality of care through woman-centred, low-cost models may address some of the health care challenges that are evolving in maternity care. A recent example is from Australia, where a caseload midwifery model was introduced in response to local workforce changes, midwives' desire to provide care and the needs of local women. The process resulted in the development of a progressive, community-focused birthing service that was a significant and positive change in the way services were provided (Tran et al., 2017).

As effective change agents, midwifery leaders need to convey both the evidence and a strong commitment to midwifery continuity of care models within the health service team. This requires them to utilise a simultaneous approach that includes a solution-driven focus in decision making about maternity services and models of care and use of their knowledge of drivers that directly and indirectly impact on midwifery service delivery (Crawshaw, personal communication, 2014). Importantly, harnessing the power of women's voices through their advocacy and sharing of experiences within maternity services is also a powerful tool for midwifery leaders to draw on when 'selling the message', as described fully in Chapter 2.

An awareness of the power dynamics and politics that exist within maternity services, including the hierarchies within the nursing and medical professions, is helpful when negotiating for change. Creating, sustaining and strengthening alliances through the formation of trusting personal relationships will go a long way to ensuring that midwifery managers are included when decisions affecting maternity care are being made in the broader health system or hospital. The key to persuasion includes the ability to think, act and communicate in such a way that others are informed, reassured and included (Sinek, 2010). Enacting this includes sharing research findings, outlining the capacity and capability of the midwives providing midwifery continuity of care, and openly exploring the financial considerations and meeting the governance requirements of the model of care. The ability to generate or influence decisions related to a reorganisation of the midwifery workforce into greater continuity is strengthened when collaboration with key stakeholders occurs. This is discussed in detail in Chapter 5.

In order to manoeuvre, negotiate and influence the prioritising of midwifery continuity of care models within a maternity service, managers need to 'sell the message' and articulate why change is important. High-level evidence clearly demonstrates the benefits of midwifery continuity of care for women (Sandall et al., 2016a), midwives (Common, 2015; Fenwick et al., 2018; Newton et al., 2014) and health services including, as described in Chapter 7 of this book, the all-important issue of cost effectiveness (Tracy et al., 2013). It has been suggested that in the presence of such overwhelming evidence it is unethical for health services *not* to offer midwifery continuity of care to women (Homer, 2016). Evidence alone, however, is rarely enough to influence change and is not always easily understood. Presenting the evidence to decision makers in health care systems in simple, easy to understand messages can be one way to address this. An example of a useful tool to guide these discussions is presented in the infographic in Fig. 4.1, developed by Jane Sandall and colleagues at a symposium in Oxford to honour the work of the late Sheila Kitzinger (Sandall et al., 2016b, p. 15).

Change in the culture of maternity services

The prevailing culture within a maternity service has the potential to impact directly on the ability to implement midwifery models of care (Brodie & Leap, 2008). In any

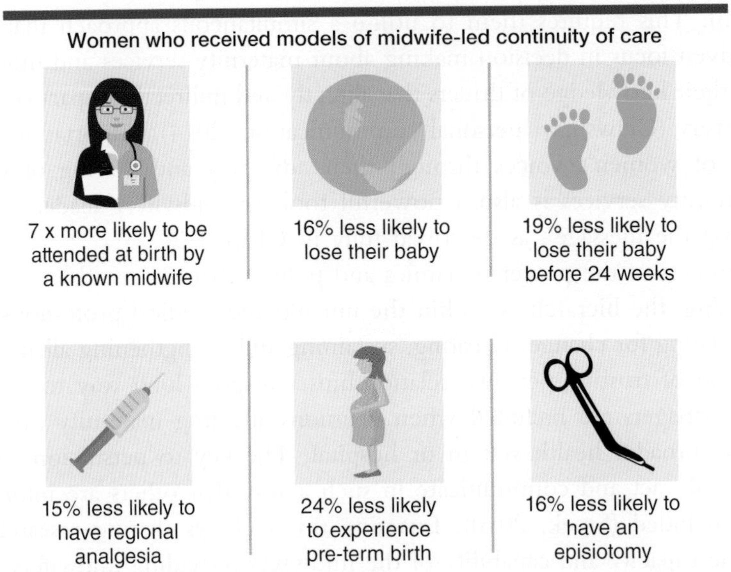

Women who received models of midwife-led continuity of care

7 x more likely to be attended at birth by a known midwife

16% less likely to lose their baby

19% less likely to lose their baby before 24 weeks

15% less likely to have regional analgesia

24% less likely to experience pre-term birth

16% less likely to have an episiotomy

Figure 4.1 *Infographic to aid discussions about the benefits of midwifery-led continuity of care (Source: Sandall J, Mackintosh N, Rayment-Jones H, Locock L, Page L (writing on behalf of the Sheila Kitzinger symposium) 2016b. The infographics were created by Nisha Mattu, Alaur Rahman and Melanie Ward in the Technology & Information team at the Health Innovation Network, the Academic Health Science Network (AHSN) for South London for Jane Sandall, NIHR CLAHRC South London)*

one environment there may be a lack of interest, vested interest in the status quo or overt expressions of opposition to innovations or change. In order to impart knowledge related to how the midwifery workforce can be reorganised, managers will need to develop a confident, steady communication style that is underpinned by consistent messaging about midwifery continuity of care and its benefits for women, midwives and the maternity service. An ability to remain resolute in the face of opposition or uncertainty about the change will be required from all those involved. Prioritisation of midwifery continuity of care also requires managers to have knowledge and awareness of their midwifery workforce's capacity and capabilities, and a confidence that the midwives working within the service are professionally prepared and ready for such a reorganisation of the midwifery workforce. This confidence in midwives' capacity should be embedded in consistent messages from midwifery managers and supported with strategies for good governance of the models as they evolve.

Successful implementation of midwifery continuity of care is characterised by early engagement with all key stakeholders from within the organisation as well as those engaged at community, regional and national levels. This is crucial to explore and build the vision, values and philosophy of midwifery continuity of care and provide opportunities for open and transparent discussion, debate and negotiation. Moving from aspiration to action provides an opportunity to demonstrate how the development of the midwifery profession, through a reorganisation of the workforce to suit the needs of the service, can improve maternity care. This unpicking of the status quo within the maternity service has the potential to create valuable building blocks for the future. In our experience, it is best undertaken through identifying the balance between what is best for women accessing the service and what will work for the midwives (Brodie & Leap, 2008; Dawson et al., 2018).

MAKING IT HAPPEN AND TAKING EVERYONE WITH YOU

Just as relationships between women and midwives are the core of midwifery, professional relationships are central to establishing midwifery continuity of care within a maternity service. Regardless of profession or position, everyone involved in maternity services has a role in supporting and strengthening maternity service reform. As discussed in Chapters 5 and 11, establishing midwifery continuity of care models will be more likely to succeed if interprofessional relationships are developed that support the planning, implementation and ongoing sustainability of the model. The manager who, at the outset, invests time and energy in building key strategic relationships with 'professional friends' will later be rewarded when these individuals become true collaborative partners and champions for the model (Brodie, 2013).

Change readiness cannot be assumed for an organisation as a whole or for individual staff at any given time. Effective change management involves working closely with individuals whose 'comfort zone' regarding practice or experience may be challenged or questioned. How individuals respond to change will vary and be expressed in a variety of ways, depending on individuals' levels of confidence about their skills and abilities. Responses may reflect entrenched views and deep-seated fears about the process of change. Seeking out those who are not completely committed to the change so that their views are listened to can be challenging. It requires time and encouragement for self-awareness and reflection. An effective manager must be perceptive and able to fine-tune messaging at times to better 'sell' the change and what it might mean to individuals as well as the team.

Organisations need to consider *all* midwives in the planning, establishment and ongoing support of the model (Sandall et al., 2016b) and early engagement with each of the different groups is an important strategy. The needs and impact of the new models on groups and individuals will vary; staff members will appreciate being included, listened to and acknowledged for their input. It may be as simple as identifying midwives willing to assume a 'link' role when midwives from the practice are not available to clarify or confirm any queries. Strategies such as this can assist in settling down any 'unrest' whilst providing an opportunity to further explore and discuss the model, including how core midwives are critical to the model's success and longevity.

Valuing core midwives

Continuity models can enhance a service by offering an option for women and midwives but, in most cases, core services are still required for the overall maternity service (National Health Service (NHS), 2017a). Core midwives are as important to a functional continuity model as the midwives working in the model itself, and for this reason, engaging and involving them through all steps of planning, implementation and evaluation is crucial. Prior to implementation of any new models, core staff can make valuable contributions that can inform decisions about how the model is to operate.

Core midwives are essential support for the model's viability and continued operation—such as when backup or cover is required by the continuity midwife, who may be overloaded and unable to provide care to all the women who have presented. These 'cover' or backup arrangements are another form of good governance and demonstrate the appropriate managing of risks or addressing excessive workload. Clearly identified and accessible arrangements to support healthy workplace practices are required by industrial regulators, who usually require service agreements to be in place (Dawson et al., 2018; NHS, 2017a). It is therefore essential that the roles and responsibilities of continuity and core midwives are explicit and that core midwives are acknowledged for the value they add to the operation of continuity models (Gilkison et al., 2017).

MEETING THE NEEDS OF THE ORGANISATION—GOVERNANCE MATTERS

An awareness of the responsibility and pressure placed on managers to sustain the profile of the maternity service and its position within the broader health service is an important component of implementing midwifery continuity of care. Many individuals working 'outside' of the maternity services may have little knowledge or interest in the benefits of the model. Ongoing discussion and respectful debate with a wide audience from both within and outside the maternity service will provide opportunities to inform and reassure whilst generating interest and a shared ownership.

Reassuring all involved across the organisation that their needs, as well as those of the women, the midwives and other staff, can be held in balance through working together is another key component. This approach helps to engender confidence that the organisation will be strengthened by having midwifery continuity of care. Interprofessional collaboration and sharing information are additional important components that are crucial to ongoing sustainability; this is examined in detail in Chapter 5 and revisited in Chapter 9. Where there is a shared understanding and transparency between managers, midwives, medical staff and the leaders of the organisation, trust and mutual respect can more readily evolve. Safe, high-quality care, consumer satisfaction and cost effectiveness are all important outcomes that will be considered as measures of success which can be shared across the wider organisation (Forster et al., 2011).

Embarking on the implementation of midwifery models of care requires the development of a suite of governance activities that will promote organisational confidence in the model. Some of the components that enable the manager to speak with confidence about the model include audit that reflects how the philosophy of midwifery care is linked to better outcomes for women and to cost effectiveness. Governance activities also need to demonstrate how midwives receive support through performance review and access to mentoring, debriefing and clinical supervision (Brodie, 2015). Innovations such as the NHS A-EQUIP (Advocating for Education and Quality Improvement) provide a platform whereby clinical supervision and personal action for quality improvement, professional development and ongoing education can support midwives to create their own continuous improvement process (NHS, 2017b).

A DIFFERENT STYLE OF MANAGEMENT

Supporting the sustainability of midwifery continuity of care may require midwifery managers to change how they have previously enacted their role. This may require a change in thinking as midwifery continuity of care models often mean that the midwives develop a primary allegiance to women rather than to the needs of the organisation (McCourt et al., 2007). As care is organised according to the needs of the women, shift-based patterns of work are usually not suitable. This can be hard to conceptualise in maternity services that are embedded within mainstream services alongside an acute health setting. Midwives providing continuity of care are also required to organise their work with a level of autonomy that differs from hospital-based care (Newton et al., 2016) and this can be challenging for managers and the health system.

The different ways of working require managers to have trust in the midwives' ability and integrity to manage their caseload of women whilst working within the practice guidelines of the organisation and the industrial framework. A critical factor is managers understanding that those working within the model need support to work flexibly and make adjustments to the way that the model is provided in order to make it personally sustainable. This can present challenges for managers who have a myriad of other pressures, some of which come from the requirements associated with being part of the acute health care services. Challenges may also arise where the midwifery workforce is overseen by a traditional hierarchy that may have limited knowledge or appreciation of contemporary midwifery practice or how continuity of care models operate (Brodie, 2002, 2004), or where the models are seen as 'alternative' (Haines et al., 2015). Managers of these models often need information, support and encouragement so that they feel able to support midwives to adapt to the different way of

> **BOX 4.1 Purpose of Weekly Midwifery Group Practice/Team Meetings**
> - Continuing to build trust and support
> - Promoting a non-hierarchical approach to working together
> - Discussing roles, responsibilities and interprofessional working
> - Working out on-call arrangements to maximise flexibility and adequate time off
> - Sharing information about current caseload and flagging issues that may need consultation and referral
> - Reflecting on practice and reviewing outcomes
> - Sharing knowledge, skills and experiences
> - Welcoming and supporting students and new graduates
> - Determining matters that require any discussion with the midwifery manager

working. They may need to harness a different leadership style—moving closer to facilitating an autonomous model of practice rather than what may previously have been a more traditional role in managing a group of individuals (Dawson et al., 2018).

Supporting midwifery autonomy

Working in a continuity model requires a different organisation of midwifery work and an understanding of autonomy of practice. Sustainable models of midwifery continuity of care require managers to step back and provide a level of support that enables midwives to self-determine how they organise their working lives and support each other. This includes supporting them to manage some of the other more personal elements of caseload work that can impact on their work and private lives (Sandall et al., 2016b).

Managers have a responsibility for enabling programmed (and paid) time for midwives in group practices or teams to meet together at least once a week in order to discuss their experiences and support each other. This is important not only for the allocation of tasks and distribution of workload but also to discuss any issues that may be affecting the way they work. In our experience, this coming together of midwives in their working groups in a safe space is an essential component of successful midwifery continuity of care models; it may also play a major role in the avoidance of burnout and isolation (Fenwick et al., 2018). The features of a weekly midwifery group practice meeting are summarised in Box 4.1.

Making it work for midwives

There is a consistent and growing body of evidence demonstrating that working in continuity has benefits for midwives and results in greater professional satisfaction (Collins et al., 2009; Fenwick et al., 2018; Newton et al., 2014, 2016) and lower levels of burnout, when compared with midwives outside of continuity models (Fenwick et al., 2018; Newton et al., 2014). The reasons for this are multifaceted, and are difficult to attribute to any one aspect of caseload work, but may include working with known women, getting feedback, working autonomously, practising to the full midwifery scope of practice, professional growth, working with midwives who share a similar philosophy and ultimately contributing to positive outcomes for women (Fenwick et al., 2018; Newton et al., 2016; Warmelink et al., 2015). Positive outcomes for midwives need to be viewed in the context of choice for midwives. Within the current organisation of most continuity models in countries like Australia and the UK, there is often self-determination of employment within continuity models—therefore those working in the models may be more satisfied because it is a model that appeals to them and they are choosing to work that way, and those who feel unsuited or choose not to work in this way are not required to do so.

Facilitating time out from working in continuity

There are times in midwives' lives where they will be more or less suited to working in a midwifery continuity of care model. The factors contributing to this are complex and relate to the nature and organisation of the work in these models, particularly when working on-call is required (Newton et al., 2016). Midwives have reported that working on-call results in a 'blurring' between personal time and work time and is unpredictable (Newton et al., 2016); therefore, suitability to this style of work is a very individual matter. Understanding that some midwives may wish to move in or out of continuity models over the duration of their career will help organisations to plan ahead for a sustainable model that harnesses and strengthens capacity of the midwifery workforce overall (Sandall et al., 2016b), without these movements being identified as a failure of either the model or the midwives.

Managers can employ a range of creative organisational strategies to reduce the potential for midwives to experience burnout in their working lives (Newton et al., 2014). This might include mixing the age range of midwives in group practices, with some having small children, and supporting newly qualified midwives to move into continuity models, with a smaller caseload of women initially. In our experience, managers who can influence the acceptance, integration and normalisation of the model into the mainstream functioning of the hospital will soon notice diminished interest from staff wishing to revert back to previous models of care as these will no longer be seen as desirable (Dawson et al., 2018).

MAKING CONTINUITY ATTRACTIVE TO MIDWIVES

Since there will be times in midwives' lives when working in continuity models may not be feasible, it is important that the model is able to attract new midwives

(Newton et al., 2016). We know that many managers and maternity services generally can be challenged to find ways to attract and support new staff to join continuity models and some have had difficulty finding adequate numbers of suitable applicants (Dawson et al., 2016; NHS, 2017a).

Innovative leaders have demonstrated enhanced success in recruitment into continuity models by providing the opportunity for midwives to have a try at working in these models without a long-term commitment. Vacancies caused by illness or periods of prolonged leave disrupt the continuity of care for women (NHS, 2017a). Thus, providing short-term relief opportunities (6–12 months) maintains the intent of the model and makes sure women receive care while providing exposure for midwives who may be considering working in continuity models but who want to test out their suitability first (Newton et al., 2016).

Addressing concerns about being 'on-call'

Ways of exposing all midwives to a realistic understanding of how continuity models operate can enhance their willingness to consider the model as a career pathway. Midwives working outside of the model may have limited exposure to the benefits that midwives report when working in this way. These benefits are often internalised (i.e. satisfaction, autonomy) and can be masked by the features of the model that are more visible, such as the unpredictable nature of on-call work (Newton et al., 2016). Most importantly, midwives need to arrange their own out-of-hours arrangements to improve sustainability (Gilkison et al., 2015).

A vignette describing 'A week in the life of a caseload midwife', published in the Royal College of Midwives' magazine (Brigante, 2017) is one example of how the lived experience of continuity work can be shared with a larger audience of potential continuity midwives of the future (Box 4.2).

Employing newly graduated midwives in continuity models

In countries where students are exposed to continuity of care as part of their preparation for practice, they report that their experience is inspirational, whilst also providing a realistic idea of the potential impact of the role on midwives' lives (Carter et al., 2015; Gray et al., 2016; Leap et al., 2017). Graduates from midwifery programs have reported being well prepared and keen to work in continuity models soon after qualification (Cummins et al., 2015; Dawson et al., 2015). Despite this, many employers limit opportunities for newly graduated (recently qualified) midwives to practise in the models until they have consolidated their experience (Dawson et al., 2015). This may be due in part to perceptions of the midwives' inexperience and inability to work autonomously and safely, as well as cultural expectations that midwives should be highly experienced in birthing before being allowed to work in continuity models (Cummins et al., 2016).

Employing and supporting newly graduated midwives in continuity models can be challenging for managers and sometimes for their experienced colleagues as well. It can also, however, be rewarding and uplifting to see how they rise to the challenge with good support and mentoring, demonstrating exemplary practice (Cummins et al., 2015, 2016). In Box 4.3 a strategy to support newly graduated midwives to move into continuity models gives some practical guidance regarding workforce succession planning and factors that contribute to sustaining midwifery continuity of care.

Self-care for managers

Meeting the needs of the organisation within a dynamic health system requires managers to remain enthusiastic, to keep 'the fire in the belly' and to access support for

---

BOX 4.2 A Week in the Life of a Caseload Midwife

Lia Brigante

Midwives can be highly satisfied when providing care in a continuity model, both from building relationships with women and families they look after and from high levels of autonomy and flexibility (Fereday et al., 2010). Working patterns can be adjusted to midwives' and service's needs, with midwives working in partnership to ensure they have adequate time off as well as a sustainable work–life balance. Factors contributing to sustainability are:

- **Autonomy in managing the caseload**—midwives can organise their workload as they see fit including working hours. Some midwives will opt for an early start and finish (scheduling visits from 8.30 am to 4.30 pm); others will prefer starting late in the morning and working through the evening depending on social commitments.
- **Self-rostering**—of days off, annual leaves and on-calls contributes to midwives' satisfaction with the on-call life as they have protected time when needed and are able to attend family events or plan a weekend getaway. The proposed rota is reviewed at team meetings to ensure there is 24/7 cover while granting requests.
- **Team support and flexibility**—being able to relay to other midwives in the team if called out to a birth or on a day off is essential. The team will cover cancelled visits and look after the colleague's caseload while she is on holiday, making sure the workload does not pile up and women are seen timely.
- **On-calls**—the team can decide which out-of-hours cover system works, determining whether on-calls should last 12 or 24 hours, how many midwives are on-call and in what order (e.g. first and second midwife on-call). Flexibility and individual arrangements should be allowed between midwives on-call on at the same time. For example, diverting the calls to a colleague for an hour or two can be extremely helpful if planning a yoga class or theatre; favours are always returned and the team's morale stays positive.
- **Job satisfaction**—being present throughout the motherhood continuum is hugely satisfying and helps midwives realise how crucial their role is for women and their families. My diary entries for a typical week illuminate how this all works in practice.

Continued

BOX 4.2 A Week in the Life of a Caseload Midwife—cont'd
A week in the life of a caseload midwife—a diary entry

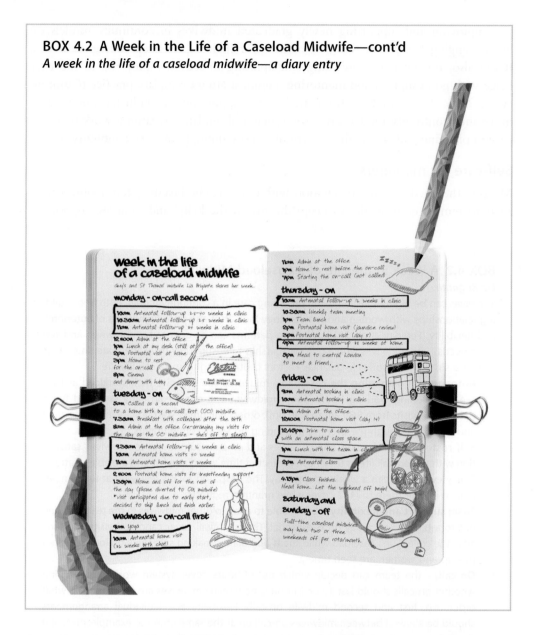

themselves from their professional connections and friends when needed (Brodie, 2015). Managers who actively seek out effective forms of self-care can strengthen their capacity to endure, remain resolute and passionate and continue being committed to the challenges ahead (Creedy et al., 2017). Managers who are self-aware and have the capacity to reflect on their actions, recognise their strengths and their weaknesses and surround themselves with people who can help 'fill in' their weaknesses are more likely to be successful in addressing challenges and difficulties as they arise.

BOX 4.3 Innovation to Enable Newly Graduated Midwives to Work in Continuity Models

Allison Cummins, Midwifery Lecturer, University of Technology Sydney, Australia

In Australia, it is estimated that only around 10% of women have access to midwifery-led continuity of care models. Midwifery managers are directed by policy and government recommendations to expand the models. One of the difficulties some managers report is the lack of midwives to staff the models.

Visionary leaders in Australia are employing newly graduated midwives to move directly into midwifery continuity of care models. This is an innovative move, as traditionally these midwives have had to complete a transition to professional practice program (or 'new grad year') for 12 months before applying for a position. The transition to professional practice program requires the midwife to rotate through a variety of wards in the maternity hospital. The midwives report that they feel prepared to work in midwifery continuity of care models on graduation, their education program having included the experience of providing continuity of care to at least 10 women. Many would prefer to work in a continuity of care model rather than undertake the transition to practice program.

Following graduation, those midwives who have had the opportunity to work in a continuity of care model state that they consolidate skills and knowledge better when they know the woman. They build a relationship of trust with both the woman and the midwives whom they work alongside and feel nurtured by the small group of midwives around them. This support, together with a reduced caseload and a longer orientation period initially, has enabled their successful transition into working in a midwifery group practice with their own caseload

Managers have found employing newly graduated midwives directly into a midwifery-led continuity of care model to be an excellent strategy for succession planning and sustaining the model in their organisations. The essential components for success are: opportunities for students and newly graduated midwives to build trusting relationships through continuity, support and mentoring, access to collaborative team meetings and finally having an approachable manager or clinical support midwife available for support. Approaches such as these will help midwifery managers to expand midwifery-led continuity of care models and increase access for women, with all the known benefits.

From time to time, managers may feel isolated within their role—the process of organisational change often heightening their sense of being somewhat removed from much of the team. This sense of isolation can be heightened if other leaders in the health service do not fully support the model, particularly if they do not understand midwifery continuity of care models or if they feel challenged from an industrial perspective.

To succeed, midwifery managers will need to take time out for regular forms of self-care whilst continuing to draw strength from their belief in midwifery continuity of care and its capacity to improve outcomes. Taking care of oneself whilst promoting the profession and the model in this way reinforces the resolve of the manager and the belief that change is possible and required. Some basic knowledge and understanding of theories of leadership are useful during these times and we have included a brief description of some of these in the next section.

THEORY TO INFORM AND ENHANCE LEADERSHIP

It is advantageous for midwifery managers to have some understanding of the dominant styles of leadership found within the change management literature. We have singled out just two examples—transformational and transactional leadership—as valuable styles that are readily applicable to the midwifery manager of today and may be useful to readers of this book. It is recognised that good leaders can demonstrate both transactional and transformational characteristics and have the ability to exercise both according to the context and needs of any given situation. A blending of both styles results in a balanced mix that enables the leader to draw on transactional and transformational abilities as needed to bring out the best in the team or the individual (Bryant, 2003).

Transformational leaders are said to be flexible, confident and capable as they move towards creating valuable and positive change. Transformational leaders motivate followers by encouraging new and deeper internal values and ideas. This leads to followers acting to ensure sustainability and the building of a collective greater good within supportive environments that encourage shared responsibility (Doody & Doody, 2012). They overtly focus on ways to emerge from being ordinary in their approach to becoming real agents of major change, empowering their followers as they move ahead together. In the process they seek to enhance morale and job performance (Burns, 1978). Transformational leaders focus on team building, motivation and collaboration to accomplish change with employees at different levels of an organisation. They set goals and incentives to push their team towards higher performance levels and provide them with opportunities for personal and professional growth (Rolfe, 2011).

In contrast, **transactional leaders** are more concerned with maintaining the norm and keeping the ship afloat (McCray, 2015). They will readily use disciplinary power and incentives to motivate employees to perform at their best. First described by Max Weber (1930), transactional leadership generally does not involve looking ahead but rather making sure everything flows smoothly as much as possible.

A maternity culture dominated by mainly transactional leadership styles will struggle to adapt and change to the extent required to make autonomous midwifery continuity of care a reality. We are nevertheless of the view that the contemporary midwifery manager may, occasionally, find the need to also enact characteristics from this style, depending on the circumstances at the time. A 'full range' model of leadership and management development (Avolio, 1996) is likely to be the most useful—depicting leadership as a 'process' that ranges from the avoidant through the transactional to the inspirational and transformational styles, which can be applied at the individual, group, organisation and community level. This approach—applied to skilled leadership that achieves changes to the workforce and models of care, and utilises a broad, all-inclusive process bringing everyone together on the journey to improved ways of providing care—is a desirable goal.

Our collective experience has highlighted the importance of the midwifery manager developing a leadership style that enables the creation of a positive working environment in which all midwives can feel both supported and safe. In such an environment, an ongoing priority will be to ensure that the philosophy of midwifery continuity of care remains linked to the best outcomes. This is why we have come to believe that, for midwives to grow and develop their practice, to feel supported in their autonomy and to meet the needs of the women, there is a need to have support from a different type of midwifery manager—one whom we shall call 'the Renaissance midwifery manager', drawing on the definition of a Renaissance man (or woman) as a person who is 'knowledgeable, educated, or proficient in a wide range of fields' (Dictionary. com definition: https://www.dictionary.com/browse/renaissance-man). The Renaissance manager understands the importance of how relationships assist in identifying and addressing the needs of both women and midwives (Brodie, 2013).

MANAGING MIDWIFERY CONTINUITY OF CARE: A CHECKLIST

Whether it be through leadership and change management theories, findings from research or experience in success (and failure) in continuity models, the checklist in Box 4.4 summarises our collective ideas about some of the important considerations in making continuity models work for managers and midwives.

CONCLUSION

In this chapter we have examined strategies for success in leading, implementing and establishing midwifery continuity of care models that 'work' for all midwives and managers. We have drawn on evidence and experience of lessons learned to illustrate that, although not without challenges, the reorganisation of maternity services to include midwifery continuity of care models is possible and beneficial not only for women, but also for midwives and health services.

The concepts discussed in this chapter outline the foundational characteristics that act as potential enablers, and set out how the manager can support progression towards the apex of successful and sustainable models of care. Maintaining a desirable equipoise between the organisation, the midwives and the midwifery managers who

BOX 4.4 Checklist for Managers: Implementing and Sustaining Midwifery Continuity of Care

1. Have an awareness of the broader context of midwifery and maternity care—professional, policy, financial and industry (theory, practice and policy interconnections).
2. Be confident in the midwifery workforce capacity and capabilities required to reorganise the workforce towards midwifery continuity.
3. Commit to building and sustaining effective relationships across the service—invest time to support opportunities to foster knowing, trust and respect.
4. Be aware of the power and politics that exist within the organisation's maternity service and the hierarchies within nursing and medicine—manoeuvre, negotiate and influence to create, sustain and strengthen alliances and create trust.
5. Be 'at the table' where decisions affecting maternity care and the profession of midwifery are made.
6. Have knowledge of the evidence and a belief in midwifery continuity of care—and be prepared to manage and dispel the myths.
7. Use data to support the model, including feedback from women.
8. Use your experience as a midwife, not necessarily within a continuity of midwifery model/homebirth, and develop an ability to share that experience with formal authority within your own role.
9. Set the agenda, hold the line and drive the agenda forward.
10. Include all levels of midwifery experience within the changed model of care.
11. Don't underestimate the value of good communication skills and emotional intelligence.
12. Be patient and keep the end goal in sight. Accept setbacks along the way; be flexible.
13. Be kind, charming and humble, and maintain your sense of humour; share it freely with your team.
14. Value midwifery as a profession, liberating midwives to ensure that their focus remains within midwifery.
15. Engage in regular self-care activities and seek out supportive relationships.

work together with a shared responsibility to support midwifery continuity of care models within their service will be an all-important balancing act.

With successful and sustainable continuity models as the 'end goal', midwives who manage can assume the role of change agents and manoeuvre, negotiate and influence whilst engaging all stakeholders. In addition, they can address the needs of the organisation—ensuring effective governance and the provision of high-quality midwifery care. Using many of the skills of effective leadership and some ideas presented in this chapter, coupled with a goodly modicum of self-care and support, the midwife who manages will be equipped to evolve into a Renaissance midwifery manager who is ready to bring fresh approaches and facilitate better services for women, midwives and the wider health system.

REFERENCES

Avolio B: What's all the karping about Down Under? In Parry K, editor: *Leadership, research and practice: emerging themes and new challenges*, Victoria, 1996, Pitman, pp 3–15.

Brigante L: Achieving work life balance—a week in the life of a caseload midwife, *Midwives magazine*, London, 2017, RCN, p 49.

Brodie P: Addressing the barriers to midwifery—Australian midwives speaking out, *Aust J Midwifery* 15(3):5–14, 2002.

Brodie P: Addressing the invisibility of midwifery: will developing professional capital make a difference? PhD thesis, 2004. Online: http://hdl.handle.net/10453/20176.

Brodie P: 'Midwifing the midwives': addressing empowerment, safety of, and respect for, the world's midwives, *Midwifery* 29:1075–1076, 2013.

Brodie P: Midwifing ourselves and each other: exploring the potential of clinical supervision, *Women Birth* 28:S8, 2015.

Brodie P, Leap N: From ideal to real: the interface between birth territory and the maternity service organisation. In Fahy K, Foureur M, Hastie C, editors: *Birth territory and midwifery guardianship*, Edinburgh, 2008, Butterworth Heinemann/Elsevier, pp 149–170.

Bryant SE: The role of transformational and transactional leadership in creating, sharing and exploiting organizational knowledge, *J Leadersh Organ Stud* 9(4):32–44, 2003.

Burns JM: *Leadership*, New York, 1978, Harper & Row.

Carter AG, Wilkes E, Gamble J, Sidebotham M, Creedy DK: Midwifery students' experiences of an innovative clinical placement model embedded within midwifery continuity of care in Australia, *Midwifery* 31:765–771, 2015.

Collins CT, Fereday J, Pincombe J, Oster C, Turnbull D: An evaluation of midwifery group practice. Part 11: Women's satisfaction, *Women Birth* 22:11–16, 2009.

Common L: Homebirth in England: factors that impact on job satisfaction for community midwives, *Br J Midwifery* 23:716–722, 2015.

Crawshaw K: Personal communication, 2014. Nursing and Midwifery Office Strategic Planning Workshop, New South Wales Ministry of Health.

Creedy DK, Sidebotham M, Gamble J, Pallant J, Fenwick J: Prevalence of burnout, depression, anxiety and stress in Australian midwives: a cross sectional survey, *BMC Pregnancy Childbirth* 17:13, 2017.

Cummins AM, Denney-Wilson E, Homer CSE: The experience of new graduate midwives working in midwifery continuity models in Australia, *Midwifery* 31:438–444, 2015.

Cummins AM, Denney-Wilson E, Homer CSE: The challenge of employing and managing new graduate midwives in midwifery group practices in hospitals, *J Nurs Manag* 24:614–623, 2016.

Dawson K, Newton M, Forster D, McLachlan H: Exploring midwifery students' views and experiences of caseload midwifery: a cross-sectional survey conducted in Victoria, Australia, *Midwifery* 31:e7–e15, 2015.

Dawson K, McLachlan H, Newton M, Foster D: Implementing caseload midwifery: exploring the views of maternity managers in Australia—a national cross-sectional survey, *Women Birth* 29:214–222, 2016.

Dawson K, Forster D, McLachlan H, Newton M: Operationalising caseload midwifery in the Australian public maternity system: findings from a national cross-sectional survey of maternity managers, *Women Birth* 31(3):194–201, 2018. doi:10.1016/j.wombi.2017.08.132.

Doody O, Doody C: Transformational leadership in nursing practice, *Br J Nurs* 21:20, 2012.

Fenwick J, Sidebotham M, Gamble J, Creedy DK: The emotional and professional wellbeing of Australian midwives: a comparison between those providing continuity of midwifery care and those not providing continuity, *Women Birth* 31:38–43, 2018.

Fereday J, Collins C, Turnbull D, Pincombe J, Oster C: An evaluation of the satisfaction of midwives' working in midwifery group practice, *Midwifery* 26:435–441, 2010.

Forster D, Newton M, McLachlan H, Willis K: Exploring implementation and sustainability of models of care: can theory help?, *BMC Public Health* 11(Suppl 5):S8, 2011.

Gilkison A, McAra-Couper J, Fielder A, Hunter M, Austin D: The core of the core: what is at the heart of hospital core midwifery practice in New Zealand?, *J N Z Coll Midwives* 53:30–37, 2017.

Gilkison A, McAra-Couper J, Gunn J, Crowther S, Hunter M, Macgregor D, et al: Midwifery practice arrangements which sustain caseloading lead maternity carer midwives in New Zealand, *J N Z Coll Midwives* 51:11–16, 2015.

Gray J, Taylor J, Newton M: Embedding continuity of care experiences: an innovation in midwifery education, *Midwifery* 33:40–42, 2016.

Haines H, Baker J, Marshall D: Continuity of midwifery care for rural women through caseload group practice: delivering for almost 20 years, *Aust J Rural Health* 23:339–345, 2015.

Homer CSE: Models of maternity care: evidence for midwifery continuity of care, *Med J Aust* 205: 370–373, 2016.

Leap N, Brodie P, Tracy S: Collective action for the development of national standards for midwifery education in Australia, *Women Birth* 30:169–176, 2017.

McCourt C, Stevens TJ, Brodie P: Working with women: continuity of carer in practice. In Page L, McCandlish R, editors: *The new midwifery: science and sensitivity in practice*, ed 2, Oxford, 2007, Churchill Livingstone, pp 141–270.

McCray J: Transactional leadership. In McCray J, editor: *Leadership glossary: essential terms for the 21st century*, Santa Barbara, CA, 2015, Mission Bell Media.

National Health Service (NHS): *Implementing Better Births: a resource pack for Local Maternity Systems*, 2017a. Online: https://www.england.nhs.uk/wp-content/uploads/2017/03/nhs-guidance-maternity-services-v1.pdf.

National Health Service (NHS): *A-EQUIP A model of clinical midwifery supervision*, 2017b. Online: https://www.england.nhs.uk/wp-content/uploads/2017/04/a-equip-midwifery-supervision-model.pdf.

Newton MS, McLachlan H, Forster D, Willis K: Understanding the 'work' of caseload midwives: a mixed-methods exploration of two caseload models in Victoria, Australia, *Women Birth* 29(3):223–233, 2016.

Newton MS, McLachlan HL, Willis KF, Forster DA: Comparing satisfaction and burnout between caseload and standard care midwives: finding from two cross-sectional surveys conducted in Victoria, Australia, *BMC Pregnancy Childbirth* 14:426, 2014.

Rolfe P: Transformational leadership theory: what every leader needs to know, *Nurse Leader* 9(2):54–57, 2011.

Sandall J, Soltani H, Gates S, Shennan A, Devane D: Midwife-led continuity models versus other models of care for childbearing women, *Cochrane Database Syst Rev* (4):CD004667, 2016a. doi:10.1002/14651858. CD004667.pub5.

Sandall J, Coxon K, Mackintosh N, Rayment-Jones H, Locock L, Page L, writing on behalf of the Sheila Kitzinger symposium: Relationships: the pathway to safe, high-quality maternity care. Report from the Sheila Kitzinger symposium at Green Templeton College. Green Templeton College, Oxford, 2016b. Online: https://www.gtc.ox.ac.uk/images/stories/academic/skp_report.pdf.

Shaw D, Guise JM, Shah N, Gemzell-Danielsson K, Joseph KS, Levy B, et al: Drivers of maternity care in high-income countries: can health systems support woman-centred care?, *Lancet* 388(10057): 2282–2295, 2016.

Sinek S: How great leaders inspire action. TED talk, 2010. Online: https://www.youtube.com/watch?v=qp0HIF3SfI4.

Sinek S: *Start with why: how great leaders inspire everyone to take action*, New York, 2011, Barnes and Noble.

Tracy SK, Hartz DL, Tracy MB, Allen J, Forti A, Hall B, et al: Caseload midwifery care versus standard maternity care for women of any risk: m@NGO a randomised controlled trial, *Lancet* 382:1723–1732, 2013.

Tran T, Longman J, Kornelsen J, Barclay L: The development of a caseload midwifery service in rural Australia, *Women Birth* 30:291–297, 2017.

Warmelink JC, Hoijtink K, Noppers M, Wiegers TA, de Cock TP, Klomp T, et al: An explorative study of factors contributing to the job satisfaction of primary care midwives, *Midwifery* 31:482–488, 2015.

Weber M: *The Protestant ethic and the spirit of capitalism*, London, 1930, Routledge.

CHAPTER 5

Building Collaborative Relationships to Support Midwifery Continuity of Care

Holly Powell Kennedy, Andrew Bisits, Pat Brodie

Contents

Maternity care is a four-voice invention. When care is given to women, four voices are singing: midwifery, obstetrics, fear, and trust. When maternity care is well delivered, these voices sing in harmony, much like Bach's three-part inventions. Each line in Bach's compositions can be played as an independent melody with its own voice, but when the lines are played together, they produce something beautiful, the result of a productive tension between the voices. If one line disappears, or if one line is played too loudly, that beauty is lost.

It's the same with maternity care. When all four voices are balanced, the result is something beautiful: a healthy baby, parents prepared for parenthood, a happy family, a satisfied caregiver, and careful and wise use of healthcare resources. But when these voices are out of balance—when fear overwhelms trust, when midwifery overwhelms obstetrics (by being too reluctant to intervene), when obstetrics overwhelms midwifery (with too much unneeded intervention)—that beauty is lost.

Raymond de Vries (2012, p. 9)

INTRODUCTION

'If only we'd talked about this ahead of time'—this is a refrain we have heard many times across our careers—the hindsight reflection that the clinical scenario would have gone smoother, or turned out altogether differently, if there had been better communication from the beginning. This chapter highlights the importance of such communication and discusses the value of building collaboration across maternity and public health communities and care providers, specifically to support midwifery continuity of care for women and families. The chapter is founded on the following assumption: collaborative relationships of mutual trust and partnering enable practitioners to work towards common goals, enhance care quality and improve health outcomes. We integrate the essential concepts of collaboration to support midwifery continuity of care with the components of the evidence-informed Quality Maternal and Newborn Care Framework presented in the *Lancet* series on midwifery (Renfrew et al., 2014).

As the authors of this chapter, we want the reader to understand the perspectives we bring to the topic. All of us are maternity care providers; Holly and Pat have over 60 combined years of experience as midwives and Andrew is an obstetrician with 30 years' experience. Holly has extensive leadership experience in developing positive alliances within the midwifery and obstetric communities in the United States while she was president of the American College of Nurse-Midwives (ACNM) (Kennedy, 2000, 2011; Kennedy & Waldman, 2012; Kennedy et al., 2009, 2018) and through her research while a Distinguished Fulbright Scholar at King's College, London. Pat has a long history of midwifery leadership having been engaged in a wide range of practice development, education, research and management roles, in Australia, Papua New Guinea and the Pacific, as well as being President of the Australian College of Midwives (ACM) (2006–10). Through this chapter, Pat shares her experiences and insights regarding the implementation of midwifery-led, collaborative models of maternity care, the development of national competency standards for midwives and the establishment of a regulatory environment that supports the profession (Brodie, 2013, 2015). Andrew, a known advocate of midwifery continuity of care and interprofessional collaboration, including the supporting of vaginal breech birth (Bisits, 2016), brings his unique perspectives from the obstetric community (Bisits, 2017; Tracy et al., 2014).

UNDERSTANDING COLLABORATION: ESSENTIAL COMPONENTS

The first essential ingredient of collaboration is communication, which is the foundation for the second: trust. Maternity care providers are socialised in different disciplines and may not always agree on how best to achieve the desired outcomes. Additionally, women and families may have different ideas and expectations, depending on their knowledge, wishes and past experiences. This is the reality of health care; it is also the rousing challenge in modern maternity service provision: to understand all perspectives and work together to set and achieve goals. Too often, however, lack of collaboration—be it within the health facility, the community or among the various professional groups—can sever the chain of continuity, reinforce stereotyped polarised views and potentially render a poor outcome. The goal of this chapter is to help the reader avoid those breaks in the chain.

Collaborative relationships across professional boundaries are discussed in the context of supporting midwifery continuity of care. We use vignettes to demonstrate examples of effective collaboration between maternity care colleagues and present a conceptual description of collaboration, including some theories about trust. The subtleties of effective relationships and professional accountabilities along with the dynamics of power, as seen in the various levels of care across institutions and organisations, will be discussed. Barriers and facilitators to effective collaboration are identified, including some practical tips for you to assess collaborative relationships in your practice. The importance of working in partnership with women and their families is highlighted as an essential element of continuity of midwifery care (Grigg & Tracy, 2013). Relationships are at the heart of all clinical interactions in maternity care provision and are particularly important if midwifery continuity of care is to flourish.

Collaboration is an essential component of all models of maternity service provision. Whether a woman is cared for in a midwifery continuity of care model, referred for consultation or transferred across practices or institutions due to changing clinical needs, collaboration among all those involved in her care is essential. Across organisations and institutions, collaboration among maternity care providers is key to supporting midwifery continuity of care and is linked to improved outcomes.

Defining collaboration

Collaboration, as defined by the Oxford English Dictionary (OED), is 'cooperation, especially in scientific work' (OED, 2018). Depending on perspective, it is also defined as, 'traitorous cooperation with the enemy'. The etymological roots are [coll] from 'college' as an organised body of persons with shared functions and privileges, and [labour], which means to work hard (Turner, 1989). Whilst collaboration can be labour intensive, when done well it can bridge many potential rifts.

In this chapter, we focus on collaboration as a dynamic, active process that leads to a purposeful relationship based on the need to either solve a problem or create something (Schrage, 1990). Collaborative efforts are often conducted within certain constraints, including varying levels of expertise, workload pressures, limited time and resources, fear of failure and the prevailing wisdom and attitudes of those involved. Additionally, collaborating partners have different skills and capabilities and may have been socialised into the dominant views and attitudes of their predecessors. These factors can be barriers or facilitators and are important to consider when embarking on a collaborative relationship.

Collaborative practice has many facets. As an example, Heatley & Kruske (2011) conducted an extensive review of interprofessional collaborative practice, examining all papers that included theoretical and empirical discussions of the concept, with a focus on maternity care. They analysed definitions, professional status and organisational factors. Although this review did not identify papers describing collaboration in the provision of midwifery continuity of care, a common principle identified was woman-centred care. This was seen as best achieved through care providers from different disciplines, but with complementary roles, working together as a team and adopting a shared decision-making approach. The authors synthesised the complexity of factors that comprise the process of maternity care professionals and women working together, and we have adopted their definition for this chapter:

> *Interprofessional collaboration is a reflexive and dynamic process that involves maternity care professionals from multiple professions* **working together with the woman** *to produce* **quality outcomes**. *Responsibility and* **accountability** *is shared in terms of appropriate level of involvement of a professional with the woman over the entire perinatal period. All involve* **trust, respect**, *understanding and foster an approach to practice which* **utilises knowledge and expertise from the various professions as required by the woman.**
>
> *(Heatley & Kruske, 2011, p. 56)*

We placed our own emphasis on a number of elements in this definition, which we believe are crucial to understanding the nature of collaborative relationships and quality maternal and newborn care. These will be further elucidated later on in the chapter.

HISTORICAL INFLUENCES ON COLLABORATION IN MATERNITY CARE

In order to make sense of current policies, practices and models of care that highlight the potential benefits of enhanced collaboration, it is wise to reflect on some historical contexts and underpinning issues that emerge at the intersection of midwifery and obstetrics. By understanding the past we can more effectively construct strategies for developing positive collaborative relationships in the future.

Sociologist Anne Witz (1992) exposed the interoccupational boundaries that exist between midwifery and medical practice, asserting that the male power (of obstetricians) has been used to limit employment aspirations of women (as midwives) since the 17th century. The resulting demarcation lines of practice continue to influence the nature and organisation of contemporary maternity service provision (Carpenter, 1993; Pringle, 1998). Using feminist and sociological concepts to explore the sources of professional power, Witz (1992) argued that class and gender have produced enduring hierarchies of power and prestige within the health care professions. Over time, the historically more independent role of the midwife was reduced to the role of obstetric nurse or handmaiden to the 'medical man' (doctor) (Donnison, 1977; Ehrenreich & English, 1973). The sphere of competence of midwives, as prescribed by the medical profession, gradually became restricted to the attendance at normal labour. In the United Kingdom, this became enshrined in the 1902 *Midwives Act* (Leap & Hunter, 2013).

Modern midwifery still reflects some of the past. McIntyre et al. (2012) conducted a discourse analysis of submissions to the Australian National Review of Maternity Services (Australian Government Department of Health, 2011) in order to interpret views about service reform from midwifery, obstetrics, general medical practice and maternity service managers. The discourse of obstetric and general medical practitioners was that their profession was the only one with the expertise to safeguard birth outcomes. 'Normal' could only be established after the birth and 'low risk' did not exist in maternity care; thus, the hierarchal positioning of doctors was explicitly asserted. The midwifery discourse reflected a philosophical stance of 'keeping birth normal', which was difficult to achieve within maternity care provided in acute care settings that potentially posed iatrogenic risks of multiple interventions (Australian Government Department of Health, 2011).

In another context, van der Lee et al. (2014) conducted an extensive review of the historical context of interprofessional collaboration in Dutch obstetric care. Although midwifery had survived as an autonomous profession over decades of change, a collaborative model was described—one in which professionals worked independently but in parallel relationships. This was thought to increase the possibility of some mistrust, which could hinder optimal collaboration. In exposing some lack of trust and power imbalances these authors identified a need for formal interprofessional governance, pointing to effective collective efforts to develop protocols and monitor quality of care (van der Lee et al., 2014, 2016).

Lane (2012) has challenged the vertical hierarchy of forced or mandated collaboration between medicine and midwifery. Amidst similar debates, the American College of Nurse-Midwives (ACNM) and the American College of Obstetricians and Gynecologists (ACOG) tackled the issue of mandated collaboration, rejecting it in favour of professional accountability to work together in the best interests of the patient (ACNM / ACOG, 2011). Their joint policy statement established that midwives and obstetricians are experts in their respective fields who can and should collaborate with one another:

> *Quality of care is enhanced by collegial relationships characterized by mutual respect and trust, as well as professional responsibility and accountability* (p. 1) *... to provide highest quality and seamless care, ob-gyns and [midwives] should have access to a system of care that fosters collaboration among licensed, independent providers.* (p. 2)

Effective collaborative relationships among key service providers, including service leaders, policy makers and maternity care professionals, are crucial aspects of safe and effective care in any setting, as discussed in Chapter 6. Effective collaboration, communication and consensus decision making are known to be central to reducing negative outcomes in maternity care (Knight et al., 2015; Lewis, 2007) and can improve experiences for both women and health professionals.

OTHER FACTORS INFLUENCING COLLABORATION

Collaboration has been studied as a process and as an intervention. To illustrate this, D'Amour et al. (2005) conducted an extensive literature review on how collaboration is conceptually defined across interprofessional health services. Elements of collaboration included sharing, partnership, interdependency and power. Broad consistent elements of collaboration were: (1) working together to address the complexity of client needs, and (2) the importance of strong teamwork that integrates the perspectives of each professional in a team who respect and trust each other (D'Amour et al., 2005, p. 127).

Australian midwife Catherine Adams conducted research to identify attributes of effective collaborators in maternity care. Using a competing values framework (CVF) (Cameron et al., 2006) to guide her analysis, she revealed the predominant culture of a maternity service as 'hierarchy', with teamwork and collaboration, innovation and flexibility not highly valued (Box 5.1).

An embedded case study by Behruzi et al. (2017) of a Quebec birth centre and its affiliated hospital is another example of the complexity of collaboration within a maternity system. Researchers interviewed administrators, nurses, midwives, obstetricians / gynaecologists and family doctors of varying levels of experience. They identified three factors that affect collaboration: interactional, organisational and systemic. Interactional factors included conflict around philosophy, autonomy and compensation. Organisational factors reflected philosophy and mission, culture, structure and resources. Systemic factors included power, status and how care was managed.

In a similar vein, a qualitative study in Canada examined models of maternity care in rural environments (Munro et al., 2013). Numerous barriers were identified, including role confusion, professional orientation, limited health resources and caseloads, differing scopes of practice and skill sets, payment inequity and lack of formal structures for shared practice models. Respect among providers and clear role definitions and responsibilities were viewed as critical to effective interprofessional collaboration. The importance of shared participation between providers and women throughout the pregnancy was also highlighted (Munro et al., 2013).

In an earlier example from Australia, an effective collaborative midwifery continuity of care model was developed, known as the 'St George Outreach Maternity Program' (STOMP). This model had a deliberate emphasis on effective collaboration between midwives and obstetricians as part of a community-based maternity service available to women of all levels of risk (Homer et al., 2000, 2001a, 2001b). Outcomes of the STOMP randomised controlled trial demonstrated a significant difference in the

---

BOX 5.1 Synergistic Working Between Organisational and Interpersonal Characteristics

Catherine Adams, Clinical Midwifery Consultant, Northern Nsw Local Health District, Australia

At the time of this work, I was the Clinical Midwifery Consultant for Northern Sydney Local Health District in New South Wales, Australia. During routine auditing at one facility I observed variations between peer hospitals that could not be explained simply by demographics. Suspecting that characteristics of the organisation could explain the difference, I commenced a process of examination of the characteristics. Below is an explanation of what I did.

The work replicates that completed in the United Kingdom (Downe et al., 2009). Two tools—Pathways to Success: A Self-improvement Toolkit. Focus on normal birth and reducing caesarean section (Baldwin et al., 2007) and the Competing Values Framework (CVF) (Cameron et al., 2006)—were used to identify the characteristics and predominant culture. Clinicians nominated peers with the attributes of effective collaborators, who were then invited to engage in an action research process.

The results of the Toolkit demonstrated a divergence in knowledge and attitudes between clinicians and those in similar units with lower rates of intervention. Using the CVF, the predominant culture of this organisation was identified as one of hierarchy. Teamwork and collaboration, innovation and flexibility were not valued highly by the organisation. Participants, however, expressed their preference for a culture that was opposite to the current one, favouring greater collaboration and innovation. They appreciated the opportunity to think critically about their service, to evaluate its characteristics and then to analyse what they would prefer the organisation to be like in order to implement change. These clinicians had not previously had such an opportunity. The nomination of 'effective collaborator' was viewed positively by those who were chosen as being the first time they had felt visible in the organisation. This contributed to achieving the necessary clinician engagement for service changes as well as providing an opportunity for strengthening teamwork and multidisciplinary collaboration.

---

caesarean section rate—with 13.3% in the STOMP group and 17.8% in the control group; this prevailed after controlling for known contributing factors to caesarean section. Women receiving STOMP care were more satisfied and costs associated with the new model were less than for standard care. Collaboration was considered by the researchers to be key to the success of this model and the outcomes (Brodie & Homer, 2009).

Another example of effective collaboration, also in Australia, was a study involving a retrospective analysis of case notes over 12 months; the aim was to assess collaboration between midwives and obstetricians in two midwifery group practice models (Beasley et al., 2012). The researchers found that consistent advice was provided and a mutual level of trust and respect was present. Clinical advice was based on current evidence, there was engagement of all team members and the interprofessional meetings

---

BOX 5.2 The 'Umbrella Theory'
Susan Bewley, Obstetrician, London, UK

This metaphor works well with women of all backgrounds but may be limited to places with unpredictable weather! When explaining uncertainty and offering reassurance with a management plan, I ask my patients '... you know how it is? If you have an umbrella it doesn't rain, and yet if you don't have an umbrella it does?' I say that my job as an obstetrician when women are experiencing complications is to listen to their fears, saying to them, 'But we've got a plan for this. The reason I'm talking about the worst-case scenario is so that it won't happen.' And quite often I see women become relieved when I say, 'Even living with the uncertainty and fears and potential dangers, if you've got a plan then maybe you can steer between that rock and hard place and maybe you can too achieve a normal delivery, even though you've got this disease.'

I describe the art of good obstetrics, just as with midwifery, as watchful waiting—knowing when to sit on your hands and when to act swiftly and competently because there is a problem. I think midwives are the rock, and support from other women who have been through it also gets women through. A lot of the doctor's role is actually to be out of the way ... not to make people frightened, and not to undermine confidence.

Trust and teamwork play a major role, especially when something goes wrong. We carry a big burden of betraying that trust, but competence and confidence and working out the communications with your other team members are the key.

---

were productive. Concepts emerging from this review suggest that communication, respect, role definition, organisational systems, skill sets, collegial relationships and alliances are all elements of effective collaboration in maternity care. Box 5.2 presents a metaphor by London obstetrician Susan Bewley to depict the roles and collaborating relationships among midwives, obstetricians and women.

COLLABORATION: IMPROVING QUALITY OF CARE

Achieving quality maternity outcomes does not happen in a vacuum; it is influenced by health systems, providers, care practices and institutions. As is often the case, no one person may have all of the skills or knowledge to care fully for all women in their caseload; thus, teamwork and partnerships are needed. We know too that health systems tend to be complex and as women cross professional boundaries they can be disconnected from the midwife who knows them best. Collaborative maternity care models should place the midwife providing continuity of care as the lynchpin to assure effective communication and care planning across the pregnancy, labour, birth and postnatal continuum.

The Framework developed as part of the *Lancet* series on midwifery for quality maternal and newborn care is useful to consider here (Renfrew et al., 2014). Fig. 5.1

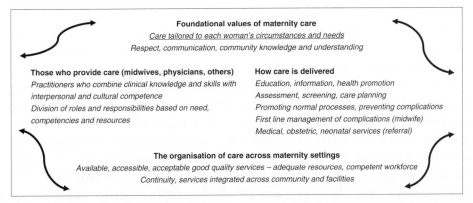

Figure 5.1 *Effective collaboration for midwifery continuity across maternity settings (Adapted from Renfrew et al. 2014 Quality Maternal and Newborn Care Framework,* Lancet *series on midwifery and Heatley & Kruske 2011 Defining collaboration in Australian maternity care,* Women Birth *24: 53-57).*

provides an adaptation of the essential elements of this framework that also reflects our adopted definition of collaborative practice (Heatley & Kruske, 2011). The figure presents the elements as interconnected; the individual woman is placed at the top to reinforce the idea that care is tailored to her individual circumstances and needs, founded on values of respect, communication, community knowledge and understanding. This quality of care has been demonstrated to be best provided through midwifery continuity of care.

Core values in collaboration: trust and respect

In any relationship, a defining element is trust between individuals and a reciprocity that assumes trust will be both given and expected (Reiger & Lane, 2009). In maternity care, trust and respect are essential if care providers are to establish and maintain effective relationships and provide care that meets each woman's circumstances. Staff in well-functioning maternity units suggest that the reasons for their successes are the well-defined roles and responsibilities between midwives and obstetricians, and a high level of trust and mutual respect (Howat & Scherman, 2005; Reiger & Lane, 2009). Establishing trust across professional boundaries is essential in assuring continuity of care, especially as some women will need to move between different care providers and types of care.

In maternity care provision, common areas of mistrust stem from different philosophical approaches. Midwives may be reluctant to communicate early on because of a concern about unnecessary intervention. Obstetricians can sometimes feel cornered when faced with a situation where it is too late to help, believing that if there had been consultation or referral earlier they could have made a difference. To illustrate this, Reiger & Lane (2009) analysed maternity units in Victoria, Australia and found that midwives valued doctors who respected them and midwifery itself, and who were willing to negotiate rather than dictate care. Likewise, doctors wanted to be respected by their midwifery colleagues and did not want to be seen as the enemy or simply as interventionists.

Another study that highlights the importance of trust examined the impact of the Advanced Life Support in Obstetrics (ALSO) course on midwives' and obstetricians' perceptions of interprofessional learning. Six weeks after the course, there were significant increases in midwives' confidence in all four aspects of interprofessional interaction. However, doctors reported a significant increase in only one aspect—increased confidence that midwives respected their decisions (Walker et al., 2015). These examples show the importance of a collaborative, cohesive team that communicates effectively, understands one another's roles and works together to provide the type of care that benefits women as well as their care providers.

In Box 5.3 a midwife in private practice, Jo Hunter, describes her role in caring for women who have complex pregnancies and the need to spend extensive time liaising with hospital staff and obstetricians to build trust and respect.

BOX 5.3 Private Midwives Caring for Women With Complex Challenges

Jo Hunter, Midwife in Private Practice Serving Women and Their Families in the Blue Mountains and Sydney Area of Australia

When the general population think of homebirth and private practice midwives (PPMs), they think that we care only for women who are considered 'low risk'. On the contrary, we work with some of *the most* traumatised women there are.

Women who have emerged from previous births suffering from physical and emotional trauma often decide that they will not re-enter the system unless absolutely necessary. This includes women who feel they were bullied and chastised into agreeing to interventions that they believe were not necessary, contributing to a cascade of interventions leading to physical and emotional trauma. Perhaps the most common instance of this I see in my practice is previous induction of labour for no medical reason other than pregnancy continuing beyond 41 weeks gestation, resulting ultimately in an unwanted caesarean section.

Other women who seek out care with PPMs include those who have experienced trauma in other parts of their lives and desperately want to maintain control over what happens to them during labour and birth—for instance, women who are survivors of sexual and/or physical abuse. It is estimated that one in three women experience physical or sexual violence in their lives. Some women choose to birth at home with PPMs so that they can select their care provider and feel safe inviting them into their domain. It is really important to these women to remain autonomous yet build a meaningful relationship with their midwife.

In all situations where women have complex pregnancies, PPMs need to spend extensive time liaising with hospital staff and obstetricians. In some cases, this involves supporting the woman who has made an informed decision to decline recommended guidelines or medical

> **BOX 5.3 Private Midwives Caring for Women With Complex Challenges—cont'd**
>
> intervention. Such situations involve the PPM in navigating systems that are in place whilst keeping the woman at the centre of care.
>
> Holding the space for a woman who has a complex pregnancy involves so much more than just clinical expertise and decision making. It involves digging deep, finding courage and really being committed to walking beside the woman, offering her emotional support, even when she makes decisions that the PPM and hospital colleagues themselves would never make.
>
> When supporting women with complex pregnancies the things that can support PPMs in their practice are:
>
> - **Good collaboration**—this means building rapport with colleagues in hospital and community settings. In my local area we organised several meetings between the senior midwifery staff at the hospital and the local PPMs. This has had invaluable consequences for me and for the women I work with. We now have great pathways for booking in, contact numbers for senior midwives who we can call on for assistance or advice and invitations to in-service training, workshops and celebrations. Building relationships with hospital staff helps them to realise that we are skilled professionals who feel passionate about our work and the women we care for.
>   We also have a productive collaborative agreement with an obstetrician; this can be used when women with higher needs wish to consult an obstetrician or give birth in hospital. It also means that we can contact an obstetrician to discuss any concerns we have or to share information.
> - **Collegial support network**—this means a network of colleagues who get it, who understand, who you can call at any time throughout the day or night and with whom you can sit down and have a good debrief. Perhaps most importantly …
> - **Providing one-to-one midwifery continuity of care**—this enables us to build a respectful and trusting relationship with the woman and her family over time. A trusting partnership means we can assist her to make informed decisions and respect and support her choices. Continuity also enables us to gain a deep understanding of the intricate needs of the woman and her family. With that knowledge we can provide culturally and socially appropriate care for each woman we work with.

Trust is also an essential element for midwives working in group practices or in small teams. Without trust, the group practice will struggle in the negotiation of schedules and flexibility as well as in providing continuity of care for women.

Trust between individuals can only be built over time and requires a level of familiarity and understanding of the other person and their capacity to perform in practice. The better people know each other and communicate, the more accurately they will be able to predict what the other will do and this predictability builds respect and enhances trust (Boon & Holmes, 1991). Thus, in midwifery continuity of care, trust takes time to develop and needs a commitment from each individual.

Strategies such as team-building days, social events and celebrations can bring all the players together so they can get to know each other and develop an understanding of one another's way of thinking and acting. Additional strategies aimed at creating a healthy culture and greater interprofessional collaboration within the maternity unit have been suggested by Hastie & Fahy (2011) and include providing an environment in which there are opportunities for midwives and doctors to come together away from direct clinical care, so that they have the opportunity to get to know, like and trust each other.

What is clear is that without trusting relationships there is no possibility of collaboration, and the potential to improve health, and maternity care outcomes in particular, will be severely limited.

Agreeing professional accountability

For most women experiencing a straightforward pregnancy, the midwife can provide care and take responsibility for decisions made. Internationally, it is recognised that educated and regulated midwives are the most cost-effective providers of maternal and newborn care. Working in partnership with women, promoting normal birth, detecting complications and accessing medical care or emergency measures as needed are the domain of the midwife (Renfrew et al., 2014).

To be safe and effective, midwives must develop collaborative relationships with others whom they may need to consult with as the woman's clinical needs change and referral to specialists may be required (Fox et al., 2018). In order for this aspect of collaboration to be effective, it is essential that the roles and responsibilities of each professional in the relationship are well defined and clearly understood.

Effective collaborative relationships reflect an integration of the roles, responsibilities, skills and competencies of each health professional, combined with a level of respect and appreciation for each other. When this does not happen, there can be devastating results. Studies examining root causes in obstetric malpractice have implicated miscommunication and poor teamwork as frequent contributors to adverse outcomes (Joint Commission, 2015). Although studies have revealed mixed views on how best to implement collaborative practice, there does seem to be agreement that the development of trusting relationships can positively influence how maternity care services work effectively (Downe et al., 2010).

Obstetrician Andrew Bisits provides a clinical example of collaborative care across these professional boundaries in Box 5.4.

In order for health professionals to trust one another it is critical that they are each personally accountable for their practice. As identified above, this requires identified and agreed upon definitions of roles, responsibilities and the parameters of working together, including agreed referral pathways. This aspect of collaboration can sometimes take the most investment by all parties. However, if this is carefully addressed,

---

BOX 5.4 An Obstetrician's Perspective on Collaboration and Midwifery Continuity of Care

Andrew Bisits, Obstetrician, Sydney, Australia

I work in a setting where there are many meaningful initiatives to foster collaboration between obstetricians and midwives. There are, however, strong remnants of the previous dominant hierarchies. The following story is a positive example of how midwifery continuity of care and positive collaboration can work well.

A 42-year-old woman having her first baby was attending a private obstetrician, whose care she valued very much. She was feeling significant pressure, however, to have an induction and possibly a caesarean because of her age.

We were able to refer her at 32 weeks gestation to a group practice with midwifery continuity of care in our setting. This midwife had previously established cooperation and collaboration with an obstetrician.

Induction of labour was offered to the woman at 40 weeks because of her age; she declined this and proceeded to have a spontaneous labour and normal vaginal birth 4 days beyond her due date.

The collaborative approach taken in the midwifery continuity of care model meant that she could discuss all the issues around her situation, but avoiding undue emphasis on risks and the anxiety accompanying this. In this situation, and many others, it is the trusting collaboration between obstetrician and midwife that enhances the confidence for women.

---

and there is personal commitment to adhere to and regularly review the agreements, the collaborative relationship will be more effective and enduring.

To return to Susan Bewley's analogy, one definition of obstetrics is to stand by— in this case, to be in the wings to step in collaboratively when needed. The Latin derivation of obstetric is to 'stand opposite to' and in modern derivation this could be interpreted as the person who 'stands by' (The Free Dictionary, 2018). One midwife described the relationship of trust that enables this to happen:

> In this practice, I have appropriate professional autonomy and respect … so I trust that my consultants are available and otherwise in a normal situation appropriately disinterested.
>
> **(Kennedy et al., 2016, p. 342)**

One effective way to address responsibility within practices is for members to identify accountability measures together, including the standards and outcomes that are important to track (Chassin et al., 2010). For example, if a midwifery group practice uses national practice guidelines, it can conduct regular audits to assure there are appropriate referrals for women with identified clinical complications. Similarly, records can be audited to confirm that when a woman is referred to a specialist there is documented communication about her plan of care with the referring midwife to assure continuity of care. Quality measurement provides a way to examine clinical workflow and outcomes (Conway et al., 2013). This approach appears to be a positive factor in contemporary Dutch midwifery (van der Lee et al., 2014) and could be applied in other contexts.

Maintaining midwifery continuity of care during consultation and referral

In Fig. 5.1, all but specialist care is the sphere of midwifery practice. When a woman does require referral to a specialist it is critical that the referring midwife remain involved. Kennedy et al. (2010) demonstrated this in an ethnography of two National Health Service (NHS) Trusts in England where the majority of births were attended by a midwife, even when there were complications present. One consultant obstetrician described why it worked (p. 264):

> What facilitates it here is the availability of midwifery care ... so that [women] never see an obstetrician, so that everything remains overtly normal. And on the obstetric side what facilitates it is a group of like-minded obstetricians who are trying to keep everything as normal as possible.

The high-risk teams were equally staffed with consultant obstetricians and midwives to assure women received the benefits of both skill sets.

As discussed in Chapter 2, women must have a voice about what is important to them in how maternity care is organised and provided. There are several foundational aspects of care in which women are partners and maternity care is co-produced (Dunston et al., 2008), including women having the right to participate in policy making that affects their care. Assuring these elements exist can enhance and improve the sustainability of a service, with care that is responsive to the changing needs of individual women in their own unique context.

Ultimately, care is enhanced when it occurs in a system that fosters seamless care, continuity and collaboration. This was a key factor identified in the *Lancet* series on midwifery (Renfrew et al., 2014). Midwifery was found to be pivotal to improved maternal and newborn health outcomes (p. 1129):

> [This] requires effective interdisciplinary teamwork and integration across facility and community settings. Future planning for maternal and newborn care systems can benefit from using the quality framework in planning workforce development and resource allocation.

An analysis by Homer et al. (2014) demonstrated that over 80% of maternal and newborn deaths could be averted if midwifery were to be universally scaled up with the addition of family planning services. Van Lerberghe et al.'s 2014 case study analysis of four countries with sustained decreases in maternal mortality provided insight on how this can be achieved. In these countries the investment included networks of service delivery and care access, competent workforce deployment, technical resources and facility birthing. The improvements went beyond singular scaling up of midwifery services to the political will of a country to commit to the health of women and babies (ten Hoope-Bender et al., 2014).

Midwives cannot function in isolation, and as a profession must create collaborative relationships within broader health systems. These include, but are not limited to, obstetrics, nursing, social work, drug and alcohol services, postnatal services, general practitioners, pediatricians and mental health services. A study by Psaila et al. (2014) of relationships between child health nurses and midwives in Australia found that the collaboration worked most effectively when both had strong professional identities, communicated well and had time to develop a trusting relationship. They described how good collaboration most often occurred when different professional groups worked to provide services and resources for vulnerable or at-risk families. The midwife in a continuity model is in a key position to enhance these relationships with other practitioners in community settings.

PRACTICAL TIPS TO IMPROVE COLLABORATION

There are no magic tricks to ensure that your collaborative efforts will be successful—other than a requirement that all parties are committed. However, there has been some excellent work to distinguish what are the specific components of successful models. Downe et al. (2009) developed a set of tools to improve collaboration between midwives and obstetricians. This included workshops, surveys and focus groups with dedicated leaders for each site. The group found that incentives and continuous encouragement were essential, in addition to having professional groups on the project steering committee. Fig. 5.2 outlines their findings on what makes a good collaborator.

In Box 5.5, Cristina Fernandez Turienzo presents a useful practice-based example of collaboration and alliance building, which was used to build a case for a midwifery caseload practice intervention to reduce pre-term birth. This work took place over a 2-year period, across professional boundaries and with key stakeholders. Within the context of supporting midwifery continuity of care, the various stages required for building these alliances and establishing stakeholder engagement are explained, as well as the dynamics, barriers and facilitators to effective collaboration.

We can learn from studying successful collaborative models. For example, Avery et al. (2012) conducted an analysis of 12 articles that described successful midwife / obstetrician collaborative models in the United States. These models reflected different clinical settings and structures. The five areas of commonality the researchers identified are relevant to many other practice contexts and are summarised as:

1. The models had a *common impetus for collaboration*. As a group, they had come together with commitment to a common goal. As you examine your collaborative relationships it is important for all involved to have their voices heard and

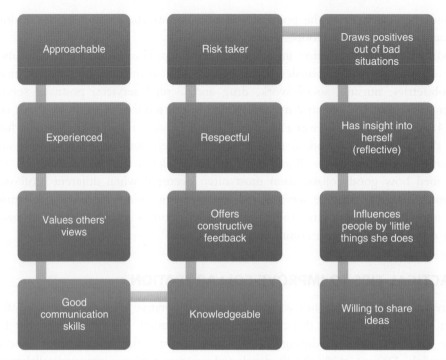

Figure 5.2 *Qualities of a good collaborator (Adapted from Downe et al. 2009 East Lancashire Childbirth Choices Project: choice, safety and collaboration. Final report. UCLan Research in Childbirth and Health (ReaCH) Research Group, University of Central Lancashire, Preston).*

BOX 5.5 The Poppie Trial: an Example of Cross-Disciplinary Collaboration
Cristina Fernandez Turienzo, Registered Nurse and Midwife and WHO Technical Advisor

The ongoing POPPIE (study of midwifery practice in pre-term birth including women's experiences) pilot trial is investigating whether a model of midwifery continuity of care for women at increased risk of pre-term birth is feasible and improves experience and pregnancy outcomes in an inner hospital in South London (UK). We describe the collaborative approach taken with an extensive set of stakeholders—spanning academia, local authorities, public hospitals and organisations, commissioning groups, the voluntary sector and parents—to develop, implement and test this complex organisational intervention. The project has recently received an award by the National Institute for Health Research (NIHR) for the 'most innovative collaboration'.

• In 2014/15 a consultant midwife in public health at the local authority approached the South London CLAHRC (Collaborations for Leadership in Applied Health Research and Care) —an organisation funded by the NIHR—to see whether there were any collaborative opportunities that could support the reduction of local pre-term births.

BOX 5.5 The Poppie Trial: an Example of Cross-Disciplinary Collaboration—cont'd

- Discussions began, led by researchers in the CLAHRC and King's College London, and actively involved key stakeholders in the Department of Public Health, maternity managerial team at the local hospital, the Children and Young People and Maternity Teams at the local cinical commissioning group, link university leads, the Maternity Voices partnership, three locally convened focus groups of parents of pre-term babies (including fathers) and other service user organisation representatives and charities (e.g. BLISS, Tommy's charity).

- After considering evidence from the Cochrane review and Better Births national policy, it was hypothesised that providing a model of midwifery continuity of care for women with risk factors for pre-term birth may potentially have an impact on local premature births.

- Three key initial strategies were used to guide the implementation process: stakeholder engagement, application for funding and development of a driver diagram to help the design and evaluation of the intervention.

- Initial meetings every 2–4 months and business cases with local stakeholders were conducted over a 2-year period to identify key barriers and facilitators to the implementation and for process mapping to identify service areas requiring improvement and possible solutions.

- Some of the barriers included workforce shortages and challenges with staff recruitment, while some of the facilitators included: stakeholders' involvement in the project, having time for piloting the model and extra funding from the commissioning group (they developed a financial formula that provided funding for 2 years for a senior midwife project manager to lead the service redesign and manage the organisational change).

- Quarterly updates on project progress, weekly brief catchups, monthly implementation meetings, seminars and events (e.g. continuity of care study day, launch), newsletters, etc. have all been essential for cultivating relationships with every partner and to build a strong coalition between local stakeholders.

- Other implementation strategies included: involving executive boards, using advisory works and workshops and conducting ongoing training.

- The collaborative planning work has already illuminated gaps in care so that the care pathway for women at risk of pre-term birth has been strengthened and issues raised by the service user groups (e.g. lack of support in neonatal units for breastfeeding) has led to a newly created infant-feeding post.

- Conversations and meetings between a wide range of partners, including parents, has illuminated contributory factors to pre-term birth such as psychological stress, domestic abuse and maternal obesity—all of which require whole-systems collaborative approaches to design interventions that work.

- The potential therefore for midwives to be pivotal innovative programs for care improvement in future through providing continuity of care is significant.

respected, and to identify achievable goals—start small and on something that is relatively straightforward; save the hard stuff for after you have established basic trust with one another.

2. The models developed *basic foundations or building blocks* on how to work with each other. Among these were how to foster good communication, guidelines for referral of clients, and developing financial structures that discouraged competition. The collective group needs to identify the processes and to follow up that these have been accomplished. Audit teams should have representatives of each of the professional disciplines.

3. The models were *committed to the partnership*. This required institutional commitment to a culture of mutual respect and trust, teamwork to solve problems together and assurance of quality. It required leadership at multiple levels. If the group is having difficulty with these steps it may be a worthwhile investment to bring in an outside facilitator to help.

4. *Care was integrated*, with providers working to their scope of practice. Clinical guidelines were developed together. Examining and interpreting evidence together within the context of your community is a positive way to establish practice priorities and viewpoints.

5. Most of the models described the *value of interprofessional health care education*, so that future practitioners learned about different professionals' scope of practice and skill sets early in their education. Although having students (e.g. midwifery, medical and nursing) in clinical practices is demanding and can affect productivity, it is essential to integrate them into the clinical setting as active members of the group. Having identified practice members representing different disciplines in charge of the educational efforts helps to streamline efforts and facilitate the teaching of collaboration.

CONCLUSION

If you think about successful collaborative relationships that you may have experienced or observed, a common thread is that they take time to build and require opportunities or the space for individuals to get to know each other; they do not happen overnight or 'on the hop'. Relationships also take patience, creativity, thoughtfulness, reflexivity and, often, tenacity. Ultimately, a strong collaborative relationship between individuals who share the common goal of achieving best possible outcomes for each woman, her baby and family is a truly rewarding experience and this contributes to building an enjoyable environment in which to work.

To finish our chapter, we share a story from the United States that illustrates how strong collaborative relationships do work and are built over time. When Holly became president of the American College of Nurse-Midwives (ACNM) the organisation was asked by the American College of Obstetricians and Gynecologists

(ACOG) to consider revising their joint statement on practice relations. They spent 2 years carefully examining every word that went into this document and eventually came to an impasse over the description of midwives and obstetricians as 'independent providers'. This terminology did not mandate collaboration, which many saw as a professional expectation. Through the 2 years of investment in the process, the presidents of each organisation began to attend the other's Board of Directors meetings, a practice that continues to today. That slow development of trust and honest, frank communication across a realistic timeframe moved them past the impasse and enabled the statement to be finalised. When the two presidents presented the final statement to a national meeting of obstetricians, one of the delegates stood up and stated how disappointed he was that a signed collaboration statement between the midwife and obstetrician was not part of the final statement. The ACOG president gave the floor to the ACNM president, who asked the obstetrician if he had a signed collaboration statement with a dermatologist to whom he referred women with skin lesions that he could not manage. He had not. Thus, the key here is that each of us holds personal professional accountability for understanding and adhering to our own scope of practice, whatever the clinical discipline. If we maintain the highest professional standards possible and communicate well across professional boundaries, the result will be a trusting, collaborative relationship that will benefit not only the woman and her family, but her health care providers as well.

REFERENCES

American College of Nurse-Midwives, American College of Obstetricians and Gynecologists (ACNM / ACOG): *Ob-Gyns and midwives seek to improve health care for women—collaborative practice statement*, Washington DC, 2011, ACNM / ACOG. Online: https://www.acog.org/-/media/News-Releases/nr2011-03-31.pdf.

Australian Government Department of Health: *National Maternity Services Plan*, Canberra, 2011. Online: http://www.health.gov.au/internet/publications/publishing.nsf/Content/pacd-maternityservicesplan-toc.

Avery M, Montgomery O, Brandl-Salutz E: Essential components of successful collaborative maternity care models. The ACOG-ACNM project, *Obstet Gynecol Clin North Am* 39:423–434, 2012.

Baldwin J, Brodrick A, Mason N, Cowley S: Maternity services. Focus on normal birth and reducing caesarean section rates, *MIDIRS Midwifery Digest* 17(2):279–282, 2007.

Beasley S, Ford N, Tracy S, Welsh AW: Collaboration in maternity care is achievable and practical, *Aust N Z J Obstet Gynaecol* 52:576–581, 2012.

Behruzi R, Klam S, Dehertog M, Jimenez V, Hatem M: Understanding factors affecting collaboration between midwives and other health care professionals in a birth center and its affiliated Quebec hospital: a case study, *BMC Pregnancy Childbirth* 17:200, 2017.

Bisits A: Risk in obstetrics—perspectives and reflections, *Midwifery* 38:12–13, 2016.

Bisits A: There is a place in current obstetric practice for planned vaginal breech birth, *Aust NZ J Obstet Gynaecol* 57:372–374, 2017.

Boon S, Holmes J: The dynamics of interpersonal trust: resolving uncertainty in the face of risk. In Hinde R, Groebel J, editors: *Cooperation and prosocial behaviour*, Cambridge, 1991, Cambridge University Press, pp 190–211.

Brodie P: 'Midwifing the midwives': addressing the empowerment, safety of, and respect for, the world's midwives, *Midwifery* 29:1075–1076, 2013.

Brodie P: Midwifing ourselves and each other: exploring the potential of clinical supervision, *Women Birth* 28:S8, 2015.

Brodie P, Homer C: Transforming the culture of a maternity service: St George Hospitals, Sydney, Australia. In Floyd RD, editor: *Birth models that work*, Los Angeles, 2009, University of California Press, pp 187–238.

Cameron K, Quinn R, Degraff J, Thakor A: *Competing values leadership: creating values in organizations*, New York, 2006, Edward Elgar Publishing.

Carpenter M: The subordination of nurses in health care. Towards a social division approach. In Weger R, editor: *Gender, work and medicine: women and the medical division of labour*, London, 1993, Sage, pp 95–130.

Chassin MR, Loeb JM, Schmaltz SP, Wachter RM: Accountability measures—using measurement to promote quality improvement, *New Engl J Med* 363:683–688, 2010.

Conway PH, Mostashari F, Clancy C: The future of quality measurement for improvement and accountability, *JAMA* 309:2215–2216, 2013.

D'Amour D, Ferrada-Videla M, San Martin Rodriguez L, Beaulieu M-D: The conceptual basis for interprofessional collaboration: core concepts and theoretical frameworks, *J Interprof Care* 1:116–131, 2005.

De Vries RG: Midwives, obstetrics, fear, and trust: a four-part invention, *J Perinat Educ* 21(1):9–10, 2012.

Donnison J: *Midwives and medical men*, London, 1977, Heinemann.

Downe S, Byrom S, Finlayson K, Fleming A, Edge E: *East Lancashire Childbirth Choices Project: choice, safety and collaboration*. Final report, UCLan Research in Childbirth and Health (ReaCH) Research Group, Preston, 2009, University of Central Lancashire.

Downe S, Finlayson K, Fleming A: Creating a collaborative culture in maternity care, *J Midwifery Womens Health* 55:250–254, 2010.

Dunston R, Lee A, Boud D, Brodie P, Chiarella M: Co-production and health system reform – from re-imagining to re-making, *Aust J Pub Admin* 68:39–52, 2008.

Ehrenreich B, English D: *Witches, midwives, and nurses: a history of women healers*, New York, 1973, The Feminist Press, City University of New York.

Fox D, Sheehan A, Homer CSA: Birthplace in Australia: processes and interactions during the intrapartum transfer of women from planned homebirth to hospital, *Midwifery* 57:18–25, 2018.

Grigg CP, Tracy SK: New Zealand's unique maternity system, *Women Birth* 26:e59–e64, 2013.

Hastie C, Fahy K: Inter-professional collaboration in delivery suite: a qualitative study, *Women Birth* 24(2):72–79, 2011.

Heatley M, Kruske S: Defining collaboration in Australian maternity care, *Women Birth* 24:53–57, 2011.

Homer CSE, Davis GK, Brodie P: What do women feel about community-based antenatal care?, *Aust N Z J Public Health* 24:590–595, 2000.

Homer CSE, Davis K, Brodie P, Sheehan A, Barclay LM, Wills J, et al: Collaboration in maternity care: a randomised controlled trial comparing community-based continuity of care with standard care, *BJOG* 108:16–22, 2001a.

Homer CSE, Matha D, Jordan LG, Wills J, Davis GK: Community-based continuity of midwifery care versus standard hospital care: a cost analysis, *Aust Health Rev* 24:85–93, 2001b.

Homer CSE, Friberg IK, Dias MAB, ten Hoope-Bender P, Sandall J, Speciale AM, et al: The projected effect of scaling up midwifery, *Lancet* 384:1146–1157, 2014.

Howat P, Scherman S: Moving towards trust and cooperation in obstetrics, *O&G Magazine* 9(2):21, 2005.

Joint Commission: Patient safety: sentinel event statistics released for 2014. Oakbrook Terrace, IL, April 2015, Joint Commission Online. Online: https://www.jointcommission.org/assets/1/23/jconline_April_29_15.pdf.

Kennedy HP: A model of exemplary midwifery practice: results of a Delphi study, *J Midwifery Women's Health* 45:4–19, 2000.

Kennedy HP: Cross-discipline and collaborative dialogue, *Quickening* 42:3, 2011.

Kennedy HP, Waldman R: The long and winding road to effective collaboration, *Obstet Gynecol Clin North Am* 39:xix, 2012.

Kennedy H, Farrell T, Paden R, Hill S, Jolivet R, Willetts J, et al: "I wasn't the only one": women's experience of group prenatal care in the military, *J Midwifery Women's Health* 54(3):176–183, 2009.

Kennedy HP, Grant J, Walton C, Shaw-Battista J, Sandall J: Normalizing birth in England: a qualitative study, *J Midwifery Women's Health* 55:262–269, 2010.

Kennedy HP, Grant J, Walton C, Shaw-Battista J, Sandall J: Perspectives on promoting primary vaginal birth: a qualitative study, *Birth* 43:336–345, 2016.

Kennedy HP, Myers-Ciecko JA, Carr KC, Breedlove G, Bailey T, Farrell M, et al: United States model midwifery legislation and regulation: development of a consensus document, *J Midwifery Womens Health* 2018. doi:10.1111/jmwh.12727. [Epub ahead of print].

Knight M, Tuffnell D, Kenyon S, Shakespeare J, Gray R, Kurinczuk JJ, editors: *Saving lives, improving mothers' care—surveillance of maternal deaths in the UK 2011–13 and lessons learned to inform maternity care from the UK and Ireland. Confidential Enquiries into Maternal Deaths and Morbidity 2009–13*, Oxford, 2015, National Perinatal Epidemiology Unit, University of Oxford.

Lane K: When is collaboration not collaboration? When it's militarized, *Women Birth* 25:29–38, 2012.

Leap N, Hunter B: *The midwife's tale: an oral history from handywoman to professional midwife*, ed 2, Barnsley, S Yorks, 2013, Pen & Sword.

Lewis G, editor: *The confidential enquiry into maternal and child health (CEMACH). Saving mothers' lives: reviewing maternal deaths to make motherhood safer—2003–2005*, The seventh report on Confidential Enquiries into Maternal Deaths in the United Kingdom, London, 2007, CEMACH. Online: http://www.publichealth.hscni.net/sites/default/files/Saving%20Mothers%27%20Lives%202003-05%20.pdf.

McIntyre M, Francis K, Chapman Y: The struggle for contested boundaries in the move to collaborative care teams in Australian maternity care, *Midwifery* 28:298–305, 2012.

Munro S, Kornelsen J, Grzybowski S: Models of maternity care in rural environments: barriers and attributes of interprofessional collaboration with midwives, *Midwifery* 29:646–665, 2013.

Oxford English Dictionary (OED): Collaboration, 2018, OED. Online: http://www.oed.com/view/Entry/5290.

Pringle R: *Sex and medicine: gender, power and authority in the medical profession*, Cambridge, 1998, Cambridge University Press.

Psaila K, Schmied V, Fowler C, Kruske S: Interprofessional collaboration at transition of care: perspectives of child and family health nurses and midwives, *J Clin Nurs* 24:160–172, 2015.

Reiger KM, Lane KL: Working together: collaboration between midwives and doctors in public hospitals, *Aust Health Rev* 33:315–324, 2009.

Renfrew MJ, McFadden A, Bastos MH, Campbell J, Channon AA, Cheung NF, et al: Midwifery and quality care: findings from a new evidence-informed framework for maternal and newborn care, *Lancet* 384(9948):1129–1145, 2014. doi:10.1016/S0140-6736(14)60789-3.

Schrage M: *Shared minds: the new technologies of collaboration*, New York, 1990, Random House.

ten Hoope-Bender P, de Bernis L, Campbell J, Downe S, Fauveau V, Fogstad H, et al: Improving maternal and newborn health through midwifery, *Lancet* 384:1226–1235, 2014.

The Free Dictionary: Obstetric, 2018. Online: https://www.thefreedictionary.com/obstetric.

Tracy SK, Welsh A, Hall B, Hartz D, Lainchbury A, Bisits A, et al: Caseload midwifery compared to standard or private obstetric care for first time mothers in a public teaching hospital in Australia: a cross sectional study of cost and birth outcomes, *BMC Pregnancy Childbirth* 24:46, 2014.

Turner G, editor: Collaboration. *The Australian Concise Oxford Dictionary*, ed 7, Melbourne, 1989, Oxford University Press.

van der Lee N, Driessen EW, Houwaart ES, Caccia NC, Scheele F: An examination of the historical context of interprofessional collaboration in Dutch obstetrical care, *J Interprof Care* 28:123–127, 2014.

van der Lee N, Driessen EW, Scheelec F: How the past influences interprofessional collaboration between obstetricians and midwives in the Netherlands: findings from a secondary analysis, *J Interprof Care* 30:71–76, 2016.

Van Lerberghe W, Matthews Z, Achadi E, Ancona C, Campbell J, Channon A, et al: Country experience with strengthening of health systems and deployment of midwives in countries with high maternal mortality, *Lancet* 384:1215–1225, 2014.

Walker L, Fetherston C, McMurray A: Perceptions of interprofessional education in the Australian Advanced Life Support in Obstetrics (ALSO) course, *Fam Med* 47:435–444, 2015.

Witz A: *Professions and patriarchy*, London, 1992, Routledge.

CHAPTER 6

Ensuring Safety and Quality

Jane Raymond, Michael Nicholl, Mandy Forrester, Donna Hartz

Contents

INTRODUCTION

The vision of the World Health Organization (WHO) is a world where 'every pregnant woman and newborn receives quality care throughout pregnancy, childbirth and the postnatal period' (Tuncalp et al., 2015, p. 1045). Quality maternity care is a multidimensional concept summarised in 'Better Births' (National Health Service (NHS) England, 2016) in a way that has resonance for all other countries (p. 8):

> *Every woman, every pregnancy, every baby and every family is different. Therefore, quality services (by which we mean safe, clinically effective and providing a good experience) must be personalized.*

Being woman centred, having high-performing teams and providing family-friendly services with access to information and individually tailored care are other terms often used to describe what is meant by 'quality maternity care'.

Safety is a key feature of quality maternity services and is enhanced by personalised care (Department of Health, 2017). As midwives working in continuity models have an opportunity to get to know the woman, they can provide quality care that is individually tailored to her needs (Sandall et al., 2016). Being aware of a woman's social situation—including her emotional and psychological responses, her expectations and aspirations—will also contribute to promoting safety, with appropriate referrals in both community and hospital settings.

The evidence-informed Quality Maternal and Newborn Care Framework in the *Lancet* series on midwifery (Renfrew et al., 2014, p. 1132) has been described and is reproduced in Chapter 5. The essential components of quality care that are identified in this framework address practice, the organisation of care and the values, philosphies, skills and attributes of care providers. As such, the framework provides a useful tool to assess and evaluate the quality of care provided in individual midwifery continuity of care models as well as in overall maternity services.

This chapter explores various processes and strategies to promote and enhance safety and quality, including how users of maternity services can be supported and protected when standards and frameworks are in place. We draw on research literature and a number of international frameworks and standards that are available online to illustrate the principles of safety and quality as well as some of the challenges associated with their implementation.

STARTING WITH TERMINOLOGY

Quality and safety literature in health uses a range of terms and definitions. Often these differ between countries and even within countries. We will start with working definitions of some of the main terms used in global evidence as these will be relevant to many countries. We recommend, though, that you look at quality and safety definitions in your own country in order to develop an understanding of how these are used in your context. Working definitions of some of the main terms used in the safety and quality literature include the following:

- **Error**—is a failure to carry out a planned action as intended, or application of an incorrect plan (World Health Organization (WHO), 2009).
- **Incident**—is an event or circumstance that resulted, or could have resulted in, unintended or unnecessary harm to a patient or consumer, or a complaint, loss or damage. An incident or potential incident that was averted and did not cause harm, but had the potential to do so, is known as a 'near miss' (Australian Commission on Safety and Quality in Health Care (ACSQHC), 2017).
- **Quality of care**—is the extent to which health care services provided to individuals and patient populations improve desired health outcomes (WHO, 2006).
- **Resilience**—is the degree to which a system continuously prevents, detects, mitigates or ameliorates hazards or incidents (WHO, 2009).

- **Risk**—is the chance of something happening that will have an impact upon objectives. It is usually measured in terms of consequences and likelihood (Standards Australia / Standards New Zealand, 2009).
- **Risk management**—includes the culture, processes and structures that are directed towards the effective management of potential opportunities and adverse effects (Standards Australia / Standards New Zealand, 2009). Clinical risk management is risk management within the clinical context, and obstetric risk management is risk management within the obstetric context. Risk management strategies, tools or controls are initiatives aimed at eliminating or minimising identified risk.
- **Safety**—is defined in terms of absence of harm in most definitions of safety within health care. The WHO describes patient safety as the reduction of risk of unnecessary harm associated with health care to an acceptable minimum (WHO, 2009).

FRAMEWORKS AND STANDARDS FOR SAFETY AND QUALITY

The goal of maternity care providers throughout the world is safe and high-quality maternity care, in whatever form this is provided (ten Hoope-Bender et al., 2014). We start by considering the ways in which safe, quality care is described in various important policy documents. We then consider some practical examples of how the principles of safety and quality frameworks are enacted in midwifery continuity of care.

The WHO describes quality of care as the extent to which health care services provided to individuals and patient populations improve desired outcomes. In order to achieve this, health care needs to be safe, effective, timely, efficient, equitable and people centred (WHO, 2006). Quality of care is therefore a multidimensional concept, within which safety is a vital feature (Tuncalp et al., 2015).

A number of global frameworks conceptualise quality maternal and newborn care. The first we will consider are the *WHO standards for improving the quality of maternal and newborn care in health facilities* (WHO, 2016). The second is the Royal College of Midwives' *The RCM standards for midwifery services in the UK* (Royal College of Midwives (RCM), 2016). We then look at how the core principles in the *Australian Safety and Quality Framework for Health Care* (ACSQHC, 2010) are enacted in midwifery continuity of care.

WHO standards for improving the quality of maternal and newborn care in health facilities

The WHO sets eight standards within a quality of care framework to define explicitly what is required to achieve high-quality care around the childbirth continuum (WHO, 2016). These standards are relevant to maternity care anywhere in the world,

---

BOX 6.1 WHO Standards for Improving the Quality of Maternal and Newborn Care in Health Facilities

- **Standard 1:** Every woman and newborn receives routine evidence-based care and management of complications during the childbirth continuum
- **Standard 2:** Use data to ensure early, appropriate action to improve the care of every woman and newborn
- **Standard 3:** Every woman and newborn with conditions that cannot be dealt with effectively are appropriately referred
- **Standard 4:** Communication with women and their families is effective and responds to their needs
- **Standard 5:** Women and newborns receive care with respect and preservation of their dignity
- **Standard 6:** Every woman and her family are provided with emotional support that is sensitive to their needs and strengthens the woman's capability
- **Standard 7:** For every woman and newborn, competent, motivated staff are consistently available to provide routine care and manage complications
- **Standard 8:** The health facility has an appropriate physical environment and resources for routine maternal and newborn care and management of complications.

(Adapted from World Health Organization, 2016)

---

including care provided within midwifery continuity of care models. The WHO encourages adaptation of the standards to the context of the country (or model of care). The document contains useful input, output and outcome measures which midwives working within continuity models can apply to monitor their practice. The WHO standards are shown in Box 6.1.

The RCM standards for midwifery services in the UK

The Royal College of Midwives standards for midwifery services in the UK (Box 6.2) have direct relevance to midwifery continuity of care (RCM, 2016). These standards were developed following reviews and reports about the quality of maternity care across the UK that consistently highlighted the need for evidence-based clinical standards to underpin improvements in service provision. The document outlines the key indicators that any midwifery service can use to measure its delivery of compassionate, well-led, evidence-based midwifery care. Continuity of carer is recognised as being crucial to promoting the physical, psychological and social wellbeing of the woman and family throughout the childbearing continuum.

Six key themes are at the heart of the RCM standards—clinical governance, communication staffing, education and accountability, family-centred care, leadership and

BOX 6.2 Royal College of Midwives Standards for Midwifery Services

Theme 1 clinical governance

Clinical governance requires that planning and organising of midwifery services take place under midwifery leadership and through multidisciplinary collaboration which supports a high-quality clinical governance framework that delivers personalised maternity services. It is important that the Director of Midwifery is placed within the organisation hierarchy that enables her/him to make decisions about the service provided.

An example of a key measurement criterion for a standard in this section

Standard	Measure	Example of evidence sources
There must be a written risk management policy, including trigger incidents, adverse incident reporting and multi-professional review.	Evidence of risk management policy.	Local arrangements and written protocols.

Theme 2 communication standard statement

Midwives must have the ability to communicate effectively with all members of the maternity team, other professionals, women receiving care and their family members. They should ensure that all information relevant to the care pathway is accessible, aids decision making and assists communication.

Effective communication is key to safety within the maternity team and with women.

An example of a key measurement criterion for a standard in this section

Standard	Measure	Example of evidence sources
The named professional responsible for the woman's care must be documented at all stages and most importantly when transfer of care takes place.	Evidence of documentation.	Local arrangements for woman held maternity notes.

Theme 3 staffing

Safe staffing levels of midwives and support staff are maintained, reviewed and audited at least six monthly. The Birthrate Plus tool is recommended (and is discussed in Ch. 9 of this book). In England, external regulators ensure that safe staffing levels are maintained.

An example of a key measurement criterion for a standard in this section

Standard	Measure	Example of evidence sources
Staffing establishments should be calculated according to a recognised workforce planning tool that ensures women have continuity of carer and one to one care from a midwife in labour.	Documented process for calculating staffing establishments.	Local arrangements and written clinical policy. Quality accounts.

Theme 4: Education and professional accountability

Midwives have a personal accountability for continuing professional development and life-long learning. The system they work in should provide a positive learning culture with

Continued

BOX 6.2 Royal College of Midwives Standards for Midwifery Services—cont'd

opportunities to fulfil these responsibilities. This statement highlights that, although it is the midwives' responsibility for professional development, the employer has to provide the opportunity for them to access opportunities.

An example of a key measurement criterion for a standard in this section

Standard	Measure	Example of evidence sources
All maternity staff should have access to courses and activities for workforce development and team building.	Evidence of workforce development and team building.	Local arrangements and written policy. Local data collection.

Theme 5: Family-centred care

Care is accessible, responsive and provided in partnership with women and their families, respecting their diverse needs, preferences and choices and in collaboration with other organisations whose services impact on family wellbeing. This statement supports a midwifery model of care that places women and their families at the centre of care and assumes pregnancy, birth and the postnatal period are normal life events for a woman and her baby. (We would suggest a modification for this theme is woman-centred care.)

An example of a key measurement criterion for a standard in this section

Standard	Measure	Example of evidence sources
Women must be fully involved in all aspects of their care enabling them to be at the centre of decision making throughout.	Evidence about women's active involvement in decision making.	Local arrangements and written policy.

Theme 6: Care and the birth environment

Care is provided in a chosen, comfortable, clean, safe setting that promotes the wellbeing of women, families and staff, respecting women's needs, preferences and privacy. The physical environment supports normality and compassionate care.

An example of a key measurement criterion for a standard in this section

Standard	Measure	Example of evidence sources
Maternity services should ensure women have access to midwifery care in all birth settings including midwifery units and home births.	Evidence of women's access to all birth settings.	Local arrangements and written clinical policy. Local published information. Local data from national survey of women's experiences.

(Examples reproduced from The RCM standards for midwifery services in the UK. RCM, London, 2016)

BOX 6.3 The Core Principles of the Australian Safety and Quality Framework for Health Care

Safe, high-quality health is always:

- **Consumer centred**—consumer centred means making sure that staff respect and respond to patients' (women's) choices, needs and values, and care is provided as a partnership between providers and recipients of care. From a maternity service perspective this means being woman centred and working in partnership with women, employing open disclosure and increasing continuity of care and carer throughout the service.
- **Driven by information**—being driven by information requires using evidence to guide decisions about care, and collecting and analysing data and then taking action to improve patients' (women's and families') experiences. From a maternity perspective, this might include the development and implementation of evidence-based guidelines, the use of quality assurance processes such as clinical audit and the monitoring of adverse incidents with an effective feedback process to bring about improvements.
- **Organised for safety**—organised for safety makes safety a central feature of how health care facilities are run, how staff work and how funding is organised. From a maternity services perspective, this might include government policy development, the implementation of risk management processes and the regulation of health care professionals. Being organised is also part of the mantra of 'the way things are done around here' where safety and quality are part of the everyday landscape and not an added extra.

care, and the birth environment—all of which are relevant to supporting continuity of carer models.

You may find the audit tool developed to assist benchmarking of midwifery services against these standards as a useful resource.

Australian safety and quality framework for health care

The core principles of the *Australian Safety and Quality Framework for Health Care* (ACSQHC, 2010) are generic to similar frameworks or approaches in other countries. The framework describes a vision for safe and high-quality health care and sets out the actions, or processes, needed to achieve this vision. Other countries work within similar structures that are designed to influence the way that care is organised locally.

The Australian framework identifies three core principles that provide a mechanism for safety and quality improvement activities; these are directly applicable to midwifery continuity of care (Box 6.3).

These principles resonate with the philosophy of midwifery care. Examples of processes or strategies within midwifery continuity of care that align with the three principles are provided in the next section.

Midwifery continuity of care is woman centred

As defined in the Introduction to this book, midwifery continuity of care is woman centred (Leap, 2009). This is a safety mechanism: when care is planned around the woman's needs she is more likely to trust her caregivers and be open to timely and relevant support.

Woman-centred approaches to decision making

An example of how woman-centred care is achieved in practice is the My Birthplace app, a computerised place of birth decision support tool developed in a process involving women and midwives (Birthplace in England Collaborative Group, 2011). The aim of the My Birthplace app was to encourage discussions between a woman and her midwife about her choice for place of birth. Information informing the app was based on the results of the Birthplace in England research program, which supported a policy of offering healthy women the opportunity to give birth in a midwifery-led unit or at home (Birthplace in England Collaborative Group, 2011).

Evaluation of the My Birthplace app demonstrated that providing women with standardised non-subjective information about place of birth appears to influence their preference and is acceptable to them (Gaskell et al., 2014). This is related to addressing health literacy, or the ability of people to understand information about their health care, which protects them from potential harm and acts as a safety mechanism (Berkman et al., 2011). Other maternity units in England and Scotland have now adopted the My Birthplace app and it is cited in the National Institute for Health and Care Excellence (NICE, 2017) guidance: Intrapartum care for healthy women and babies.

The My Birthplace app was designed to facilitate discussions between women and their midwives, based on a generic 'shared decision-making model' (Elwyn et al., 2012). Decision making in partnership between women and midwives is not, however, a simple process of providing information and then expecting women to be able to make choices. Highly complex social, cultural and familial influences, including values, beliefs and vulnerabilities for both parties, will affect conversations where women are facing making choices (Noseworthy et al., 2013). The values and opinions of the person providing the information (in this case the midwife) are likely to affect the decisions women make (Leap & Edwards, 2006). For midwives, there might be the tension that often exists working in a culture dominated by risk management processes (Ménage, 2016a; Symon, 2006). Ménage (2016b) provides a new model for evidence-based decision making in midwifery—one that is informed by the woman, the midwife, resources and research—that also takes into account the environment affecting all of those influencing factors, including societal values and culture.

Undoubtedly, midwifery continuity offers the opportunity for a relationship to develop that facilitates decision making and quality care. Ménage (2016a, p. 46) suggests that:

It is the quality of this relationship that determines the quality of the midwifery care in terms of the woman's safety, empowerment and satisfaction with care.

Ménage proposes that decision making with women requires the midwife to have emotional intelligence and self-awareness drawing on: knowledge and skills, experience, judgement, intuition, empathy and compassion, and professionalism guided by regulation and standards (Ménage, 2016b).

Midwifery continuity of care is driven by information

One example of the way that midwifery continuity of care is driven by information is the use of evidence-based consultation and referral guidelines; these have been developed in several countries to support midwifery clinical decision making. The Netherlands first developed such guidelines in 1998 (The Royal Dutch Association of Midwives, The National Association of General Practitioners and The Dutch Association for Obstetrics and Gynaecology, 1998). Guidelines for consultation and referral were developed in Australia (Australian College of Midwives (ACM), 2017), Canada (College of Midwives Ontario, 2014) and New Zealand (NZ Ministry of Health, 2012) as midwifery-led continuity of care models were developed and a need for professional clarification was identified regarding the roles of midwives and the midwifery scope of practice.

The main purpose of all of these guidelines is to promote safety and quality and confidence in services for service users and practitioners. The ACM National Midwifery Guidelines for Consultation and Referral (ACM, 2014, reprinted May 2017 with amendments) are now a key component in the development and implementation of midwifery continuity of care models in Australia. Midwives are able to use these guidelines in any location in which they provide care including, for example, in a woman's home or in a remote location.

Using such evidence-based guidelines upholds midwifery skills and promotes effective collaborative care. Guidelines for consultation and referral promote collaborative care based on effective communication, trust and respect; these qualities are are seen as central to effective risk management for midwifery-led services (Monk et al., 2014) and particularly where midwives provide continuity of care to women of 'all risk' at major referral hospitals (Tracy et al., 2013). The use of such guidelines is an essential part of the risk assessment and early preparation for starting a midwifery continuity of care model, as discussed below.

Midwifery continuity of care and risk assessment processes

Care that is organised for safety means taking action to prevent or minimise harm through risk assessment. International standards on risk management have been developed in the past two decades. In 2018, an updated international standard on risk management priniciples was published by the International Organization for

Standardization (ISO, 2018). These standards are designed to be locally adopted, and the previous version was adapted for the Australian and New Zealand context as *AS/NZS ISO 31000:2009 Risk management—principles and guidelines* (Standards Australia/Standards New Zealand, 2009).

A specific risk assessment framework has been used over a number of years in New South Wales (NSW) as a positive change management strategy to help design and implement models of midwifery continuity of care. A *Midwifery continuity of carer model tool-kit* was published by the NSW Ministry of Health in 2012 (NSW Health, 2012) to assist managers and clinicians working in NSW public maternity services to develop and implement such models. The Tool-kit describes AS/NZS ISO 31000:2009 as the standard in NSW to risk assess changes in maternity services, whether small or large. There is a detailed risk assessment plan in the document which describes how to undertake a gap analysis and assess the risks associated with changes to clinical work processes in line with AS/NZS ISO 31000:2009.

Box 6.4 identifies how the risk assessment process was used in the implementation of the Ryde Midwifery Group Practice (MGP), the story of which is told by Professor Sally Tracy in Chapter 2, Box 2.9. Ryde MGP provides 24-hour midwifery-led care for women having uncomplicated pregnancies. There are no on-site obstetric services. The initial risk assessment process was undertaken in 2004 by a team of midwifery and medical professionals, led by the NSW Health Department's insurer.

Over the intervening years this rigorous process has been employed to incorporate new developments and this has contributed to the Ryde MGP remaining as safe as the nearby tertiary referral hospital (Monk et al., 2014). In 2015, the service was perceived by women in the state of New South Wales to be one of the best public hospitals in NSW (Bureau of Health Information, 2017).

The first part of this chapter has outlined some of the specific safety and quality frameworks and standards in maternity care that benefit women and families. The next section explores some of the challenges associated with implementing and ensuring safety and quality.

CHALLENGES TO SAFETY AND QUALITY

Perceptions of risk

Perhaps the biggest challenge to safety and quality in maternity service provision is the individual or, in some cases, collective perception of risk. The word 'risk' generally has a negative connotation. When we think of risk, we usually think of some danger, jeopardy, peril, hazard, menace or threat. When discussing the risks associated with pregnancy with women, many clinicians invariably focus on the negative or unwanted outcomes first. Compounding this, individual practitioners can sometimes

BOX 6.4 An Example of a Risk Assessment Process: Implementing the Ryde Midwifery Group Practice

Step 1: Process map the work flow of the existing and the new model

Each facet of current and proposed care was mapped from antenatal presentation to postnatal discharge through the Ryde maternity service.

Differences in care and necessary modification in service delivery were identified.

Step 2: Identify the risks/threats to change

The group utilised 'brainstorming' to identify the risks and threats to the women, the midwife and the service.

Step 3: Risk rank the threat by consequence/likelihood (Severity Assessment Code)

The risks were ranked utilising the New South Wales Health Department's Severity Assessment Code (SAC) scoring system. This system is a method for quantifying the level of risk associated with an incident depending on what the consequences of the risk could be and the likelihood of this occurring. Each risk is assigned a numerical rating from 1 to 4, with 1 being the highest risk rating.

Step 4: Identify current controls and possible additional controls

Example of controls identified or developed include:

- ACM national midwifery consultation and referral guidelines for all clinical review and assessment
- clearly defined organisational and clinical pathway/algorithms
- multidisciplinary clinical case reviews—in early pregnancy and for women with emerging health concerns
- 24-hour on-call telephone liaison/consultation with a tertiary referral centre
- peer review—prospective audit using specific clinical indicators for continuous clinical practice improvement.

Step 5: Identify priority risks and priority controls

Risks that were ranked extreme and high risks (SAC 1 and 2) were given priority for risk management and for controls to be implemented. For example, all midwives undertook advanced maternal and neonatal monitoring and resuscitation training to mitigate the risk of maternal and neonatal morbidity and mortality.

modify their own perception of risk (Dahlen, 2010); these modifications can broadly be described in three categories:

- Firstly, perception of risk can be heightened or exaggerated. Everyone has their own particular fears, sometimes based on what happened yesterday in clinical practice or what is doing the rounds in the media. This is especially so if one is confronting something new. A situation that is very normal can be 'pathologised' and fear can be whipped up quite quickly.

- Secondly and conversely, perception of risk can be blunted or trivialised. Something pathological can be 'normalised', which leads to a lack of identification and therefore poor escalation. We see this sometimes in maternity care as most women are healthy and everything progresses normally—we almost will ourselves that all is still normal even when it may not be.
- Thirdly, the perception of risk may be in itself pathological. Many years of experience in clinical practice can make clinicians either immune to risk or even more anxious—and both states of being are a risk in themselves. As clinicians, our own perceptions and experiences in terms of risk can clearly bias the information-sharing process with women.

There is a tendency to avoid thinking of risk in its broadest sense—best described as 'the chance of something happening that will have an impact on objectives' (Standards Australia / Standards New Zealand, 2009). Clearly, under such a definition, impacts can be both positive and negative. This is perhaps best evidenced in the financial world where the perception of risk that drives activity is generally a positive one. Clinical risk is commonly considered in terms of an adverse event and the sequelae of that event, and is most commonly quantified in terms of the consequence of the event and its likelihood.

Dealing with risk is also subject to the same biases. With such negative connotations associated with 'risk', risk avoidance is generally the preferred method rather than the management of risk. All too often there is a decision not to become involved in, or to withdraw from, a situation associated with risk. Equally, this may result in defensive clinical practice to avoid being exposed to any possibility of risk, however small, even if the alternative also carries risk. Indeed, the perceived risk in some clinical specialties is sometimes blamed for workforce shortages as individuals move away from areas where personal or professional risk is perceived as high. It is conceivable that women may themselves decide not to pursue pregnancy if they perceive the risk to themselves personally, professionally or financially, to be too great.

Introducing midwifery continuity of care models has been impacted on by this perception of risk and indeed by how risk is dealt with. Any change to service delivery models in maternity care has associated clinical, organisational, personal, professional, community, societal, financial and environmental risks and these can challenge an already stretched organisation or health system. How such risks are addressed will determine the success or otherwise of the change in service delivery to midwifery continuity of care.

Clinical decisions and engaging with uncertainty

Clinical risk management is a subset of risk management. Every action or inaction in clinical decision making may be associated with positive and negative effects. The complexity of some clinical situations means that not all risks can be anticipated or

BOX 6.5 Fundamental Challenges for Services and Clinicians

- What are the risks?
- What risks should be discussed?
- How should risk be discussed with the woman?
- Qualitative vs quantitative probability?
- Quantitative expressions for risk
- Patient errors in risk estimation
- Reconciling the average and the individual
- Patient preference and frameworks for decision

known. However, even in more straightforward clinical scenarios—for example, whether to have a particular test or not—risk may not be adequately discussed because of gaps in knowledge or simply uncertainty about how much and what information should be communicated. Midwives, particularly those working in midwifery continuity of care models, confront this regularly in antenatal care provision. Box 6.5 outlines some of the fundamental challenges in discussing clinical risk in health care generally. These need to be adapted to the context of midwifery continuity of care.

Discussing clinical risk, however, is not straightforward. Midwives, like other clinicians, are operating in an environment of considerable uncertainty and this can be responded to in a number of ways. Hall explored clinician responses to uncertainty and described four main responses: denial, the tendency to do what peers are doing or would do, stress and action rather than inaction (Hall, 2002). The net result of clinical decision making under uncertainty is that low probabilities are overweighted and moderate and high probabilities are underweighted—i.e. the tendency to treat all cases the same and thus not manage the risk appropriately. Scamell & Alaszewski (2012) refer to this as 'an ever-narrowing window of normality' and offer a precautionary approach to the management of uncertainty through risk management approaches. It may be helpful for practitioners to tackle the three sources of uncertainty in clinical practice: technical, personal and conceptual.

- **Technical sources of uncertainty**—relate to the lack of data or information regarding the efficacy or value of proposed treatment plans. In order to overcome such uncertainty, service providers and educators must provide the workforce with tools to understand better and interpret the available research evidence. Clinicians must acknowledge uncertainty in their conversations with women and share decision making with them. Service providers and educators must improve the risk literacy of their workforce through a better understanding of relative risk reduction and baseline risk, and better numeracy skills, as well as presenting risk in a way that allows women to make informed choices.

- **Personal sources of uncertainty**—arise from the human interaction between clinicians and the woman. Services can improve such interactions by role modelling good communication, mentoring junior clinicians and being active listeners to women's voices.
- **Conceptual sources of uncertainty**—arise from the complexity of the clinical environment. This environment needs to be made simpler. Services should divest themselves of low-value interventions and change the behaviours of the next generation of clinicians by routinely reporting the harm from commonly performed interventions.

Human error factors

Despite everyone's best efforts, things still go wrong occasionally. One of the most frequent contributors to adverse events is human error, which is estimated to be implicated in up to 80% of adverse clinical events in health care. Human error is usually reflective of system complexity which results in multiple gaps in care (NHS England, 2013; Palmieri et al., 2008). In reality, adverse events are the result of humans working in complex sociotechnical systems with differing cultures (Jensen, 2008).

Unsafe acts caused by human error in maternity care generally fall into two broad groupings: errors and violations (Box 6.6).

James Reason (1990) suggested that there are four levels of human failure, each having an impact on the next. In the so called 'Swiss cheese' model he described active failures or unsafe acts at the final point of task execution, which were preceded by a series of latent failures including preconditions for such unsafe acts, unsafe supervision and organisational influences (see below).

Reason (1995) also described two types of error: **failures of execution** (slips and lapses) and **failures of planning or problem solving** (mistakes). Failures of execution can result from the plan being adequate but the associated actions not going as intended (i.e. there is a failure of task execution); in failures of planning the actions may go as intended but the plan is inadequate (i.e. the failure occurs at a higher level). Failures of execution most commonly occur during the automatic performance of a routine task in familiar surroundings. It is easy to see how this could happen in maternity care; the most commonly identified in adverse event analysis are failure to recognise, loss of situational awareness or attentional failure due to distraction or preoccupation, memory failure resulting in skill-based errors, or selection failures with wrong diagnosis or treatment. Personal conditions such as fatigue, sleep deprivation, hunger, pain, etc. may contribute to such failures. Without mitigation processes, midwifery continuity of care models may be prone to such personal conditions, owing to their very nature.

Mistakes, on the other hand, are generally either rule based or knowledge based. Rule-based mistakes have a lot to do with how clinicians deal with uncertainty. In

BOX 6.6 Unsafe Acts in Maternity Care

Errors

- Failures of execution (slips and lapses):
  - failure to recognise
  - loss of situational awareness or attentional failure:
    - distraction
    - preoccupation
  - memory failure resulting in skill-based errors
  - selection failures:
    - wrong diagnosis
    - wrong treatment
- Failures of planning or problem solving:
  - rule-based mistakes
  - knowledge-based mistakes

Violations

- Unintentional
- Intentional
  - routine violations
  - situational violations
  - optimising violations
  - exceptional violations

complex clinical situations, cognitive dissonance and bias flourish. As part of intuitive decision making in complex situations, clinicians develop heuristics (loosely established knowledge built from actual past events rather than theory, i.e. 'rules of thumb'). In many situations using heuristics can result in accurate predictions and reflect a highly adaptive and efficient response to decision making in the real world; however, they can be a source of cognitive and informational bias and subsequent error. Making more 'personal' decisions is quicker than analysing the clinical situation, drawing on the available evidence and effecting a patient centred response. Generally, clinicians are less able to accept new evidence that challenges their established ways of working. Such behaviours are reinforced by the need to 'belong' in the clinical work space. Being forced to challenge a long-held belief or beliefs threatens an individual's sense of competence and professionalism.

Violations are different from errors in that they are deviations from well-established policies, guidelines, practices, rules or standards. Violations are usually conceptualised in terms of their presumed causes (e.g. unintentional or intentional). Unintentional violations happen when a work instruction or protocol is not clear, not simple or confusing. For example, a midwife may exceed her/his safe work hours after misinterpreting a complicated rostering tool. Such violations are very similar to 'mistakes' as described above.

On the other hand, intentional or deliberate violations come in many forms: routine violations, situational violations, optimising violations and exceptional violations. Routine violations happen when clinicians develop 'work arounds' which become the routine way of working (i.e. they are skill based). Situational violations are generally rule based whereby clinicians do what they think just to get the task done or where the 'rules' (procedures, guidelines) are seen to be inappropriate for the present clinical situation. Optimising violations occur when clinicians are seeking personal rather than goal- or woman-based outcomes. Exceptional violations tend to occur at the knowledge-based level as they occur in unique and unfamiliar circumstances that are not explicitly covered in existing 'rules'.

In the model by Reason (2000), unsafe acts in maternity care are almost always preceded by a series of **latent failures** including preconditions for such acts, unsafe supervision and organisational influences (i.e. active failures are usually preceded by latent failures). Such latent failures arise from decisions made by designers, builders, procedure writers and top-level management (Reason, 2000). Latent failures have two kinds of adverse effect: they can translate into conditions encouraging error within the local workplace (e.g. time pressure, understaffing, inadequate equipment, skill mix) or they can create long-lasting work environments with untrustworthy performance indicators, unworkable procedures, poor workplace design, etc. Latent conditions may lie unrecognised within a workplace for many years before they combine with active failures and local triggers to create the environment for an adverse clinical incident. However, whilst active failures cannot be predicted, latent failures can be actively sought and corrected in a proactive rather than a reactive manner.

Working in midwifery continuity of care models can be demanding. The provision of high-quality safe maternity care is constantly challenged by the hidden latent failures in the systems in which midwives work. At a model level, such failures must be proactively identified and eliminated by managers. At a personal level, minimising error by understanding its potential sources and avoiding violations will reduce the human contribution to adverse events.

This section has explored challenges to safety and quality in the workplace and some of the theories underpinning risk assessment. Individual perception of risk, uncertainty and human error can contribute to destabilise the processes described at the beginning of the chapter. The next section describes a number of mitigation strategies designed to maximise safety, reliability and consistency in practice.

Moving from risk management to resilience

Understanding how errors occur enables significant opportunities to improve quality and safety in maternity care. This realisation has led to a shift of focus from the traditional 'what went wrong' and 'how many times did it go wrong' to 'how can we prevent this happening again'. As a result we can move to redesign in order to reduce recurrence (Jeffcott et al., 2009).

In moving away a little from the traditional risk management framework, health care is beginning to focus on the concept of 'resilience'. Whereas risk management focuses on the elimination of risk, a resilience framework proposes the identification of gaps in model capacity (Carthey & DeLeval, 2001). This refers to the ability to understand how failures are avoided and how success can be achieved. It is how people learn and adapt to create safety in settings that are frequently fraught with gaps, hazards, trade-offs and multiple goals (Cook et al., 2000).

In terms of emerging theory, resilience can be considered as having three different but related levels: (1) personal or knowledge based, (2) group or team based and (3) whole of service based. A resilience framework adds a temporal component to risk management by moving from preparing for adverse clinical events to dealing with or absorbing them when they occur, recovering from them, and adapting to prevent them from occurring in the future (Carthey & DeLeval, 2001).

In the context of midwifery continuity of care, moving from a risk management framework to a resilience one not only reduces the chances of error but also allows models to become more sustainable and rewarding to work in, as it reduces a significant amount of stress in the work environment. Research exploring resilience in midwifery suggests that various coping strategies are used by midwives in relation to challenges and adversity; these include: a strong sense of professional identitiy and love of midwifery, an ability to access support, self-awareness and the ability to draw on personal resources, work–life balance, a sense of autonomy and self-efficacy, recognising warning signs and taking pre-emptive action to avoid adversity (Hunter & Warren, 2013, 2014, 2015).

When looking at midwifery continuity of care from a resilience perspective, there are four main domains that need to be considered: the physical, the informational, the cognitive and the social. Each of these domains needs to be supported across the course of a disruptive event (e.g. an adverse clinical event) in order for resilience to be maximised. The physical domain refers to the physical resources and the capabilities and the design of those resources. The information domain refers to information and information development about the physical domain. The cognitive domain refers to the use of the information and physical domains to make decisions. The social domain refers to the model structure and communication for making cognitive decisions.

Table 6.1 describes some potential elements when considering a resilience framework for midwifery models of care. These elements describe the model functions through the course of an adverse event. Each element can be scored based on the ability of that element to achieve its intended aim. The whole matrix of elements can be scored to give a snapshot of overall midwifery continuity of care model resilience.

Table 6.1 Elements to consider when developing a resilience framework for midwifery models of care

	Prepare	Absorb	Recover	Adapt
Physical	Support services Workforce Equipment	Networked arrangements Model downtime procedures Demand management	Model business continuity plan	Investment where required
Information	Clinical indicator program Benchmarking activities Adverse events monitoring	Clinical data collection Incident notifiction	Analysis and multidisciplinary review of data and incidents	Refinement of data collection and dissemination of information
Cognitive	Service model	Escalation pathways	Model review Individual performance reviews	Model service planning Model redesign
Social	Professional development Culture	Staff support Complaints management Staff survey	Feedback to staff	Policy / procedure change Education updates Cultural change

Such a matrix can be compared over time or compared with similar models of care. The most obvious advantage of such a tool is that gaps in the model of care are identified and can be monitored over time.

Resilience theory offers a system-based approach, assisting midwives in models that provide continuity of care to understand both what sustains and what hinders their ability to adapt to changing pressures, or how to learn to stay 'safe' or 'protect the model'. Resilience theory looks proactively rather than reactively. It does not assume that individuals degrade an otherwise safe model. Rather, resilience aligns with a 'new view of human error' as described by Dekker (2006), who sees humans as a primary source of resilience in creating safety.

Communication to enhance safety in midwifery continuity of care

The framework for quality maternal and newborn care developed by Renfrew et al. (2014) describes the care and services that childbearing women and newborn infants need in all settings. These authors identify midwives as being pivotal to the provision of quality maternal and newborn care, supported by the necessary clinical knowledge and skills, interpersonal and cultural competence, appropriate values and a shared philosophy that strengthens women's capabilities.

Ensuring that midwives are well supported in their work, and are able to access continuing professional development, is central to the provision of high-quality care. Regular communication, both formal and informal, is especially important in midwifery continuity of care models where midwives often work in small teams and rely on their colleagues for support and 'cover' over busy periods. Having agreed expectations—for example, in relation to working hours, systems for backup and for providing a 'fresh set of eyes'—can help to relieve fatigue and, in turn, prevent errors. These aspects should be regularly discussed in group practice / team or department meetings.

There are specific aspects of working in midwifery continuity of care models that can increase stress (when adverse incidents occur, for example). Supporting individual midwives through a structured program of self-care, such as clinical supervision, can be a proactive strategy for building individual resilience. Ideally, clinical supervision should be an integral component of midwifery continuity of care models, both to encourage a reflective approach to practice and as a means of enhancing quality of clinical care through increased awareness and empathy (Brodie, 2015; NSW Health, 2012). Different models of supervision and peer review exist internationally. For example, in the UK, the professional midwifery advocate (PMA) has replaced the Supervisor of Midwives to provide clinical support and in Australia, a peer review system known as Midwifery Practice Review is designed to support safe, quality practice (Griffiths & Homer, 2008).

CONCLUSION

In keeping with other service models, and no matter where in the world they are developed, models of midwifery continuity of care require robust safety and quality strategies and frameworks to ensure that necessary standards are met. Such strategies and frameworks put the safety of women and babies at the centre of care, and can help to create organisational and consumer trust, confidence and support.

This chapter has shown how various initiatives have been introduced to address the challenges faced worldwide by maternity care providers in regard to reducing the risk of potential harm to women and babies. These initiatives have often been adapted to suit local requirements and the individual needs of the various models of care. Where the principles of safety and quality remain the priority, the agreed standards will ultimately depend on the needs of women accessing the service and the commitment of all those involved in ensuring the highest quality of care.

Safety and quality is a complex area and one that has a range of competing issues, cultures, viewpoints and approaches, which are at times expressed in what might seem to be quite dense theory. In this chapter we have considered a number of these complexities and sought to explain how they can be applied to models of midwifery continuity of care. Some readers will have differing views on the best ways to ensure a safe maternity service. We acknowledge these debates and challenges, and encourage you to read widely and think broadly to ensure you can argue your own view clearly. We believe that all safety and quality initiatives in midwifery continuity of care and the wider maternity service must uphold the principles of woman-centred care and be part of an informed discussion with women, key care providers and others engaged in the systems in which we work.

REFERENCES

Australian College of Midwives (ACM): *National midwifery guidelines for consultation and referral*, ed 3, issue 2, 2014 (reprinted May 2017 with amendments). Online: https://issuu.com/austcollegemidwives/docs/consultation_and_referral_guideline.

Australian Commission on Safety and Quality in Health Care (ACSQHC): *Australian safety and quality framework for health care*, Sydney, 2010, ACSQHC. Online: https://www.safetyandquality.gov.au/wp-content/uploads/2012/04/Australian-SandQ-Framework1.pdf.

Australian Commission on Safety and Quality in Health Care (ACSQHC): *National model clinical governance framework*, Sydney, 2017, ACSQHC. Online: https://www.safetyandquality.gov.au/wp-content/uploads/2017/11/National-Model-Clinical-Governance-Framework.pdf.

Berkman N, Sheridan S, Donahue K, Halpern D, Viera A, Crotty K: Low health literacy interventions and outcomes: an updated systematic review, *Ann Intern Med* 155(2):97–107, 2011.

Birthplace in England Collaborative Group: Perinatal and maternal outcomes by planned place of birth for healthy women with low risk pregnancies: the birthplace in England national prospective cohort study, *BMJ* 343:d7400, 2011.

Brodie P: Midwifing ourselves and each other: exploring the potential of clinical supervision, *Women Birth* 28:S8, 2015.

Bureau of Health Information (BHI): *Patient perspectives: experiences of maternity care in NSW public hospitals*, Sydney, 2017, BHI. Online: http://www.bhi.nsw.gov.au/BHI_reports/patient_perspectives/experiences_of_maternity_care_in_nsw_public_hospitals.

Carthey J, DeLeval M: Institutional resilience in healthcare systems, *Qual Saf Health Care* 10:29–32, 2001.

College of Midwives Ontario: *Consultation and transfer of care*, 2014. Online: http://www.cmo.on.ca/wp-content/uploads/2015/11/Standard-Consultation-and-Transfer-of-Care-Nov.-2015.pdf.

Cook R, Render M, Woods D: Gaps: learning how practitioners create safety, *BMJ* 320:791–794, 2000.

Dahlen HG: Undone by fear? Deluded by trust? Commentary, *Midwifery* 26:156–162, 2010.

Dekker S: *The field guide to understanding human error*, London, 2006, Ashgate.

Department of Health: *Safer maternity care: the national maternity safety strategy: progress and next steps*, London, 2017, Department of Health and Social Care. Online: https://www.gov.uk/government/publications/safer-maternity-care-progress-and-next-steps.

Elwyn G, Frosch D, Thomson R, Joseph-Williams N, Lloyd A, Kinnersley P, et al: Shared decision making: a model for clinical practice, *J General Int Med* 27:1361–1367, 2012.

Gaskell E, Walton G, Forrester M, Westwood G, Grosvenor M, Phillips D: My birthplace – an app to support shared decision making, *Int J Integrated Care* 18:8, 2014.

Griffiths M, Homer C: Developing a review process for Australian midwives: a report of the midwifery practice review project process, *Women Birth* 21:119–126, 2008.

Hall K: Reviewing intuitive decision-making and uncertainty: the implications for medical education, *Med Educ* 36:216–224, 2002.

Hunter B, Warren L: *Investigating resilience in midwifery. Final report*, Cardiff, Wales, 2013, Cardiff University. Online: https://orca.cf.ac.uk/61594/1/Investigating%20resilience%20Final%20report%20 oct%202013.pdf.

Hunter B, Warren L: Midwives' experiences of workplace resilience, *Midwifery* 30:926–934, 2014.

Hunter B, Warren L: Caring for ourselves: the key to resilience. In Byrom S, Downe S, editors: *The roar behind the silence. Why kindness, compassion and respect matter in maternity care*, London, 2015, Pinter & Martin, pp 111–115.

International Organization for Standardization (ISO) *ISO 31000:2018 Risk management—guidelines*, 2018. Online: https://www.iso.org/standard/65694.html.

Jeffcott S, Ibrahim J, Cameron P: Resilience in healthcare and clinical handover, *BMJ Qual Saf* 18:256–260, 2009.

Jensen C: Sociology, systems and (patient) safety: knowledge translations in healthcare policy, *Sociol Health Illn* 30:309–324, 2008.

Leap N: Woman centred care or women centred care: does it matter?, *Br J Midwifery* 17(1):736–740, 2009.

Leap N, Edwards N: The politics of involving women in decision making. In Page LA, Campbell R, editors: *The new midwifery: science and sensitivity in practice*, ed 2, London, 2006, Churchill Livingstone, Ch. 5, pp 97–123.

Ménage D: Part 1: A model for evidence-based decision-making in midwifery care, *Br J Midwifery* 24(1):44–49, 2016a.

Ménage D: Part 2: A model for evidence-based decision-making in midwifery care, *Br J Midwifery* 24(2):137–143, 2016b.

Monk A, Tracy M, Foureur M, Grigg C, Tracy S: Evaluating midwifery units (EMU): a prospective cohort study of freestanding midwifery units in New South Wales, Australia, *BMJ Open* 4:10, 2014.

National Institute for Health and Care Excellence (NICE): *Intrapartum care for healthy women and babies: Clinical guideline CG190*, London, 2017, NICE. Online: https://www.nice.org.uk/guidance/cg190.

National Health Service (NHS) England: *Human factors in healthcare. A concordat from the national quality board*, London, 2013, NHS England. Online: https://www.england.nhs.uk/wp-content/uploads/ 2013/11/nqb-hum-fact-concord.pdf.

National Health Service (NHS) England: *Better Births: improving outcomes of maternity services in England—a five year forward view for maternity care. National maternity review*, London, 2016, NHS England. Online: https://www.england.nhs.uk/wp-content/uploads/2016/02/national-maternity-review-report.pdf.

Noseworthy DA, Phibbs SR, Benn CA: Towards a relational model of decision-making in midwifery care, *Midwifery* 29:e42–e48, 2013.

NSW Health: *Midwifery continuity of carer model tool-kit*, Sydney, 2012, Government of NSW. Online: http://www.health.nsw.gov.au/nursing/projects/Publications/midwifery-cont-carer-tk.pdf.

NZ Ministry of Health: *Guidelines for consultation with obstetric and related medical services (referral guidelines)*, Wellington, 2012, Government of New Zealand. Online: https://www.health.govt.nz/system/files/ documents/publications/referral-glines-jan12.pdf.

Palmieri P, DeLucia P, Ott T, Peterson L, Green A: The anatomy and physiology of error in averse healthcare events, *Adv Health Care Manag* 7:33–36, 2008.

Reason J: *Human error*, New York, 1990, Cambridge University Press.

Reason J: Understanding adverse events: human factors, *BMJ Qual Saf* 4:80–89, 1995.

Reason J: Human error: models and management, *BMJ* 320:768–770, 2000.

Renfrew M, McFadden A, Bastos H, Campbell J, Channon A, Cheung N, et al: Midwifery and quality care: findings from a new evidence-informed framework for maternal and newborn care, *Lancet* 384:1129–1145, 2014.

Royal College of Midwives (RCM): *The RCM standards for midwifery services in the UK*, London, 2016, RCM. Online: https://www.rcm.org.uk/sites/default/files/RCM%20Standards%20for%20 Midwifery%20Services%20in%20the%20UK%20A4%2016pp%202016_12.pdf.

Sandall J, Soltani H, Gates S, Shennan A, Devane D: Midwife-led continuity models versus other models of care for childbearing women, *Cochrane Database Syst Rev* (9):CD004667, 2016. doi:10.1002/14651858. CD004667.pub4.

Scamell M, Alaszewski A: Fateful moments and the categorisation of risk: midwifery practice and the ever-narrowing window of normality during childbirth, *Health Risk Soc* 14(2):207–221, 2012.

Standards Australia / Standards New Zealand: *Risk management—principles and guidelines (AS / NZS ISO 31000:2009)*, 2009. Online: https://www.standards.org.au/standards-catalogue/sa-snz/other/ob-007/as-slash-nzs–iso–31000-2009.

Symon A: Risk and choice: knowledge and control. In Symon A, editor: *Risk and choice in maternity care: an international perspective*, London, 2006, Churchill Livingstone, pp 159–165.

ten Hoope-Bender P, de Bernis L, Campbell J, Downe S, Fauveau V, Fogstad H, et al: Improving maternal and newborn health through midwifery, *Lancet* 384:1226–1235, 2014.

The Royal Dutch Association of Midwives, The National Association of General Practitioners, The Dutch Association for Obstetrics and Gynaecology: *Obstetric manual:* final report of the Obstetric Working Group of the National Health Insurance Board of the Netherlands (abridged version), 1998. Online: http://www.kastanis.org/uploads/0000/0590/Nr.16.OBSTETRIC_MANUAL.pdf.

Tracy S, Hartz D, Tracy M, Kildea S, Allen Y, Forti A, et al: Caseload midwifery care versus standard maternity care for women of any risk: M@NGO, a randomised controlled trial, *Lancet* 382:1723–1732, 2013.

Tuncalp O, Were W, MacLennan C, Oladapo O, Gulmezoglu A, Bahl R, et al: Quality of care for pregnant women and newborns—the WHO vision, *BJOG* 122:1045–1049, 2015.

World Health Organization (WHO): *Quality of care: a process for making strategic choices in health systems*, Geneva, 2006, WHO. Online: http://www.who.int/management/quality/assurance/QualityCare_B.Def.pdf.

World Health Organization (WHO): *Conceptual framework for the international classification for patient safety, version 1.1: final technical report*, Geneva, 2009, WHO. Online: http://www.who.int/patientsafety/taxonomy/icps_full_report.pdf.

World Health Organization (WHO): *Standards for improving quality of maternal and newborn care in health facilities*, Geneva, 2016, WHO. Online: http://www.who.int/maternal_child_adolescent/documents/improving-maternal-newborn-care-quality/en/.

CHAPTER 7

Is Midwifery Continuity of Care Cost Effective?

Roslyn Donnellan-Fernandez, Vanessa Scarf, Declan Devane, Andy Healey

Contents

INTRODUCTION

There is no consistency regarding the costs and funding of maternity care services. Variation between, and within, high-, medium- and low-income countries shows funding can be provided publicly, privately, by health insurance schemes or through a combination of methods. In this chapter, we consider the cost effectiveness of midwifery continuity of care, predominately in publicly funded systems. With growing emphasis on value-based health care, models of maternity care that are demonstrated to be clinical and cost effective are of increasing importance to funders, providers and consumers. Identifying the specific cost benefits associated with midwifery continuity of care that will reduce chronic disease in mothers and babies is an important public health issue and should be a priority area for all health systems.

This chapter provides an overview of existing evidence for some of the cost effectiveness of midwifery continuity and identifies areas where further investigation is warranted. First, we cover the definition of cost effectiveness and the essential features of what, when and how to cost. This includes some of the challenges and limitations of current economic evaluations of models of maternity care. We then discuss evidence that supports the cost effectiveness of midwifery continuity of care. This includes care for women with a healthy pregnancy and cost efficiencies associated with birth in home, hospital and birth centre settings. Following this, we examine some cost considerations in models of midwifery continuity where women and their babies have complex needs. Factors to be taken into account when planning and undertaking an economic evaluation are considered—including place of birth, geographical catchment, population profile, health service configuration, health workforce and patterns of work, industrial requirements, finite budgets, financing models and time horizon. Additional important considerations related to childbearing and the perinatal period that also influence cost may include long-term health outcomes across the life course.

WHAT IS COST EFFECTIVENESS AND WHY DOES IT MATTER?

In general, an activity is usually considered to be cost effective if it is good value for the amount of money paid. In health economics, the term 'cost-effectiveness analysis' (CEA) refers to a specific form of economic analysis that compares the relative costs and outcomes (effects) of different courses of action. The purpose of CEA is to provide information that will help inform decisions on the most effective care options to provide in relation to cost and outcomes. CEA is usually conducted alongside or piggy-backed onto a randomised trial as this is considered the most robust form of evidence when evaluating the effects of health care interventions (Drummond et al., 2005). Comparisons in CEA may include different models of care, a new intervention compared with an existing intervention or no intervention, and / or alternative treatments—for example, surgeries and pharmaceutical drug trials. To date, many economic evaluations of maternity care have not fulfilled the specific criteria required for CEA. Studies have instead utilised a variety of methods of economic analysis, thus making robust comparison of maternity models, including different midwifery models, challenging (Donnellan-Fernandez, 2016a; Donnellan-Fernandez et al., 2018).

Resourcing effective maternity services is an important priority for all health systems and governments (Homer et al., 2014). Health care systems face increasing demands within limited resources, and controlling cost while improving quality produces competing tensions and challenges for health care providers and funders. Setting of priorities requires judgement and decisions about clinical effectiveness and the relative costs of alternative services and treatments (Callander & Fox, 2017, 2018). These judgements and decisions do not occur in a vacuum; rather, they are influenced by broader societal values and goals (Porter, 2015, 2017). Transparency, participation and justice are three key civil society requirements. Therefore, even when decisions are supported by robust evidence, they may be the subject of multiple competing demands that are context specific. Many countries are introducing systems and decision-making tools to assess 'value for money' to aid prioritisation of health service provision. Value-based health care—that is, how institutions, governments and health authorities incorporate societal values into decision making to allocate scarce resources—is essential to address growing health inequity and sustainable service solutions across the globe (International Consortium for Healthcare Outcomes

---

BOX 7.1 Bundled Pricing for Maternity

Sally Tracy, Professor of Midwifery and Women's Health, University of Sydney, Australia

One of the most powerful levers for change in any industry is the response to rising pressures of cost. The 'childbirth industry' is no different. In the 1960s and 1970s, as a result of their dissatisfaction with the medical establishment and with the rising cost of medical care, various groups of women began calling for minimal medical intervention in birth. What followed was the introduction of low(er)-cost birth centres. More recently the move to access continuity of midwifery care has become bogged down in the arguments about how costly it is for health services to introduce caseload care into mainstream maternity services.

In Australia one of the recent positive blips on the maternity horizon is the proposed introduction of 'bundled pricing' for maternity. (Bundled pricing is where a single price is determined to cover a full package of care over a defined period of time, spanning multiple events and settings of care.) It is hoped that this approach will make resources and funding easier for hospitals to manage, to allow financial flexibility in order to encourage improved models of care and drive better service delivery. Utlimately, the aim is that these elements will lead to better outcomes and lower costs in the longer term.

The plan was to provide hospitals with a single price for the cost of treating a pregnant woman across the continuum of her pregnancy care. It was hoped that, by introducing bundled pricing in maternity care, managers and policy leaders would be able to better promote midwifery group practice care within the public hospital system and move away from the current reliance on payment for each occasion of service to fund maternity care. (This current payment system carries with it an inherent perverse disincentive to reduce rates of surgical birth because the price for a caesarean section is higher than that for a vaginal birth.)

Maternity care service volumes and outcomes are relatively predictable and there is huge potential for savings. So bundling the payments for maternity would allow each health service to plan and encourage the provision of maternity care in a way that would not penalise attempts to introduce less interventionist, less costly and clever maternity care. Through a bundled pricing model the majority of women in any maternity service could be offered caseload midwifery without penalising the funding stream offered to each service.

Measurement (ICHOM), 2017; Littlejohns, 2017). Box 7.1 provides an Australian example of an attempt to find a new way of funding maternity services that is in line with the evidence on cost effectiveness.

Multiple definitions of midwifery continuity of care and the heterogeneity of outcomes measured have made it difficult to generalise about the cost of providing these models of care in different contexts (Devane et al., 2007). This is further confounded by economic evaluation methods that have applied divergent funding mechanisms for calculating maternity service costs. In different countries, these might include national tariffs and activity-based funding / diagnostic-related group (DRG) classifications, 'bundled pricing' or provider charges in fee-paying systems. Clear definitions, therefore, are crucial for robust evaluation of costs associated with any model of maternity care including midwifery continuity of care. In Australia, recent adoption of a national Maternity Care Classification System (MaCCS) that clearly defines the provider/s, scope and pattern of care delivered in different maternity models, as well as common terminology in describing outcomes to be compared, should improve both transparency and reliability of future service evaluation including comparative cost-effectiveness analysis (Donnolley et al., 2016). This system has been well described in Chapter 3. Similarly, use of international measures and benchmarks such as the ICHOM Standard Set for Pregnancy and Childbirth (ICHOM, 2017) and of core outcome sets in evaluating models of maternity care (Devane et al., 2007; Smith et al., 2017) will enable more meaningful future cross-country comparison.

IMPACT OF MIDWIFERY CONTINUITY OF CARE ON COSTS

It has been assumed that woman-centred care including midwifery continuity is likely to cost more than standard maternity care (Shaw et al., 2016). However, an increasing body of international evidence shows that relational midwifery continuity may cost no more and can even cost less than other models without such continuity (Begley et al., 2011; Janssen et al., 2015; Kenny et al., 2015; Ryan et al., 2013; Sandall et al., 2016; Schroeder et al., 2017; Toohill et al., 2012; Tracy et al., 2013). A number of factors contribute to savings in the model. Firstly, midwives providing continuity of care work flexibly, responding to the care requirements of individual women, in contrast to 'staffing an institution'. Midwives' time is therefore more effectively deployed as they work—that is, time is not used in the maternity unit 'waiting' for women to come into the health facility. Consequently, the number of caseload women per midwife (based on modelling hours of direct care) is provisionally more than in standard care (Australian College of Midwives (AGM), 2017; Ryan et al., 2013). Moreover, intervention rates, length of stay and re-admission rates are reduced, which in turn reduces costs significantly (National Health Performance Authority (NHPA), 2014; National Institute for Health and Care Excellence (NICE), 2014; Petrou & Khan, 2013; Sandall et al., 2016).

One of the challenges in costing midwifery continuity of care is that the relationship between continuity of care, mode of birth and the long-term health consequences, including linked cost consequences, have not been examined in systematic studies. Although there are still only limited studies that address the costing of midwifery continuity of care, and specifically caseload models as compared with alternative maternity models, these are gradually increasing.

Two early models of midwifery continuity of care that examined the cost implications were the Australian Ryde midwifery group practice (MGP) evaluation (Tracy & Hartz, 2006) and the United Kingdom one-to-one MGP evaluation (Page et al., 2001). Both services were established as public midwifery models in which a primary midwife provided antenatal, labour and postnatal care for a defined annual caseload of women (40 women / FTE). Professional standards guided consultation, referral and transfer with other services and providers. In the caseload model, midwives are paid an annualised salary and each primary midwife is supported with a partner / backup midwife for cover and time off within a small group practice of four to six midwives.

The Ryde MGP evaluation included a cost analysis that examined the impact on direct costs and included salaries, activity, transfer and goods and services both before and after implementation of the new model of care—that is, 'bottom up' costing. The analysis indicated a significant saving per woman of $A927 (19.0%) in 2004–05 terms, which equated to an absolute saving of $A259,000 on the basis of 280 women per year. Savings accrued as a result of increases in midwifery productivity (i.e. an increase in woman-to-midwife ratio from 23 women / midwife to 33 women / midwife), as well as reductions in length of hospital bed stay postnatally (30% reduction between 2003 and 2005) and medical costs (85% reduction) after implementing the midwifery model (Tracy & Hartz, 2005). Similarly, in the UK one-to-one midwifery care model ($n=1400$), which included women with high- and low-risk pregnancies, women had a reduced rate of caesarean sections (18% versus 29%, $p<0.01$) (the crude caesarean cost ratio is at least 2.5 times the cost for uncomplicated vaginal birth) and also were less likely to be admitted to hospital during the antenatal period. As well as experiencing higher rates of vaginal birth (70% versus 57%, $p<0.01$), women also had a shorter length of hospital bed stay (3.05 versus 3.87 days, $p<0.01$) further reducing institutional costs. Moreover, modelling based on bed occupancy and bed usage showed that increasing one-to-one care to 75% of the maternity service's workload would result in fewer inpatient beds being needed (Piercy et al., 2001).

Earlier and more recent studies internationally also have highlighted both the economics of current maternity service provision and short- and longer-term health outcomes for women, their babies and families within different midwifery service models (Bernitz et al., 2012; Gao et al., 2014; Hitzert et al., 2017; Howell et al., 2014; Hundley et al., 1995; Janssen et al., 2015; Kenny et al., 2015; O'Brien et al., 2010; Schroeder et al., 2012, 2017; Stone et al., 2000). These studies demonstrate cost savings associated with the implementation of publicly funded models of midwifery care that complement high rates of clinical effectiveness—in particular optimising physiological vaginal childbirth and reducing interventions (Sandall et al., 2016).

A number of economic evaluations conducted alongside randomised controlled trials have compared the costs of team midwifery with standard hospital care in the same setting (Begley et al., 2011; Homer et al., 2001a, 2001b; Kenny et al., 1994; Rowley et al., 1995) whereas others have specifically evaluated continuity of care models—for example, caseload midwifery and MGP (McLachlan et al., 2012; Tracy et al., 2013). In a team model, the level of continuity varies more than that in caseload or MGP models. The cost evaluations of team midwifery cited have included women of all-risk status and, in the MIDU study in Ireland, although the women included were low risk at booking, many women developed specialised needs during the course of care (Kenny et al., 2015).

A recent cost analysis, the M@NGO study ($n=1748$) was undertaken across two states in Australia and aimed at assessing the clinical and cost outcomes of caseload midwifery care for women irrespective of risk factors. This study included pregnant women of all-risk status and demonstrated that caseload midwifery care cost an average AU$566.74 (95% confidence interval (CI) 106.17–1027.30; $p=0·02$) less per woman than standard care (Tracy et al., 2013). The cost savings were attributed to flexible care delivery, an increase in the spontaneous labour rate with consequent reductions in obstetric interventions, decreased length of bed stay and re-admission rates, and improved retention of workforce due to increased staff satisfaction (ACM, 2017, p. 36). Internationally validated cost ratios for mode of birth have also been successfully applied to population data to model the projected cost of birth intervention in public caseload midwifery care compared with standard care and private obstetric care (Tracy et al., 2014).

Findings from economic analyses vary depending on the structure of health care within a given country, including the factors used in any modelling (Sandall et al., 2016). For example, economic analysis to assess cost effectiveness in relation to continuity and midwifery workforce configuration in the UK demonstrate that volume and caseload are critical to cost effectiveness (Ryan et al., 2013). Ryan et al. (2013) showed that the mean cost saving for eligible women in the study was estimated to be £12.38 (sterling). The conclusion was that an aggregate cost saving of £1.16 million per year would be possible if midwife-led services were expanded to 50% of all eligible women in the UK. However, the study also showed using sensitivity analyses that the cost changes per maternity episode could vary from a saving of £253.38 to a cost increase of £108.12 depending on the assumptions used. Therefore, the more women who receive this type of care, the more the cost efficiency is maximised.

A number of other studies have examined the cost implications of 'new' models of midwifery care, although none of these exclusively focused on caseload midwifery. All suggest a cost-saving effect in intrapartum care, and one study suggested a higher cost of postnatal care when midwifery-led care is compared with standard maternity care. Although there is a lack of consistency in estimating maternity care costs between studies, there seems to be a trend towards the cost-saving effect of midwife-led care in comparison with standard care (Sandall et al., 2016).

It seems evident that 'more intervention' costs more than 'less intervention', and economic studies have demonstrated that uncomplicated normal birth costs significantly less than caesarean section in terms of immediate costs as well as community midwifery, re-admissions and general practitioner care. An overview of the health economic implications of elective caesarean section has been undertaken by Petrou & Khan (2013), who reviewed 12 studies published since 2000 that used a decision analytic model and included a caesarean section comparator. This review concluded that, although some economic evaluations have shown planned caesarean section to be a cost-effective mode of delivery in selected clinical contexts, elective caesarean section overall (or caesarean as a whole) appears to be costlier than either spontaneous or instrumental vaginal birth in low-risk or unselected populations. Australian research has that shown the relative cost of birth increases by up to 50% for low-risk primiparous women and by up to 36% for low-risk multiparous women as labour interventions such as induction, use of epidural and birth using instruments and surgery accumulate (Tracy & Tracy, 2003; Tracy et al., 2014). Research from other countries has also examined the cost effectiveness of early postnatal discharge and midwifery home visits compared with a traditional postnatal hospital stay and found that early postnatal discharge combined with midwifery home visits resulted in significant cost savings (Petrou et al., 2004).

In the UK, the NICE (2014) intrapartum care guidelines identified the importance of cost effectiveness in maximising health gain within scarce health care resources and suggested the use of a decision-analytic approach. One way to apply this is to use a 'decision tree' modelling framework to assess cost effectiveness of place of birth (Schroeder et al., 2014). Decision tree modelling frameworks are commonly used by health economists as an method for determining cost effectiveness. In the example provided we are simply applying it to place of birth. Using this framework, data on birth outcomes by place of birth can be compared against the relevant national tariffs (National Health Service (NHS), 2017). As part of a CEA that used both 'bottom-up' and 'top-down' costing methods to examine the cost effectiveness of alterative planned places of birth in woman at low risk of complications, the Birthplace National Prospective cohort study in the UK ($n=64,538$) incorporated relevant tariffs that demonstrate incremental cost increase per woman related to birth setting (total unadjusted mean costs were £1066, £1435, £1461 and £1631 for births planned at home, in freestanding midwifery units, in alongside midwifery units and in obstetric units respectively (equivalent to €1274, AU$1701; €1715, AU$2290; €1747, AU$2332; and €1950, AU$2603 respectively) (Schroeder et al., 2012). In Australia, the federal government also applies standard costs based on DRGs to calculate the average expenditure per public hospital admission for mode of birth. For example, in 2011–12 the average cost per public hospital admission for vaginal birth without complications was AU$4600 (range AU$2200–6500). In contrast, during the same period, the average cost for caesarean surgery without complications was AU$8800 (range AU$5500–15,300) (NHPA, 2015, pp. 28–9).

MIDWIFERY CONTINUITY IS A COST-EFFECTIVE MODEL

International literature largely demonstrates a cost saving where women with a low-risk pregnancy are cared for in a midwifery model of care, which includes continuity

(Hitzert et al., 2017; Kenny et al., 2015; McLachlan et al., 2012; Schroeder et al., 2017; Tracy et al., 2013, 2014). Savings may be further enhanced by place of birth—for example, free-standing midwifery unit, alongside midwifery-led unit (both also commonly referred to as 'birthing centre') or home as compared with obstetric consultant-led unit in hospital (Janssen et al., 2015; Kenny et al., 2015; Schroeder et al., 2017). Whereas a free-standing midwifery unit is located separately to hospital facilities, an alongside midwifery led-unit or birth centre is co-located with or beside a hospital. See Table 7.1 for a summary of comparative model of care costs calculated in various economic evaluations of midwifery models, including birth setting.

Table 7.1 Summary of economic evaluations of midwifery-led care

Author country (date)	Model of care comparison	Events measured	Cost outcomes (average)	Mean difference
Begley et al. Ireland (2009)	MLU vs CLU	Antenatal, birth, postnatal, neonatal, transport	MLU: €2545.13 CLU: €2877.93	+€332.80
Bernitz et al. Norway (2012)	MLU vs SCU	Labour and birth	MLU: €1672 SCU: €1950	+€278
Gao et al. Australia (2014)	MGP (caseload) vs baseline care (MW, Dr, AHW)	Antenatal, birth, postnatal, neonatal, transport	MGP: AU$ 12,955 Baseline: AU$13,658	+AU$703
Hitzert et al. Netherlands (2017)	Community MW care at home vs birth centre vs hospital	Labour, birth up to 7 days postnatal	Home: €2998 BC: €3327 Hospital: €3330	+€329 +€332
Homer Australia (2001a)	MGP vs standard care (MW, Dr)	Antenatal, birth, postnatal, neonatal	MGP: AU$2578.70 Standard: AU$3482.79	+AU$904.09
Howell et al. USA (2014)	FSBC vs usual care (Dr, MW)	Average birth cost	FSBC: US$6055 Usual: US$7218	+US$1163
Hundley et al. UK (1995)	MLU vs CLU	Labour and birth	Net increase per women £40.71 in MW-led unit	
Janssen et al. Canada (2015)	MW care homebirth MW care hospital birth Physician hospital birth	Antenatal, birth, postnatal, transport	MW HB: Can$2275 MW Hosp: Can$4613 Phys hosp: Can$4816	+Can$2338 +Can$2541

Table 7.1 Summary of economic evaluations of midwifery-led care—cont'd

Author country (date)	Model of care comparison	Events measured	Cost outcomes (average)	Mean difference
Kenny et al. Ireland (2015)	MW care in BC MLU vs CLU in hospital	Antenatal, birth, postnatal, accommodation	MLU: €2598 CLU: €2780	+€182
O'Brien et al. Canada (2010)	MW care vs physician hospital care	Prepregnancy, antenatal, labour and birth, up to 6 months postnatal.	MW: Can$2450 Physician: Can$5617	+Can$3167
Schroeder et al. UK 2012	MW care at home vs AMU vs FMU vs OU	Labour, birth, postnatal, transfer	Home: £1066 AMU: £1435 FMU: £1461 OU: £1631	+£369 +£395 +£565
Schroeder et al. UK 2017	MW care in FMU vs MW care in hospital	Labour, birth, postnatal, transfer	FMU: £1296.23 Hospital: £2146	+£850
Stone et al. USA (2000)	MW care in FSBC vs MC	Antenatal, birth, postnatal, accommodation	MW: US$6087 MC: US$6803	+US$716
Toohill et al. Austraia (2012)	MGP vs standard care (MW, Dr, GP)	Antenatal, birth, postnatal, neonatal	MGP: AU$4722 SC: AU$5641	+AU$919
Tracy et al. Australia (2013)	MGP vs standard care (MW, Dr, GP)	Birth	MGP: AU$5497.34 SC: AU$5903·67	+AU$566·74
Tracy et al. Australia (2014)	MGP vs PO vs standard care (MW, Dr, GP)	Antenatal, birth, postnatal, neonatal	MGP: AU$3904.64 PO: AU$5299.52 SC: AU$5839.86	+AU$ 1394.88 +AU$ 1935

AMU=alongside maternity unit; AHW=Aboriginal health worker; BC=birth centre; CLU=consultant-led unit; FMU=free-standing maternity unit; FSBC=free-standing birth centre; HB=homebirth; MC=medical care; MGP=midwifery group practice—caseload midwifery care; MLU=midwife-led unit; MW=midwife; OU=obstetric unit; PO=private obstetrics.

Few studies, however, have consistently assessed or measured the cost effectiveness of midwifery continuity of care compared with other models of maternity care. In the Cochrane systematic review of midwifery-led continuity models versus other models of care, Sandall et al. (2016) reported cost findings narratively to emphasise this lack of consistency in the measurement and assessment of costs of various maternity models. To date, the most robust economic evaluation studies of midwifery continuity models have been piggy-backed onto randomised controlled trials investigating clinical effectiveness outcomes.

In the Cochrane systematic review by Sandall et al. (2016), only seven of 15 randomised trials included in the review incorporated an economic evaluation. Among these seven studies there were varying degrees of midwifery continuity provided, as both caseload and team midwifery models were included (Begley et al., 2011; Flint et al., 1989; Homer et al., 2001b; Kenny et al., 1994; Rowley et al., 1995; Tracy et al., 2013; Young et al., 1997). Although a trend towards a cost-saving effect was identified for the midwifery continuity of care models compared with other care models, there was also inconsistency in the way the cost outcomes were reported. Consistent adoption of methods of economic analysis and a standard set of indicators for cost measurement, alongside core clinical outcome sets, will greatly assist future evaluation of cost effectiveness of midwifery continuity models compared with other maternity models.

Cost savings for women with healthy pregnancies

The broad drivers of cost in maternity services have been identified as workforce, mode of birth, birth setting and length of stay (Sandall et al., 2011). The capacity of midwifery continuity models to reduce unnecessary hospitalisation and resource use across the childbearing continuum is an important public health objective that optimises utilisation of resources and services where women experience healthy pregnancy and childbirth. Hospital admissions and bed stay are variables commonly associated with increased intervention in childbirth, especially surgical birth (Scarf et al., 2018). Interventions and complications that arise from these procedures cause iatrogenic effect, increase requirement for hospital staffing and incur additional costs (Duckett et al., 2015; NHPA, 2014, 2015). Elective caesarean surgery and other childbirth interventions are not cost neutral when compared with uncomplicated vaginal birth (Petrou & Khan, 2013; von Gruenigen et al., 2013). Ineffective treatment—for example, elective caesarean in the absence of medical indication—result in poorer outcomes (e.g. increased pre-term birth rate and increased admission to special care baby nurseries for respiratory compromise) with resultant increases in cost and resource use (Kok et al., 2014; Signore & Klebanoff, 2008; Tracy et al., 2007).

Table 7.1 summarises the available economic evaluations of midwifery-led care. While many of these studies include midwifery continuity of care, it is not possible to say they are costings of continuity of care per se. Many of these studies are also related to different places of birth (home, birth centre, hospital), which highlights the close relationship between model of care and birth setting, particularly for women with a healthy pregnancy (Scarf et al., 2016). What is evident in all except one paper (Hundley et al., 1995) is that midwifery-led units and therefore midwifery-led care confer cost savings for health services, even when the women give birth in a hospital setting (Begley et al., 2011; Gao et al., 2014; Hitzert et al., 2017; Janssen et al., 2015; Schroeder et al., 2012; Tracy et al., 2013).

Cost impact when women and their babies have complex needs

The negative long-term transgenerational effects of programming experienced during the perinatal period (developmental origins of health and disease, DOHaD), including disruption of the human microbiome at birth, is recognised as a challenge that has immediate and enduring costs for all health systems and societies (Babenko et al., 2015; Dunlop et al., 2015; Moore et al., 2017; Peters et al., 2018). An additional challenge in many high-resource settings is the increasing number of childbearing women with pre-existing co-morbidities and those who are experiencing pregnancies with more specialised and complex needs (e.g. obesity, perinatal mental health compromise). These examples, and other factors such as age and use of assisted reproductive technology, and social determinants like poverty that impact on health, can contribute to complex pregnancy. Such factors predispose the women in these populations to higher levels of intervention and resource use.

The clinical and cost benefits that accrue when women with healthy pregnancies are provided with midwifery continuity of care may deliver additional longer-term health and cost dividends for women and vulnerable groups experiencing complex pregnancies related to physical, emotional or socioeconomic factors (Bertilone & McEvoy, 2015; Gao et al., 2014; NHS, 2017; Rayment-Jones et al., 2015; Yelland et al., 2015). However, caution is advised when attributing the outcomes of continuity of care for women with healthy pregnancies to women who experience complexity, as the effect of the model of maternity care may be context and population specific. As further evaluation of the cost benefit of midwifery continuity of care for women who experience complex pregnancy is warranted, it is important that economic analysis built into trials where women are randomised to models of care at point of booking includes costs for women who develop complex needs.

A recent example of retrospective data base analysis and evaluation of women with complex pregnancies in South Australia showed suboptimal quality outcomes between two models of care for women with 'moderate-risk' pregnancies ($n=12,406$). In this study, significant cost savings and efficiency were found for women allocated to integrated caseload continuity (MGP model) in a tertiary hospital compared with women who received standard hospital care (SHC). The cost was calculated across a 7-year period and was sustained; it was AU\$863.92 less per woman in midwifery care (MGP) in the adjusted model ($\beta=0.79$; 95% CI 0.76–0.82) (Donnellan-Fernandez, 2016b). The savings may be attributed to reductions both in admissions (i.e. maternal hospital antenatal admissions and admissions to special care baby nursery) and in birth intervention for women with complex pregnancies who received midwifery continuity—woman in the MGP were 1.5 times more likely to achieve a spontaneous vaginal birth (95% CI 1.40–1.65) and less likely to experience routine interventions and childbirth morbidity such as postpartum haemorrhage (≥ 500 mL), elective caesarean section, induction of labour, use of epidural and episiotomy. The babies of women who received the midwifery caseload continuity service also showed significantly different characteristics from the babies in standard care. They were more likely to have a gestation greater than 37 weeks and a birth weight greater than 3000 grams. In this study, the demographic characteristics of women who did and those who did not access the midwifery continuity model differed significantly; women with the highest socioeconomic disadvantage were overrepresented in the standard care group and had least access to midwifery continuity of care.

PLACE OF BIRTH AND COST EFFICIENCIES IN ALTERNATIVE BIRTH SETTINGS

When considering the cost of birth in different settings there are many factors that contribute to the measurement and allocation of resources. Admission to hospital to give birth is the primary reason for acute hospital admission. Internationally, the availability of options other than birth in hospital varies depending on the availability of midwifery care (however, homebirth in some countries is available through the care of general practitioners or family care physicians) (Benoit et al., 2005). Legislation, social norms and cultural values also affect women's access to midwifery care and place of birth (Vedam et al., 2018). Cost is a considerable driver of maternity care in high-income countries (Shaw et al., 2016) and transferring the cost of place of birth could result in cost savings through a reduction in admission to hospital, a reduction in interventions (Allen et al., 2006; Birthplace in England Collaborative Group, 2011) and a shorter length of stay, particularly for women with a healthy pregnancy (Scarf et al., 2018).

A systematic review examined costs associated with alternative birth settings for pregnant women at low risk of complications (Scarf et al., 2016). The studies included were from Australia, Canada, Ireland, the Netherlands, Norway, United States (USA) and the UK. Of the 11 studies included, four compared costs between homebirth and the hospital setting and seven focused on the cost of birth centre care and the hospital setting. The maternity care services in countries of included studies varied somewhat, with midwifery care common in the UK through the NHS, in the Netherlands with its extensive primary health care service (midwives and general practitioners), and in Norway and Australia. In Canada, the regulation of midwives in 1994 expanded the options for women to give birth at home or in a birth centre and now these choices are offered in six of the 13 provinces (Hutton et al., 2009; Janssen et al., 2015). The USA has complex midwifery regulatory and credentialling laws that vary between states and this is reflected in the availability of homebirth and birth centre choices for women in a number of states (Alliman & Phillippi, 2016; MacDorman et al., 2014; Vedam et al., 2018).

Eight of the 11 studies reviewed reported a cost saving associated with giving birth at home ($n=3$) or in a birth centre ($n=5$), two reported no significant difference and one found it was more costly to provide care in a birth centre owing to increased midwifery staffing levels and setup costs. Of all the birth settings reviewed, home was the least costly as the resources mainly included midwifery time and consumables, compared with the hospital group where accommodation, the fixed costs of facility use and variable costs including staff time, consumables and interventions increased the cost considerably. The savings for women giving birth in birth centres centred around fewer interventions and procedures and shorter stays in the birth centre facility, whether alongside or free-standing. Unsurprisingly, hospital admission for childbirth carries the highest cost and, considering the spontaneous birth rate in women with a healthy pregnancy (around 50% in Australia (Homer, 2016) and 69% in Ireland (Begley et al., 2011)), this level of care is not necessary for all women. If we consider the factors that increase the cost of giving birth—namely accommodation, interventions and staffing—it follows that birth in a midwifery-led model, and therefore birth in a setting outside a hospital, would be likely to confer cost savings on the health services.

STUDYING THE ECONOMICS OF MIDWIFERY SERVICES AND MATERNITY MODELS

Quantification of the resource and cost impact of introducing midwifery continuity of care is integral to evaluating whether it represents a cost-effective approach to service delivery compared with standard practice. In planning an economic evaluation as part of a randomised trial or other study designs, consideration needs to be given to three core aspects: study perspective, resource use / clinical activity measurement and unit costing.

Deciding on the study perspective is important as economic evaluations can vary in terms of the scope of resource impacts and the costs captured. These can range from a narrow health care provider perspective through to a broader 'societal' evaluation of resource impacts that capture impacts on services within and beyond those delivered directly as part of maternal care pathways—for example, use of primary care and other community-based health services that may be paid for and provided by other agencies. The approach taken will partly depend on who is commissioning the research and who will use the end results. Early clarity on the perspective to be taken is important so that plans can be made for measurement of resource use and costs that reflect the desired perspective in specific cases. Costs associated with medical and midwifery staffing are significant drivers of any costing model. Pregnancy and birth are temporal in nature (i.e. ante-, intra- and postnatal components) and some women will, based on emerging (or resolving) clinical need, require transfer care between models of care and probably receive specific tests and interventions (such as ultrasonography and cardiotocography) that will incur costs. It is important, therefore,

Table 7.2 Identifying relevant medical resource items for economic evaluation

Identify clinical care pathways	Resource measures
Identify different clinical care pathways that could be followed from the first antenatal appointment to hospital discharge including the different medical resources that could be utilised for different pathways followed, e.g. women with 'low-' or 'higher-'risk complications of pregnancy Identify areas of the maternal care pathway most likely to be affected through delivery of continuity of care, plus The medical resource items expected to be impacted on Prioritise accurate quantification of items with the greatest resource and cost implications	Measure frequency and type of service contact (e.g. midwife- versus consultant-led antenatal appointments) Log incidence of hospital and neonatal intensive care admission Calculate exposure to tests, procedures and method / route of birth Can be informed by current evidence from existing economic evaluations, and / or Theory of change and logic models underpinning the application of continuity of care approaches in midwifery Hospital admissions more important to capture than low-cost, infrequent intervention that is unlikely to affect conclusions regarding cost effectiveness

Table 7.3 Quantifying clinical activities undertaken

• Quantifying 'units' of clinical activity delivered over the course of a pregnancy is most reliably done through extraction of data from electronic hospital information systems; these also draw on records from clinical case notes including the entries of medical and midwifery staff	• Most reliable data source
• Patient retrospective self-report is also an option (where appropriate), e.g. can be used retrospectively to collate information on use of services, exposure to different procedures and interventions over the course of a pregnancy and postnatal period	• Valuable and informative where data is required on resource use outside of the hospital setting, e.g. in primary care services • More likely to be susceptible to recall bias • Works most reliably when requesting people to report major items of resource use, i.e. frequency of antenatal appointments, hospital admissions experienced, type of birth and postnatal and neonatal admissions

that costs and resource use are mapped against the potential care pathways women will take through their pregnancy and birth. Table 7.2 identifies aspects of medical resource use including clinical care pathways and resource measures that should be determined when planning an economic evaluation.

Table 7.3 focuses on two approaches to quantifying clinical activity related to continuity of care: electronic data extraction or self-report, summarising the advantage

Table 7.4 Unit costs for economic evaluation

• Unit costs for economic evaluation should fully reflect the value of all resources allocated to the delivery of units of service delivery and interventions.	Examples: • cost per antenatal appointment • cost per night spent in neonatal intensive care • cost per ultrasound scan. Includes:
• In economic terms these values should approximately equate to the opportunity cost of resources consumed, i.e. the value of a resource in its next best alternative use, in the delivery of units of clinical activity.	• cost of clinical time • cost of medical equipment • cost of consumables • cost of organisational overheads (able to reasonably be apportioned out). Example:
• Unit-based costs for hospital-based health care are often used to support financial resource allocation in health care systems and available for public use. These costs will typically be linked to diagnostic or prespecified health resource grouping (HRG) codes.	• National Health Service (NHS) in England publishes national 'Reference Costs', i.e. specific items of use across all medical specialities, including maternal care.
• Care should be taken when interpreting these costs for use in economic evaluation as they can often reflect guidelines around tariffs that providers of health care should charge commissioners for patient care.	• current fixed tariffs for antenatal care in England are specified for low- and higher-risk pregnancies. These broadly reflect differentials in resource use in each risk grouping but will not vary with the number of appointments, tests and procedures carried out, and are therefore less useful for economic evaluation where identification of variation in activity levels and actual resource use is important.
• Published health economic evaluations conducted to accepted methodological standards are a good additional source for unit costs data. Where bespoke estimation of unit costs becomes necessary because of gaps in health system data or published evaluations, a 'bottom-up' approach to developing unit costs is recommended.	All resource inputs to an activity are measured and valued using relevant pricing information, e.g. staff salaries and 'on-costs' for valuation of clinical time.

and limitation of each. Whichever approach is adopted (patient records or self-report) the 'units' of resource use measured need to be compatible with available data on unit costs (see Table 7.4) so that the two can be combined (multiplied together) to estimate the total cost of care delivered across individual pregnancies.

Table 7.4 provides an overview of unit costs that can be used for economic evaluation. Examples of data commonly collected to provide information on unit costs for hospital-based health care that utilise 'top-down' or 'bottom-up' costing are shown. This may include estimation where there is a gap in available health care data.

Other specific considerations additional to those identified in Tables 7.2–7.4 may be important in an economic evaluation. These can be context dependent—for example, implementation and setup costs and service efficiency. A post-hoc evaluation of models of continuity of care delivered in specific contexts also provides an opportunity for estimating costs linked to activities and processes that are integral to successful implementation. This will include the costs of training staff in the new ways of working and accounting for resources allocated to monitoring care quality and safety on an ongoing basis.

Although not usually of direct relevance to a cost-effectiveness evaluation (where the focus is on evaluating incremental costs and benefits / outcomes of changes to existing practice in delivery of maternity care), consideration should also be given to efficiency impacts defined more broadly. In a continuity of care context, this could involve assessments of the impact of midwifery continuity of care on clinical caseloads, of the extent to which changing practice is linked to observed impacts on use of interventions and procedures over the care pathway (as measured in a cost-effectiveness evaluation) and of whether the maintenance of anticipated throughputs of pregnancies will have wider workforce implications.

CONCLUSION

There is mounting pressure on health care systems around the world to deliver safe, cost-efficient services. This chapter includes ample evidence of the safety of midwifery continuity of care for childbearing women—not only those women with a healthy pregnancy, but also those experiencing complexities. Economic evaluations of interventions such as midwifery continuity of care are difficult to perform, and in this chapter we have outlined some of the facilitators and challenges to effectively evaluating the cost of midwifery continuity of care. There is a logical link between favourable outcomes for women in continuity models and the reduced comparative cost when factors such as interventions and hospital accommodation are included.

The cost implications of optimising pregnancy and birth outcomes for women and babies is not only applicable to the immediate birth episode but can also have a long-term impact on the health care system. This is an area in need of further investigation, particularly in relation to continuity of care models. We have provided some guidance for the conduct of research into economic evaluations, particularly relating to midwifery. We have outlined the steps to collecting meaningful data on the resources required to sustain a continuity model in order to evaluate its efficacy.

REFERENCES

Allen VM, O'Connell CM, Baskett TF: Cumulative economic implications of initial method of delivery, *Obstet Gynecol* 108:549–555, 2006.

Alliman J, Phillippi JC: Maternal outcomes in birth centers: an integrative review of the literature, *J Midwifery Womens Health* 61:21–51, 2016.

Australian College of Midwives (ACM): *Delivering midwifery continuity of care to Australian women. A handbook for hospitals and health services*, ed 3, Canberra, 2017, ACM.

Babenko O, Kovalchuk I, Metz G: Stress-induced perinatal and transgenerational epigenetic programming of brain development and mental health, *Neurosci Biobehav Rev* 48:70–91, 2015. doi:10.1016/j.neubiorev.2014.11.013.

Begley C, Devane D, Clarke M: *An evaluation of midwifery-led care in the health service executive north eastern area: the report of the MidU study*, Dublin, 2009, School of Nursing and Midwifery, Trinity College Dublin, Health Service Executive (HSE).

Begley C, Devane D, Clarke M, McCann C, Hughes P, Reilly M, et al: Comparison of midwife-led and consultant-led care of healthy women at low risk of childbirth complications in the Republic of Ireland: a randomised trial, *BMC Pregnancy Childbirth* 11:85, 2011.

Benoit C, Wrede S, Bourgeault I, Sandall J, Vries RD, Teijlingen ER: Understanding the social organisation of maternity care systems: midwifery as a touchstone, *Sociol Health Illn* 27:722–737, 2005.

Bernitz S, Aas E, Oian P: Economic evaluation of birth care in low-risk women. A comparison between a midwife-led birth unit and a standard obstetric unit within the same hospital in Norway. A randomised controlled trial, *Midwifery* 28:591–599, 2012.

Bertilone C, McEvoy S: Success in Closing the Gap: favourable neonatal outcomes in a metropolitan Aboriginal Maternity Group Practice Program, *Med J Aust* 203:262.e1–262.e7, 2015.

Birthplace in England Collaborative Group: Perinatal and maternal outcomes by planned place of birth for healthy women with low risk pregnancies: the Birthplace in England National Prospective Cohort study, *BMJ* 343:d7400, 2011.

Callander E, Fox H: What are the costs associated with child and maternal healthcare within Australia? A study protocol for the use of data linkage to identify health service use, and health system and patient costs, *BMJ Open* 8(2):e017816, 2017. doi:10.1136/bmjopen-2017-017816.

Callander E, Fox H: Changes in out-of-pocket charges associated with obstetric care provided under Medicare in Australia, *Aust N Z J Obstet Gynaecol* 58(3):362–365, 2018. doi:10.1111/ajo.127602018.

Devane D, Begley C, Clarke M, Horey D, Oboyle C: Evaluating maternity care: a core set of outcome measures, *Birth* 34:164–172, 2007.

Donnellan-Fernandez RE: Proceed with caution—the strength and weakness in reported cost data in South Australia, Women's Healthcare Australasia Annual Benchmarking Meeting, Northside Conference Centre, Sydney. In *Enhancing performance and cost effectiveness in maternity and women's healthcare*, Canberra, 2016a, Women's Healthcare Australasia.

Donnellan-Fernandez R: MGP versus SHC: a cost and resource study of women with complex pregnancy, PhD thesis, Adelaide, 2016b, Flinders University. Online (Flinders Digital Thesis Repository): https://flex.flinders.edu.au/file/c1ad3c98-90fd-4d6a-8ae0-7af681b7158b/1/THESIS_Final%20Print%20Version%20Post%20Exam_RozDF_2016.pdf.

Donnellan-Fernandez R, Creedy D, Callander E: Cost-effectiveness of continuity of midwifery care for women with complex pregnancy – a structured review of the extant literature, *Women Birth* 31(1):S46–S47, 2018. doi:10.1016/j.wombi.2018.08.139.

Donnolley N, Butler-Henderson K, Chapman M, Sullivan E: The development of a classification system for maternity models of care, *Health Inf Manag* 45:64–70, 2016.

Drummond MF, Sculpher MJ, Torrance GW, O'Brien BJ, Stoddart G: *Methods for the economic evaluation of health care programmes*, ed 3, Oxford, 2005, Oxford University Press.

Duckett S, Breadon P, Romanes P, Fennessy P: *Questionable care: avoiding ineffective treatment*, Melbourne, 2015, Grattan Institute.

Dunlop AL, Mulle JG, Ferranti EP, Edwards S, Dunn AB, Corwin EJ: Maternal microbiome and pregnancy outcomes that impact infant health: a review, *Adv Neonatal Care* 15:377–385, 2015.

Flint C, Poulengeris P, Grant A: The 'Know Your Midwife' scheme—a randomised trial of continuity of care by a team of midwives, *Midwifery* 5:11–16, 1989.

Gao Y, Gold L, Josif C, Bar-Zeev S, Steenkamp M, Barclay L, et al: A cost-consequences analysis of a Midwifery Group Practice for Aboriginal mothers and infants in the Top End of the Northern Territory, Australia, *Midwifery* 30:447–455, 2014.

Hitzert M, Hermus M, Boesveld I, Franx A, van der Pal-de Bruin K, Steegers E, et al: Cost-effectiveness of planned birth in a birth centre compared with alternative planned places of birth: results of the Dutch Birth Centre Study, *BMJ Open* 7:e016960, 2017.

Homer C: Models of maternity care: evidence for midwifery continuity of care, *Med J Aust* 205:370–374, 2016.

Homer C, Matha DV, Jordan LD, Wills J, Davis GK: Community based continuity of midwifery care versus standard hospital care: a cost analysis, *Aust Health Rev* 1:85–93, 2001a.

Homer C, Davis G, Brodie P, Sheehan A, Barclay L, Wills J, et al: Collaboration in maternity care: a randomised controlled trial comparing community-based continuity of care with standard hospital care, *BJOG* 108:16–22, 2001b.

Homer C, Friberg IK, Dias MAB, ten-Hoope Bender P, Sandall J, Speciale AB, et al: The projected effect of scaling up midwifery, *Lancet* 384:1146–1157, 2014.

Howell E, Palmer A, Benatar S, Garrett B: Potential Medicaid cost savings from maternity care based at a freestanding birth center, *Medicare Medicaid Res Rev* 4:E1–E13, 2014.

Hundley V, Donaldson C, Lang GD, Cruickshank F, Glazener C, Milne J, et al: Costs of intrapartum care in a midwife-managed delivery unit and a consultant-led labour ward, *Midwifery* 11:103–109, 1995.

Hutton EK, Reitsma AH, Kaufman K: Outcomes associated with planned home and planned hospital births in low-risk women attended by midwives in Ontario, Canada, 2003–2006: a retrospective cohort study, *Birth* 36:180–189, 2009.

International Consortium for Healthcare Outcomes Measurement (ICHOM): *Pregnancy and childbirth data collection reference guide* (version 1.0.3), 2017. Online: http://www.ichom.org/downloads/ichom-reference-guides/.

Janssen PA, Milton C, Aghajanian J: Costs of planned home birth vs hospital birth in British Columbia attended by registered midwives and physicians, *PLoS ONE* 10(7):e0133524, 2015.

Kenny C, Devane D, Normand C, Clarke M, Howard A, Begley CA: Cost comparison of midwife-led compared with consultant-led maternity care in Ireland (the MidU study), *Midwifery* 31:1032–1038, 2015.

Kenny P, Brodie P, Eckermann S, Hall J: *Westmead Hospital Team Midwifery Project Evaluation final report*, Sydney, 1994, Centre for Health Economics Research and Evaluation, University of Sydney.

Kok N, Ruiter L, Hof M, Ravelli A, Mol BW, Pajkrt E, et al: Risk of maternal and neonatal complications in a subsequent pregnancy after planned caesarean section in a first birth, compared with emergency caesarean section: a nationwide comparative cohort study, *BJOG* 121:216–223, 2014.

Littlejohns P: *Creating sustainable health care systems through the application of evidence and shared values*, Menzies Health Institute Queensland and Data Sciences Seminar, Gold Coast University Hospital. London, 2017, National Institute for Health Research Collaboration for Leadership in Applied Health Research and Care. Online: https://wileymicrositebuilder.com/trends/wp-content/uploads/sites/13/2017/11/Otago_talk_2017-2.pdf.

MacDorman MF, Mathews TJ, Declercq E: *Trends in out-of-hospital births in the United States, 1990–2012*, National Center for Health Statistics data brief no. 144. Hyattsville, MD, 2014, NCHS. Online: https://www.cdc.gov/nchs/data/databriefs/db144.pdf.

McLachlan H, Forster DA, Davey MA, Farrell T, Gold L, Biro M, et al: Effects of continuity of care by a primary midwife (caseload midwifery) on caesarean section rates in women of low obstetric risk: the COSMOS randomised controlled trial, *BJOG* 119:1483–1492, 2012.

Moore TG, Arefadib N, Deery A, West S: *The first thousand days, an evidence paper*, Parkville, Melbourne, 2017, Centre for Community Child Health, Murdoch Children's Research Institute.

National Health Performance Authority (NHPA): *Healthy communities: child and maternal health in 2009–2012*, Sydney, 2014, NHPA.

National Health Performance Authority (NHPA): *Hospital performance: costs of acute admitted patients in public hospitals in 2011–2012*, Sydney, 2015, NHPA.

National Health Service (NHS): *Implementing Better Births: a resource pack for Local Maternity Systems*, London, 2017, NHS. Online: https://www.england.nhs.uk/wp-content/uploads/2017/03/nhs-guidance-maternity-services-v1.pdf.

National Institute for Health and Care Excellence (NICE): *Intrapartum care: care of healthy women and their babies during childbirth (CG190)*, London, 2014, NICE.

O'Brien B, Harvey S, Sommerfeldt S, Beischel S, Newburn-Cook C, Schopflocher D: Comparison of costs and associated outcomes between women choosing newly integrated autonomous midwifery care and matched controls: a pilot study, *J Obstet Gynaecol Can* 32:650–656, 2010.

Page L, Beake S, Vail A, McCourt C, Hewison J: A comparative cohort study of clinical outcomes and maternal satisfaction with one-to-one midwifery practice, *Br J Midwifery* 9:700–706, 2001.

Peters L, Thornton C, de Jonge A, Khashan A, Tracy M, Downe S, et al: The effect of medical and operative birth interventions on child health outcomes in the first 28 days and up to 5 years of age: a linked data population-based cohort study, *Birth* 2018 Mar 25. doi:10.1111/birt.12348. [Epub ahead of print].

Petrou S, Boulvain M, Simon J, Maricot P, Borst F, Perneger T: Home-based care after a shortened hospital stay versus hospital-based care postpartum: an economic evaluation, *BJOG* 111:800–806, 2004.

Petrou S, Khan K: An overview of the health economic implications of elective caesarean section, *Appl Health Econ Health Policy* 11:561–576, 2013.

Piercy J, Page L, McCourt C: Economic study. In Beake S, McCourt C, Page L, editors: *Evaluation of one-to-one midwifery: second cohort study*, London, 2001, Thames Valley University, pp 77–86.

Porter M: *Values based healthcare delivery: strategy for health care leaders*, Boston, 2015, Harvard Business School.

Porter M: The strategy to transform health care and the role of outcomes, OECD Policy Forum, People at the Center: The Future of Health. Paris, 2017, OECD. Online: https://www.oecd.org/health/ministerial/policy-forum/Michael-Porter-Presentation-OECD-Health-Forum-2017.pdf.

Rayment-Jones H, Murrells T, Sandall J: An investigation of the relationship between the caseload model of midwifery for socially disadvantaged women and childbirth outcomes using routine data—a retrospective, observational study, *Midwifery* 31:409–417, 2015.

Rowley MJ, Hensley MJ, Brinsmead MW, Wlodarczyk JH: Continuity of care by a midwife team versus routine care during pregnancy and birth: a randomised trial, *Med J Aust* 163:289–293, 1995.

Ryan P, Revill P, Devane D, Normand C: An assessment of the cost-effectiveness of midwife-led care in the United Kingdom, *Midwifery* 29:368–376, 2013.

Sandall J, Homer C, Sadler E, Rudisill C, Bourgeault I, Bewley S, et al: *Staffing in maternity units: getting the right people in the right place at the right time*, London, 2011, The King's Fund. Online: https://www.kingsfund.org.uk/sites/default/files/staffing-maternity-units-kings-fund-march2011.pdf.

Sandall J, Soltani H, Gates S, Shennan A, Devane D: Midwife-led continuity models versus other models of care for childbearing women, *Cochrane Database Syst Rev* (4):CD004667, 2016.

Scarf V, Catling C, Viney R, Homer C: Costing alternative birth settings for women at low risk of complications: a systematic review, *PLoS ONE* 11:e0149463, 2016.

Scarf V, Rossiter C, Vedam S, Dahlen H, Ellwood D, Forster D, et al: Maternal and perinatal outcomes by planned place of birth among women with low-risk pregnancies in high income countries: a systematic review and meta-analysis, *Birth* 62:240–255, 2018. doi:10.1016/j.midw.2018.03.024.

Schroeder E, Petrou S, Patel N, Hollowell J, Puddicombe D, Redshaw M, et al: Cost effectiveness of alternative planned places of birth in woman at low risk of complications: evidence from the birthplace in England national prospective cohort study, *BMJ* 344:18, 2012.

Schroeder E, Petrou S, Hollowell J, Redshaw M, Brocklehurst P: *Birthplace cost-effectiveness analysis of planned place of birth: decision analytic model. Birthplace in England research programme*, Final report part 7. NIHR Service Delivery and Organisation Programme, London, 2014, HMSO.

Schroeder E, Patel N, Keeler M, Rocca-Ihenacho L, Macfarlane AJ: The economic costs of intrapartum care in Tower Hamlets: a comparison of cost between the cost of birth in a freestanding midwifery unit and hospital for women at low risk of obstetric complications, *Midwifery* 45:38–45, 2017.

Shaw D, Guise JM, Shah N, Gemzell-Danielsson K, Joseph K, Levy B, et al: Drivers of maternity care in high-income countries: can health systems support woman-centred care?, *Lancet* 388:2282–2289, 2016.

Signore C, Klebanoff M: Neonatal morbidity and mortality after elective caesarean delivery, *Clin Perinatol* 35:361–371, 2008.

Smith V, Daly D, Lundgren I, Eri T, Begley C, Gross MM, et al: Protocol for the development of a salutogenic intrapartum core outcome set (SIPCOS), *BMC Med Res Methodol* 17:61, 2017.

Stone P, Zwansiger J, Walker P, Buenting J: Economic analysis of two models of low-risk maternity care: a freestanding birth center compared to traditional care, *Res Nurs Health* 23:279–289, 2000.

Toohill J, Turkstra E, Gamble J, Scuffham PA: A non-randomised trial investigating the cost-effectiveness of Midwifery Group Practice compared with standard maternity care arrangements in one Australian hospital, *Midwifery* 28:e874–e879, 2012.

Tracy SK, Hartz D: *The quality review of Ryde Midwifery Group Practice, September 2004 to October 2005.* Final report. Sydney, 2006, Northern Sydney and Central Coast Health. Online: https://www.uts.edu.au/sites/default/files/ryde-midwifery-caseload-practice.pdf.

Tracy SK, Tracy M: Costing the cascade: estimating the cost of increased obstetric intervention in childbirth using population data, *BJOG* 110:717–724, 2003.

Tracy SK, Sullivan ES, Tracy MK: Admission of term infants to neonatal intensive care: a population based study, *Birth* 34:301–307, 2007.

Tracy SK, Hartz DL, Tracy MB, Allen J, Forti A, Hall B, et al: Caseload midwifery care versus standard maternity care for women of any risk: M@NGO, a randomised controlled trial, *Lancet* 382:1723–1732, 2013.

Tracy SK, Welsh A, Hall B, Hartz D, Lainchbury A, Bisits A, et al: Caseload midwifery compared to standard or private obstetric care for first time mothers in a public teaching hospital in Australia: a cross sectional study of cost and birth outcomes, *BMC Pregnancy Childbirth* 14:46, 2014.

Vedam S, Stoll K, MacDorman M, Declercq E, Cramer R, Cheyney M, et al: Mapping integration of midwives across the United States: impact on access, equity, and outcomes, *PLoS ONE* 13:e0192523, 2018.

von Gruenigen V, Powell D, Sorboro S, McCarroll ML, Unhee K: The financial performance of labor and delivery units, *Am J Obstet Gynecol* 209:17–19, 2013.

Yelland J, Riggs E, Small R, Brown S: Maternity services are not meeting the needs of immigrant women of non-English speaking background: results of two consecutive Australian population based studies, *Midwifery* 31:664–670, 2015.

Young D, Lees A, Twaddle S: Professional issues: the costs to the NHS of maternity care: midwife managed vs shared, *Br J Midwifery* 5:465–472, 1997.

CHAPTER 8

How to Monitor and Evaluate Midwifery Continuity of Care

Helen Cheyne, Sue Kildea, James Harris

Contents

INTRODUCTION

In this chapter we introduce monitoring and evaluation of midwifery continuity of care. We discuss why these are essential aspects of successful sustained implementation in practice and we suggest some strategies and tools that may be helpful in planning and undertaking real-world evaluations.

The chapter is not intended to be prescriptive. Midwifery care is complex, situated within maternity and health care systems that are also complex comprising a large number of interacting components—of which midwifery continuity of care is only one of its many interwoven elements. Health care systems in turn are situated within the wider political, societal and cultural frameworks of the countries in which they operate. Each of these contextual layers impacts in some way on midwifery practice. This means that midwifery continuity of care cannot easily be evaluated in isolation. People and organisations will be at different starting points in relation to the organisation of midwifery care, in the implementation of midwifery continuity of care and in the outcomes that may be anticipated. Organisations in diverse settings will have very different resources and requirements for evaluation. Our purpose is to offer some guiding principles, to stimulate thinking about evaluation and to offer those planning, implementing and working with midwifery continuity of care some ideas and tools to assist them in considering how robust, timely and useful information may support successful sustained implementation of midwifery continuity of care.

In this chapter, we introduce and discuss some models and frameworks that may be helpful to provide structure and guide the evaluation process. We then discuss approaches to data collection and data collection tools that may be used to collect information about continuity of care in real-world maternity care settings. We provide some advice on evaluation pitfalls, and how to avoid them, and give some practical examples that we hope will provide ideas and possibly inspiration for stimulating creativity in evaluating midwifery continuity of care. A number of online resources exist that might also be useful. Some of these are presented in Box 8.1.

DO WE NEED MORE EVIDENCE?

This chapter builds on earlier chapters that have presented and discussed the evidence for midwifery continuity of care. The evidence base for midwifery continuity of care has come a long way since the first edition of this book was published in 2008. At that time, although models of midwifery continuity of care had been tested in several randomised controlled trials (RCTs), the evidence was still somewhat disparate and the chapter on evaluation in the first edition had a focus on the need to generate more robust RCT evidence of effectiveness; it also introduced the ideas of complex interventions and realist evaluation—concepts that have now become much more widely accepted in research and evaluation methods. However, as Chapter 1 of this edition makes clear, the evidence base for the effectiveness of continuity of care has grown, with several new trials and systematic reviews demonstrating the benefits of midwifery continuity of care models (Sandall et al., 2016).

The research now needed is to explore the scaling up and the sustainability of midwifery continuity models and to look at their adaptation in low-income countries, or with women who have previously been excluded from trials—for example, women who are socially disadvantaged or who have significant medical or obstetric complexity in pregnancy (Homer, 2016). Although there is still a need for more large-scale research, continued evaluation work on implementation sustainability and scaling up

BOX 8.1 Useful Online Resources to Support Monitoring and Evaluation

Monitoring and evaluation methods:

Online logic model builder: https://cyfar.org/build-your-own-logic-model

Guide to developing logic models: http://www.evaluationsupportscotland.org.uk/media/uploads/resources/supportguide1.2logicmodelsjul09.pdf

Using the RE-AIM framework: http://re-aim.org/resources-and-tools/re-aim-online-module-training/.

Designing and conducting PDSA cycles: https://improvement.nhs.uk/resources/pdsa-cycles

Conducting a realist evaluation: https://www.odi.org/publications/8716-realist-impact-evaluation-introduction

Guides to implementation and evaluation:

Introduction to implementation science: http://www.bmj.com/content/347/bmj.f6753

WHO guide to reporting standards for programs in maternal and family health: http://www.who.int/maternal_child_adolescent/documents/programme-reporting-standards/en/

Evaluability assessment: a systematic approach to deciding whether and how to evaluate programs and policies: https://www.scribd.com/document/349118798/WWS-Evaluability-Assessment-Working-Paper-Final-June-2015

The Health Foundation guides: http://www.health.org.uk/collection/improvement-projects-tools-and-resources?origin=lookingfor_topnav

Undertaking a stakeholder analysis

Stakeholder mapping tool: http://personcentredcare.health.org.uk/resources/stakeholder-mapping-tool

Stakeholder mapping and analysis tool: http://www.health.gov.au/internet/main/publishing.nsf/content/ocp-mat

must be ongoing. This should not be viewed as solely the domain of researchers; rather it should be seen as essential to inform successful implementation in practice and to demonstrate the value of continuity of midwifery care in the complex landscape of competing demands in modern health care systems. For these reasons this chapter is focused on the needs of midwives, service managers and policy makers, rather than those of researchers and academics.

Well-designed monitoring and evaluation has the potential to:

- explain variation and inequity
- demonstrate links between activity and outcomes
- provide evidence of value for money
- identify progress towards longer-term goals as well as blocks and barriers
- celebrate success
- identify whether resources are being used as planned
- check that the intervention or program is reaching the right people

- identify problems early on to establish what is being encountered, and by whom, and seek solutions
- ask 'How can this work better?'
- determine whether anticipated improved outcomes are being achieved and, *most importantly*, determine whether the intervention is making a positive difference (Raine et al., 2016; The Health Foundation, 2015).

Before getting started with evaluation, there are a number key issues that need to be considered—in particular, identifying key stakeholders and deciding who to involve, considering the local context and developing common understandings of midwifery continuity of care.

IDENTIFYING KEY STAKEHOLDERS AND DECIDING WHO TO INVOLVE

Interventions do not *in themselves* bring about change; rather they provide opportunities and resources that may *enable* change if they are appropriate for the contexts into which they are introduced and are understood, taken up and used by all the relevant stakeholders (Pawson & Tilley, 2005). For this reason it is vital to think about who should be involved in planning and undertaking an evaluation (stakeholder mapping). This should include all those who may be impacted by implementation of midwifery continuity of care, either positively or negatively.

Maternity services are complex systems with networks of influence and authority. Involvement of strategic, senior stakeholders is key to successful evaluations. Failure to do so at an early stage may result in frustration due to lack of adequate resource provision to undertake the evaluation and to subsequent lack of authority to act on findings. As discussed in Chapter 2, it is equally important to engage representatives of all the relevant clinical, managerial and service user groups who have the essential 'on the ground' knowledge of how care delivery works, the barriers and enablers, and how continuity of care is experienced. There are a number of resources available to assist in undertaking a stakeholder analysis (see Box 8.1).

CONSIDER THE CONTEXT

Context is important. There is considerable evidence from a wide range of health care domains of interventions which have proven to be effective in one setting but which fail in another (Robert & Fulop, 2014) and of well-intentioned health care policies that are never applied in practice (Molloy et al., 2016). There are many reasons for this; one is that trials often fail to define adequately or to describe the intervention that has been tested, making it difficult to replicate. Recent guidance on trial reporting may lessen this problem in future trials (EQUATOR Network, 2018). Secondly, researchers, policy makers and service managers often fail to take account of the effects that local contexts will have on intervention effectiveness. It is inevitable that even large-scale multicentre trials are relatively context specific. Although more recent trials often aim to be 'pragmatic' and test the intervention in the 'real-world' setting (Loudon et al., 2015), some degree of control is intrinsic to their design. This means that those tasked with planning and implementing continuity models will almost always be faced with tailoring and adapting them to a wide range of service contexts that may be very different from those informing research (see Ch. 1).

In planning an evaluation it is important to recognise that context is never a neutral backdrop for implementation—a blank canvass on which continuity of care is played out as planned. Much has been written about the fundamental ways in which context—the physical, political, financial, environmental, resource, people and historical factors particular to care locations—interact in both positive and negative ways with a planned intervention or program (Robert & Fulop, 2014)—in this case, midwifery continuity of care The resultant outcomes may be very different from those that had been anticipated on the basis of RCT evidence.

Staff in some care settings may have travelled some way towards adopting midwifery continuity of care models and may have existing successful examples to draw on, meaning that service planners may be 'pushing on an open door'. Other settings may be more hostile towards changes, with long and deeply held negative opinions about midwifery continuity of care; in this case, implementation is likely to be considerably more challenging and the short- and medium-term outcomes (at least) are likely to be very different from those imagined. For example, the realist evaluation of normal birth pathways in Scotland (Cheyne et al., 2013) found that some NHS boards had already adopted a social model of care and many aims of the normal birth pathways had already been achieved, whereas other boards displayed deeply entrenched medical approaches to care and this exerted a powerful influence that was highly resistant to change, resulting in different outcomes from those hoped for.

DEFINING THE MIDWIFERY CONTINUITY OF CARE MODEL

Continuity of care is, superficially, a straightforward, easily understood concept; however, it can be deceptively complex to define and therefore to evaluate in practice. As discussed in Chapter 3, one issue is the lack of agreed terminology to describe the diverse models of midwifery care that have proliferated over the last two decades (Donnolley et al., 2016). This potential diversity applies where continuity models may seem superficially similar but potentially differ in important aspects, for example:

- **the number and configuration of midwives working in the model**—is there one primary midwife, midwives working in pairs or with partners, or a team / group practice? How large is the team? How are part-time midwives incorporated?

- **the women receiving care**—does the model involve low-risk women only or are high- and low-risk women included? How large is each midwife's caseload?
- **care pathways**—are all stages of the maternity care journey (antenatal, intrapartum and postnatal) included? What about planned versus unplanned episodes of care?

Although it is important to tailor models of care to local needs, the lack of agreed and recognised terminology for different models may make evaluation difficult and comparison of outcomes across services prone to misinterpretation and error. Over-arching definitions of midwifery continuity of care are available (Donnolley et al., 2016)—as described in Chapter 3—but locally agreed definitions need to be discussed, refined and understood by all stakeholders before evaluation and monitoring can be undertaken. Regional and nationally agreed terminology for the range of models of maternity care will be required for robust evaluation at national level.

One efficient method of engaging stakeholders, identifying the characteristics of contexts and agreeing operational definitions of continuity is to have an all-inclusive workshop, for example using a World Café-type setting (The World Café, 2018), in which all the stakeholders come together. Such a workshop affords the opportunity to provide an overview of best evidence, including existing local data, and get buy-in for the aims and methods of the evaluation; stakeholders can provide valuable input into designing the new model and plans for subsequent actions based on the findings (Kildea et al., 2018). An example of how this has been used in practice is given in Box 8.2.

EVALUATION PROCESSES

The field of implementation science considers the methods and strategies to bring evidence-based guidelines into routine practice. It aims to improve health care by bringing best practice directly to patient care. It examines what works, for whom and under what circumstances, and how interventions can be adapted and scaled up in ways that are accessible and equitable (Bauer et al., 2015). It is therefore an inherently useful approach to introducing and evaluating practice innovations such as midwifery continuity of care. This section takes teachings from this approach and demonstrates how they could usefully be applied when evaluating models of care.

When thinking about evaluating a midwifery continuity of care model, decision makers may want to consider the following broad questions:

1. Is the model being implemented as it was planned?
   a. Is there fidelity to the planned care model?
   b. Is there progress towards longer-term goals?
   c. Are resources being used as planned?
2. Are anticipated improved outcomes being achieved (including physical, psycho-logical and sociological outcomes)?

BOX 8.2 Engaging Stakeholders Using a World Café-style Workshop
Sue Kildea, University of Queensland and The Mater Mother's Hospital, Australia

We used a World Café-style workshop to enable dissemination of the results of an evaluation of an Aboriginal antenatal clinic and to engage stakeholders in service planning and redesign. We had been approached to conduct the service evaluation by the staff working in the clinic who believed it was underresourced to meet demand. We invited service users, community members, Aboriginal Elders, service providers and health policy representatives and it was co-facilitated by myself and the Director of Community Engagement at the Institute of Urban Indigenous Health. The day commenced by presenting evaluation findings and the overarching aim, which was to explore ideas for strengthening and integrating tertiary and primary care services and improving outcomes during pregnancy, birth and the first year of life.

Participants rotated through nine roundtables to discuss topics drawn from the evaluation: cultural competency in the health workforce; a new model of care; community engagement; family-centred care; vulnerable families and social services; and communication, collaboration and information sharing. Each table was facilitated and participants were rotated after 25 minutes. The new group built on the last group's progress and every participant had the opportunity to discuss each topic and was asked to 'aim for the sky'. Recommendations were fed back to the group and later compiled into a report for dissemination.

The workshop evaluation found this to be a successful and popular strategy with stakeholders that resulted in the development of a multiagency partnership between the tertiary hospital and two Aboriginal community-controlled organisations. Together they joined resources to establish a new model of care based on the workshop recommendations and successfully applied for funding for a community-based Mums and Bubs Hub and an evaluation. A program logic was developed based on participants' recommendations and partner inputs. See Kildea et al. (2018) for more details.

---

3. Is it acceptable and sustainable for midwives and others who may be impacted by new care models?

4. Is there evidence of value for investment of resources?

The next section of this chapter will consider some tools to aid evaluation of midwifery continuity of care models. The decision about tools used will be dependent on individual context, with some being more appropriate than others. Four different approaches are presented in order of potential complexity, starting with 'easier' evaluations and moving on to processes that require a greater amount of work and expertise.

Logic models

A logic model is a pictorial representation of a project or service that outlines how it is supposed to work and helps to identify explicitly the activities that will bring about change and expected results. It provides a systematic and visual presentation of the relationships between the resources (inputs), the planned activities and the expected results of a program or service; this often includes shorter-term outcomes, indicators for measuring and anticipated longer-term impacts (McCawley, 2001).

There are a variety of different formats, and these can have alternative names such as 'conceptual maps' and 'program theories', but the purpose of the model is to outline specific factors of the issue under investigation. These factors can include:

- inputs (the resources required for the service)
- context (the climate that the service operates in)
- activities (the actions that will be taken with the identified resources)
- outputs (the evidence that the activities were performed as planned)
- effects (the changes that occurred as an effect of the activities).

Many researchers also include a clear statement on the purpose of the initiative, along with identified assumptions, which may or may not be tested, and external factors that could influence the effects.

Fig. 8.1 illustrates a logic model developed for the POPPIE trial. The POPPIE trial aims to test the impact of a midwifery continuity of care model on women at risk of pre-term birth. The pilot trial aims to test the implementation (fidelity, acceptability to staff and women, reach, cost) of the model alongside the impact on maternal and neonatal outcomes.

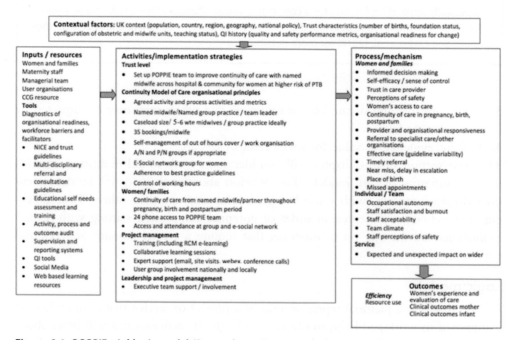

Figure 8.1 *POPPIE trial logic model (Source: https://www.medscinet.net/POPPIE).*

You can see that the trial team have spent time identifying key elements of their program, including wide-ranging **inputs** comprising people such as service commissioners (identified as 'CCGs', Clinical Commissioning Groups within the UK's NHS) and 'tools' such as local and national guidelines and education activities. These feed into **activities,** including core principles of the care model, a section on the potential **mechanisms** of action for the model (a key research question for this trial) and the potential **outcomes**. This model has helped the team to identify what to evaluate, and why, to see whether the trial has been successful.

Evaluation Support Scotland has provided a useful guide to creating a logic model for your own service: http://www.evaluationsupportscotland.org.uk/media/uploads/resources/supportguide1.2logicmodelsjul09.pdf and an online logic model builder has been created by the University of Minnesota: https://cyfar.org/build-your-own-logic-model.

Improvement science including process mapping and the PDSA cycle

Improvement science is the scientific field that explores how to undertake quality improvement in a systematic way (Improvement Science Research Network, 2018). It is a developing field that has identified a number of theories, models and frameworks that can be utilised to assess and evaluate how a service is performing. We will explain two of these simple tools here, and readers are further directed to the resources developed by The Health Foundation for other examples (The Health Foundation, 2018).

In the UK a project called NHS Improvement (2018) aims to improve the care that service users receive in the NHS. The NHS Improvement website recommends the use of a 'model for improvement' that provides a sequential process for developing, testing and implementing changes that lead to improvement. This model encourages services to identify first what is currently happening, including the processes that service users and staff follow, to enable identification of what needs to be improved: https://improvement.nhs.uk/search/?q=model+for+improvement.

Process mapping

A process is a series of connected steps or actions to achieve an outcome (Van der Waldt, 2004). It can be a prolonged process that takes significant time and resources to complete—for example, the process of a woman selecting a maternity care provider to provide all care until she is discharged from maternity services—or a short one, such as the details of an initial booking visit that includes a midwife appointment, a visit to a phlebotomist and an ultrasound scan. By plotting the process that an individual goes through, stakeholders can identify potential problems that require improvements. This is a powerful way for teams to appreciate problems from the service user's perspective. It helps to identify areas that can be improved, provide an overview of the complete process and discover where the service is failing. A process map should consider the number of stages a service user is required to take to complete a process: the total time required and how many times they are referred to another care provider, the time required for a task and any waiting, and whether or not each of these stages have value.

PDSA cycles

Once the process that a service user undertakes is clearly identified, change can be instigated to improve care. It is common for service providers to be overwhelmed by the amount of change required. The Plan, Do, Study, Act (PDSA) cycle enables people to take this improvement process in stages; the impact of small changes can be measured and built upon in small cycles until the ultimate goal of sustainable improvement is achieved. An online guide to conducting these cycles can be found at: https://improvement.nhs.uk/resources/pdsa-cycles/. Fig. 8.2 identifies the process that is required to complete a PDSA cycle. The analogy of 'how does one eat an elephant' applies here—with one small chunk at a time, improvement can be effectively measured, but also sustained.

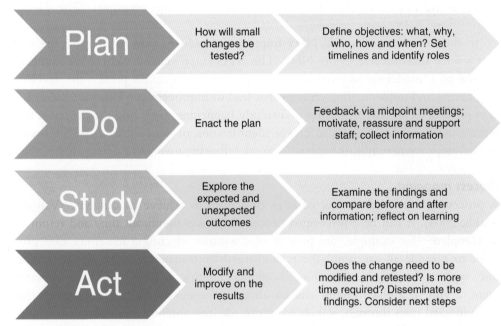

Figure 8.2 *Plan, Do, Study, Act cycle (Adapted from: http://re-aim.org/resources-and-tools/re-aim-online-module-training/).*

RE-AIM

There are a vast number of different resources to aid implementation including:

- implementation frameworks (a list of determinants that have been found to influence implementation outcomes)
- models (a guide to the process of translating research into practice)
- theories (both classic theory and specific implementation theories that suggest outcomes based on a series of empirical studies).

Nilsen (2015) provides a useful summary of these different resources. We focus here on a commonly used framework designed specifically for evaluation purposes. The RE-AIM framework was first created as a tool to test the impact of health promotion interventions, but is now used more widely to encourage service providers, policy makers and commissioners to consider essential elements of a service in order to achieve sustainable adoption and implementation of evidence-based interventions (RE-AIM, 2018).

RE-AIM is an acronym of five required areas to facilitate sustainable change—reach, efficacy / effectiveness, adoption, implementation and maintenance. Each of these elements is explained in Fig. 8.3. RE-AIM is designed to aid translation of research into practice and it provides standardised ways of measuring key factors in evaluation of health impacts. It can be used both to plan a service and to evaluate an ongoing one. The tool enables each of the five areas to be 'scored', thereby identifying areas to work on to improve the model. Readers interested in conducting a RE-AIM analysis of their care model may wish to complete the helpful online training manual, which can be found at: http://re-aim.org/resources-and-tools/re-aim-online-module-training/.

Realist evaluations

Although less-detailed evaluations may be useful in many instances, there are times when greater detail is required. A model of care may not be getting the expected results, or a small-scale introduction may require greater justification for a larger investment to achieve nationwide scaling up. In these situations, understanding the mechanisms of action while being mindful of specific contextual factors is useful. Realist evaluation can help this process.

Realist evaluation is a theory-driven approach to evaluating an intervention. It argues that for evaluations to be useful they need to adopt the framework developed by Pawson & Tilley (2005), who highlight the importance of exploring what works, for whom, in what respects, to what extent, in what contexts, and how. Realist evaluation is theoretically based on the assumption that an intervention works (or does not work) because individuals make particular decisions in response to that intervention. The 'reasoning' of the actors in response to the opportunities provided by the intervention is what causes the outcomes (Pawson, 2013). A realist evaluation has three stages:

Tools & Resources

Measures

Questions to Ask about RE-AIM Dimensions When Evaluating Health Promotion Programs and Policies

Caption: RE-AIM Dimensions and Template Questions for Evaluating Health Education and Health Behavior Research

RE-AIM Dimension	Questions
Reach (Individual Level)	What percent of potentially eligible participants a) were excluded, b) took part and c) how representative were they?
Efficacy or Effectiveness (Individual Level)	What impact did the intervention have on a) all participants who began the program; b) on process intermediate, and primary outcomes; and c) on both positive and negative (unintended), outcomes including quality of life?
Adoption (Setting Level)	What percent of settings and intervention agents within these settings (e.g., schools/educators, medical offices/physicians) a) were excluded, b) participated and c) how representative were they?
Implementation (Setting/agent Level)	To what extent were the various intervention components delivered as intended (in the protocol), especially when conducted by different (non-research) staff members in applied settings?
Maintenance (Individual Level)	What were the long-term effects (minimum of 6-12 months following intervention)? b) What was the attrition rate; were drop-outs representative; and how did attrition impact conclusions about effectiveness?
Maintenance (Setting Level)	a) To what extent were different intervention components continued or institutionalized? b) How was the original program modified?

Figure 8.3 *Questions to ask about RE-AIM dimensions when evaluating midwifery continuity models (Source: http://re-aim.org/wp-content/uploads/2016/09/questions.pdf).*

1. **Development of initial program theory**—this identifies how the mechanisms of the intervention interact with specific context issues to lead to expected outcomes. These can be developed through previous research, knowledge and / or experience. For example, if a woman has midwifery continuity of care with someone whom she identifies with, then she is able to build a trusting relationship.

2. **Choosing the evaluation methods**—realist evaluations are method neutral and can use quantitative data (e.g. birth outcome data), qualitative data (e.g. interviews to test satisfaction) or a combination. The method chosen should be guided by the program theories that are being tested. Most commonly, a mixed-methods approach is used.

3. **The realist data analysis approach**—the analytical approach takes a similar approach to qualitative thematic analysis, but rather than developing themes the aim is to develop 'context–mechanism–outcome' statements—for example, 'In a large health care setting, provision of a continuity of care model for socially

---

BOX 8.3 A Realist Evaluation of Midwifery Continuity of Care Models for Socially Vulnerable Women

Hannah Rayment-Jones, PhD Candidate, King's College London

Social vulnerabilities lead to health inequalities. Women living in areas of highest poverty are over 50% more likely to experience a stillbirth or neonatal death in the UK. They are also subject to increased rates of premature birth, low birth weight and maternal death.

Evidence suggests that women with socially complex lives who receive relational continuity of care have better birth outcomes, less clinical interventions, shorter hospital stays and increased liaison with support services. However, we do not yet know what specific models of care work best for socially vulnerable women, or what the mechanisms of action are for these models.

I am currently undertaking a doctoral study using realist evaluation methodologies to try to address these questions. It aims to identify, for women with low socioeconomic status living complex lives, what model of care works to improve their outcomes and how it works. The project will be undertaken in two distinct phases: identifying program theories and conducting a realist evaluation.

The program theories will be identified through two reviews: one identifying what works for this group of women, and another exploring how these women experience their care. These theories will then be tested via an ethnographic comparison of two differing models of care: one that takes a geographical approach, located in an area of significant health inequality, and another that provides a specialist approach where women are referred to the team based on inclusion criteria of social risk factors.

Through immersion in the settings I will test the mutual influence of the context and care delivered within each model, and its impact on outcomes such as practitioner–mother interactions, clinical outcomes and cost effectiveness. Other methods will include interviews and focus groups along with quantitative measurements of engagement and birth outcomes.

It is hoped that, following completion of this work, services will be in a better position to tailor their services to meet the needs of the women at greatest risk of negative outcomes during their pregnancy.

---

vulnerable women enabled a building of trust between woman and midwife generating better birth outcomes'.

A more detailed introductory guide to realist evaluation can be found at: https://www.odi.org/publications/8716-realist-impact-evaluation-introduction.

The vignette in Box 8.3 shows how realist evaluation is being used in an ongoing study of midwifery continuity care models for women in vulnerable situations in the UK.

Economic evaluations

Economics clearly has an important role in any service provision (Shiell et al., 2002). Not only will commissioners want to see value for money, but those providing services will also want to ensure a sustainable model with adequate staffing.

BOX 8.4 An Example of a Cost Analysis for a Midwifery Continuity of Care Model

Yu Gao, Obstetric and Health Economics, University of Queensland, Australia

Maternity care uses significant resources within the health care system with resource usage increasing across the world as more births become medicalised. With limited resources the policy makers need to consider not only the efficacy but also the cost when designing and implementing a new maternity service. There are four types of economic evaluations, which differ according to the measurement costs and consequences.[a] A cost–consequences analysis reports the costs of resources used in the delivery of maternity care and the clinical outcomes (e.g. caesarean section rates, % of babies admitted to neonatal nursery). The cost-effectiveness analysis compares costs with a single clinical outcome that may differ between the alternative programs. The cost–utility analysis compares costs with a generic outcome, usually expressed as quality-adjusted life-years. Cost–benefit analysis requires program benefits to be valued in monetary units to examine the 'willingness-to-pay' for the health outcomes (e.g. by individual, insurance, agencies or government).

In 2014, we published a health economic evaluation using a cost–consequences analysis technique to compare midwifery group practice (MGP) with standard care.[b] The new program aimed at improving the maternal and infant health outcomes of Aboriginal women and their infants in the Northern Territory of Australia. A MGP was established and women and their infants were followed for 1 year to investigate whether the MGP service was cost-effective from the NT Department of Health perspective. The results showed that women who received MGP care had significantly more antenatal care, had more ultrasound scans, were more likely to be admitted to hospital antenatally and had more postnatal care. The MGP cohort had significantly reduced length of stay for infants admitted to special care nursery. The study found a non-significant cost savings of $703 for the MGP cohort for the whole antenatal–birth–postnatal episode. The study demonstrated that the new MGP model is a cost-effective maternity service, where women received better care with equivalent birth outcomes at lower cost.

[a]Drummond MF, Sculpher MJ, Torrance GW, O'Brien BJ, Stoddart GL 2005 *Methods for the economic evaluation of health care programmes.* Oxford University Press.
[b]Gao Y, Gold L, Josif C, Bar-Zeev S, Steenkamp M, Barclay L, et al. 2014 A cost–consequences analysis of midwifery group practice for Aboriginal mothers and infants in the top end of the Northern Territory, Australia. *Midwifery* 30(4): 447-455.

Health economics provides a set of analytical techniques to test whether a service is *efficient*—achieving its aims with an appropriate amount of resources—and *equitable*—ensuring that services are fair (not necessarily equal) for all. Efficiency may consider technical elements (testing how to maximise positive outcomes of continuity models for least cost) or allocative elements (how many women should receive a continuity model without there being no increase in benefits). Equity may consider horizontal elements—ensuring equal access for equal need—and vertical equity—how many more resources do socially vulnerable women need over those without vulnerability? Chapter 7 provides greater detail on economic evaluations. Box 8.4 provides as example of how an economic evaluation was used in an Australian study (Gao et al., 2014).

Tools for evaluation of continuity of care

The previous section has introduced different approaches and frameworks to help structure effective monitoring and evaluation of midwifery continuity of care. These will help you to identify clearly your objectives, think about realistic outcomes and identify points in the process where information should be collected, analysed and fed back into the system to facilitate change. We have highlighted the importance of involving key stakeholders and informants at the early stages of planning for implementation and evaluation. However, once you have an overarching strategy you then need to think about the ways of collecting the information you need.

No one source of information will be enough for a robust and useful evaluation. Just as a craftsman uses different tools for different tasks, a range of data collection tools are needed, with the choice of tool dictated by the type of information required and the sources of that data—for example, you may want to use data from individual case records, maternity service level data on clinical outcomes or workforce, or the views and experiences of staff or service users. These sources of data all require different tools for data collection. In this section we discuss different sources of data and types of data collection tools addressing the evaluation questions we posed earlier.

Is the model being implemented as it was planned?
Dimensions of continuity

Continuity of care has three dimensions: relational, informational and management (Haggerty et al., 2003; Saultz, 2003; Saultz & Lochner, 2005) (Fig. 8.4). **Relational** or **interpersonal continuity** incorporates the notion of *relationship* experienced by an individual woman and her care providers *over time*. In this book, midwifery continuity of care is further defined as care that is provided throughout the antenatal, labour and birth and postnatal continuum by a named or primary midwife or small group of midwives whom the woman gets to know during pregnancy (continuity of carer). How this definition is interpreted and operationalised in your maternity policy and service will be central to decisions about what data to collect in assessing whether continuity of care has been provided as planned over time and whether positive relationships between a woman and her midwife / midwives have been established as a result.

Informational continuity is concerned with consistency of information giving across care providers whereas **management continuity** relates to seamlessness in coordinating different services or in management of different health care problems. It is important to consider these aspects of continuity as they are important to women (i.e. women often report receiving conflicting advice, and disconnection between

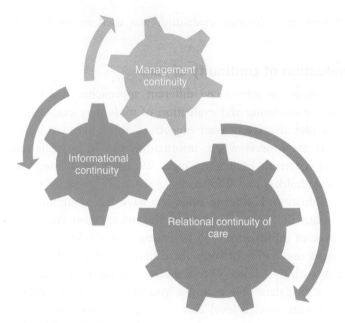

Figure 8.4 *Dimensions of continuity*

home and hospital care and in referrals to other services, such as neonatal care or family doctors). Many problems in these dimensions of continuity may be ameliorated by effective relational continuity of care; however, the provision of safe maternity care requires the involvement of or transfer between wider health care and social systems, and seamless coordination between services and consistency of information are optimal so they do need to be assessed in any evaluation.

Assessing fidelity to relational continuity of care models

Assessing fidelity (i.e. the extent to which relational continuity of care is being implemented as planned) can be undertaken in two main ways: auditing clinical records sources, either individual records or maternity data systems, and asking women about their experience of care.

Here we describe two indices / measures of relational continuity based on work by Jee & Cabana (2006):

- **Density**—is the proportion of care provided by the main care provider, in this case the primary midwife or caseload holder. The denominator is the total number of care contacts during a defined period. This might be the complete maternity care journey including antenatal, intrapartum and postnatal care or defined portions of that journey. Density is calculated as the number of care episodes provided by the caseload holder / primary midwife as a proportion of total care episodes.
- **Dispersion**—is a measure of the total number of staff involved relative to the total number of care episodes.

Combining these two measures may be the most useful approach—that is, how many different care providers were there in total *and* what proportion of care was given by the primary midwife. However, this may be tricky in practice and there are some additional things to think about. Maternity care is a relatively discrete care journey with a broadly defined length (although there may be some local differences—e.g. in duration of postnatal care) so it is generally possible to determine the total number of planned care episodes. This is important as, for example, meeting three different midwives in a total of 15 care episodes is very different from meeting three midwives in four care episodes. The majority of care episodes may be planned or semi-planned. However, there will also be some unplanned episodes of care that fall outside the pathway (e.g. attendances at daycare or ultrasound clinics, antenatal education group sessions and drop-in days) and some women will have complex coexisting medical, obstetric or social conditions that may also require involvement of midwives within the wider multidisciplinary team.

Taking these issues into account, before embarking on an audit you need to:

1. Define the denominator (total care episodes) and ensure everyone involved understands and agrees.
   a. Decide what constitutes a 'care episode', and whether to include or exclude unplanned care episodes.
   b. Decide on which periods of care are involved (i.e. antenatal care, intrapartum care, hospital postnatal care, community-based care or the total maternity care pathway).
2. Define 'care provider': is this the midwife who provides a primary task at a particular point on the care pathway (e.g. an antenatal or postnatal assessment), does it include other midwives who provide additional care and does it involve other members of the maternity care team?

The sources of data for audit are at the individual level. The advantage of audit is that it provides relatively objective data on adherence to planned care pathways. However, data may be very labour intensive to collect, and it can often be difficult to define and distinguish care providers; defining care episodes can also be tricky and interpreting findings may be difficult. For example, there might be a situation where the primary midwife may have been attending a woman in labour for 12 hours and has gone home an hour before the birth.

Data collection forms or spreadsheets (often known as proforma) may need to be developed locally to reflect local case records or information systems and care pathways. Proforma are familiar in many health care situations; they may be in paper- or computer-based formats and they standardise the data to be collected and the format of that data for each case. It may be most efficient if midwives audit their own caseload, or each undertakes audit of a small number of cases (see Box 8.5 for an example).

Data collected should be anonymised and secure storage of computer- and/or paper-based records will be essential and must comply with local ethics and governance procedures.

BOX 8.5 Auditing Continuity of Carer to Enable Change

Jaki Lambert, Consultant Lead Midwife from Argyle and Bute in NHS Highland

Argyle and Bute in the West of Scotland includes many remote and rural communities. There are five free-standing community maternity units (CMU) all serving distinct and distant communities. With 23 inhabited islands the midwives' journey for one appointment can entail a 3-day round trip from the islands, with the west coast weather always playing a part. The nearest consultant unit is 137 miles from the furthest CMU and 22 miles (with a ferry ride) from the nearest.

On average, 500 women annually receive their care from the five midwifery teams. Each team has a minimum of five whole-time equivalent midwives in order to provide 24/7 services; some are larger depending on caseload numbers. Caseloads are smaller than those in urban areas but it may take a day to provide one visit in Argyle and Bute and this has influenced how the service has developed. The midwife teams have built a strong, resilient network that provides mutual support, agreed standards, shared learning, cross-cover and a shared identity. Weekly huddles and monthly video-linked clinical supervision sessions help create a community of practice.

The results of a local survey in 2016 indicated that many more women wanted to give birth locally and that they wanted continuity of care and were dissatisfied with long waits for visits. A baseline review showed that levels of antenatal continuity of carer ranged from 36% to 85%. The team leads sat down to define what they regarded as continuity and agreed that it was care from the named midwife for planned care, birth and postnatal care.

Each team then took ownership of meeting with local stakeholders, developing driver diagrams and action plans for their own services and deciding what they would aim for in terms of continuity and how they were going to achieve it. Teams have the freedom to identify local solutions, but all the data and outcomes are entered onto a database on a shared drive monthly. The database includes a range of information about each woman including transfers, births and outcomes. The results are shared with all of the teams.

Just by increasing the focus on the value of continuity and by collecting data, change was possible. The process of development and ongoing audit enabled midwives to influence and make decisions about how care is provided and they are better able to support women to exercise choice. It is wonderful to hear midwives taking pride in how they are supporting the women and families in their communities, but where this is most successful it is built on the teams working together to find local solutions and help each other out.

Over 70% of women in the survey wanted continuity of consultant. It is taking time but we are nearly there with a telehealth solution to appointments, which allows the midwife to be with the woman on the island and link into the consultant on the mainland. The hardest part is finding solutions to the continuity for the over 60% of women who were high risk at term and where local birth is not a preferred option. Realistic solutions that improve incrementally from where we are now are being considered to enable cross-board working. There is enthusiasm for following women, especially the more vulnerable women, to the hub unit as a means of gaining clinical exposure in the hub unit.

Continuity of care from the perspective of the woman

The three dimensions of continuity (relational, information and management) may be assessed by asking women about their experiences of care; indeed, this may be the most effective and efficient approach. Although women may not be able to remember precisely how many midwives they met, they will remember whether they saw the same midwife most of the time, whether they saw too many (or too few) midwives) and whether they saw a midwife who was known to them at key points of their maternity care journey. Informational and management community and many of the outcomes associated with continuity of care are strongly related to women's experiences and may be assessed only by asking women about their experiences—for example, did they experience: confidence, trusting and supportive relationships with their midwife/midwives; consistency of information giving and advice; or receiving care from someone who knew them and who took their personal circumstances into account? Women will also be able to provide information about negative aspects of continuity—for example, experiencing poor communication, having a midwife whom they did not like or form a relationship with, or experiencing instances where care was fragmented.

Women's experiences of continuity of care may be elicited through questionnaires or interviews. Interviews are more likely to be used for research than for local evaluation; while superficially straightforward to undertake, conducting useful interviews is a skilled research task and, unless interviewers not directly involved in the women's maternity care are used, biases may be introduced that may make findings meaningless.

Questionnaires may be more useful and avoid some of the opportunities for bias. They have the advantage of asking standard, predetermined questions of all women surveyed. They are a relatively inexpensive and efficient method of gathering data from large numbers of women. However, the lack of flexibility can be a disadvantage. It may be difficult to create questions that are relevant to all women in any maternity care setting, in particular the cross-cultural or multilingual contexts, and response rates can be low with systematic non-reponse by some groups. Questionnaires also require some level of literacy and this may disadvantage some groups of women.

It is also important to consider the timing of questionnaire administration. If questionnaires are administered too close to (or during) maternity care, or administered by care providers, women may feel obliged to give positive or desirable answers. If they are administered at a point too distant from maternity care then it may be more difficult to make contact as many women move home after giving birth or may move to stay with relatives. Ideally, questionnaires should be administered between 2 and 6 months following the birth, with options for completion methods (paper, online, via telephone or other face-to-face contact) and with facilities for translation into at least the main local languages. Evaluators need to consider costs of post and payments (e.g. paid-return envelopes) as well as issues of confidentiality and data protection. Ethics approval may also be required.

In general, it is advisable to use or adapt pre-existing questionnaires as these have the advantage of having undergone robust processes of development and testing, and in some cases are validated to ensure that they do assess the construct/idea that they aim to (in this case, dimensions of continuity of care) and that they are understandable and straightforward to complete.

There are many examples of such questionnaires and we suggest some here. There are a few points to be aware of, however. Some questionnaires are free to access and use whereas others need to be purchased. All published questionnaires will be subject to copyright and their use will need to be acknowledged. It may be necessary to seek permission of the author to adapt the questionnaire to local context.

The UK national maternity surveys undertaken in England and Scotland have used the Care Quality Commission (CQC) maternity survey questionnaire (the version used in Scotland has been adapted slightly to the local context). These questionnaires include some questions about relational continuity—for example, 'If you saw a midwife for your antenatal check-ups, did you see the same one every time?' (CQC, 2018)—and informational continuity—for example, 'Did you feel that midwives and other health professionals gave you consistent advice about feeding your baby?' (NHS Scotland, 2015). These questionnaires have the advantage of extensive testing and successful use in successive large-scale surveys. However, although they are useful in providing benchmark measures of experience of continuity across a maternity service, they are designed to capture a large amount of general information about maternity care experience rather than to address the multidimensional nature of continuity specifically.

Many questionnaires have been developed and validated to assess continuity of care (Uijen et al., 2011) in a range of patient or disease groups; however, many of these do not readily adapt for maternity care contexts as, for example, they may focus on information and management continuity across diverse care providers. One potential exception is the Nijmegen Continuity Questionnaire (NCQ), which is a generic measure for continuity of care (Uijen et al., 2011). It was developed in the Netherlands and is designed to measure perceptions of relational, team and cross-boundary continuity; it is not specific to care setting and is validated for general health populations. An English language version is freely available from the lead author (Uijen) on request; however, the questionnaire does require some further refinement and validation for use in English language maternity care settings. Another useful example of a questionnaire is the one used in the COSMOS trial to assess whether women knew midwives who cared for them in labour; several questions address the potential complexity of this issue (Forster et al., 2016).

Are anticipated improved outcomes being achieved (including physical, psychological and sociological outcomes)?

Midwifery continuity of care has been associated with a number of important clinical and psychosocial outcomes, as described in earlier chapters. Although it will always be important to monitor and assess these outcomes as part of evaluating the implementation and long-term impacts of continuity of care models into routine practice, some caution must be exercised in interpreting findings, in particular in assuming causation from associations. This means that, although particular outcomes may be observed at the same time that midwifery continuity of care models are introduced, it does not also mean that the model has *caused* the observed outcomes, which is particularly important when assessing outcomes that are relatively rare (although very important) including serious events such as stillbirth or pre-term labour. Randomised controlled trials are designed to take account of rarer events and often have data-monitoring committees that investigate the occurrence of adverse events occurring in the course of a trial. In undertaking an evaluation of midwifery continuity of care models it is important to monitor serious but rare events; however, common errors of thinking—described as heuristics and biases—can result in wrong conclusions being drawn from assuming cause and effect and in extrapolating from small numbers of occurrences. It may be more useful to assess the circumstances surrounding the occurrence of serious adverse outcomes using locally agreed clinical governance procedures that are able to take local contextual factors into account.

Most of the clinical outcomes that are reported to be associated with continuity of care will be readily available through routine maternity care data systems. Others, in particular outcomes relating to women's experiences of care and longer-term health outcomes, will need to be collected using questionnaires, as discussed below.

Women's experience of care

As described above, asking women about the care they have experienced is an important means of assessing process (i.e. is it happening?) issues. However, women's experience is also an important source of information on outcomes associated with midwifery continuity of care models. Surveys such as the UK CQC questionnaire (CQC, 2018) include questions useful for assessing women's experience of specific elements of care that relate to care quality (safe, effective, person centred, timely, equitable) (Institute of Medicine, 2001) and many of these elements are also important outcomes that are associated with midwifery continuity of carer (e.g involvement in decision making, having confidence and trust in those providing care, experiencing good communication).

The CQC and other similar questionnaires do not, however, generally assess women's satisfaction with their care. 'Satisfaction' is an often-used but poorly defined term (Sawyer et al., 2013). It is related to care experience but is also partly related to the health and wellbeing of the mother and her baby (Waldenström et al., 2004) and also to individual expectations of care (Ware et al., 1983); this means that it is possible for a woman to be satisfied with care that may not have been high quality if her expectations of care were low. Women's satisfaction should not be used as the only measure of care quality; nevertheless women's satisfaction with their maternity care is an important outcome that is frequently associated with continuity of care models.

A comparative review (Sawyer et al., 2013) examined nine measures of women's satisfaction with labour and birth and recommended three options: the intrapartal-specific Quality from the Patient's Perspective questionnaire (QPP-I) (Wilde-Larsson et al., 2010) was considered useful for in-depth measure of satisfaction with labour and birth; for more brief measures the review suggested either Six Simple Questions (SSQ) (Harvey et al., 2002) or Perceptions of Care Adjective Checklist (PCACL-R) (Redshaw & Martin, 2009).

The Childbirth Experience Questionnaire (Dencker et al., 2010) is a valid and reliable measure of childbirth experience; it was initially developed in Sweden and was recently validated for use in UK maternity services (Walker et al., 2015). It uses 22 closed questions (Likert scale and visual analogue scales) across four domains: own capacity (e.g. 'I felt capable during labour and birth'), professional support (e.g 'My midwife understood my needs'), perceived safety (e.g. 'I have many positive memories from childbirth') and participation (e.g. 'I felt I could have a say in deciding my birthing position'). This questionnaire has been validated for use in UK maternity services. It is recognised, though, that many of the existing tools to measure women's experiences appear to be designed to assess fragmented models of care rather than midwifery continuity of care. It is likely that new tools will be developed in future years to enable better benchmarking and quality improvement (Perriman & Davis, 2016).

A number of tools and instruments exist to assess mental health and psychological wellbeing. These include the following.

- The **Edinburgh Postnatal Depression Scale** (Cox et al., 1987)—is a commonly used tool to screen for symptoms of depression. It is estimated to take approximately 5 minutes and we would recommend that referral pathways are in place for women scoring high on this scale if it is not anonymous. Women must be informed of this prior to answering these questions.
- The **Kessler Psychological Distress Scale** (Kessler et al., 2002) is a 10-item scale that takes only 3 minutes to complete. It has been shown to be a sensitive screen for anxiety and mood disorders and has been validated for use with First Nations peoples in Canada (Bougie et al., 2016) and Aboriginal and Torres Strait Islander people in Australia (McNamara et al., 2014), although neither were in childbearing populations.
- The **Warwick–Edinburgh Mental Wellbeing Scale** (Warwick Medical School, 2015) is a validated tool for assessing mental wellbeing (it is not a screening tool for mental illness) and may be useful as part of evaluations of interventions or

programs that may have an impact on mental wellbeing. It comprises a 14-item scale in which all items are worded positively, making analysis straightforward, and is summed to provide a single score ranging from 14 to 70.
- The **Depression, Anxiety and Stress Scale–21** (Lovibond & Lovibond, 1995) uses three self-report scales (of 7 items each) to measure negative emotional states of depression, anxiety and stress. Scoring is classified into categories of normal, mild, moderate, severe and extremely severe.

When deciding on which scale to use and how to analyse and report the findings, we suggest seeking advice and support from a researcher in this field before you start collecting any data. In particular, you will need to think through what referral mechanisms you have in place to manage timely and sensitive referral.

Is the model sustainable?

The above sections have looked at ways of assessing whether midwifery continuity of care is being implemented as planned and whether its anticipated benefits are being achieved by women and babies. This section discusses ways of assessing the sustainability of midwifery continuity of care programs. This really relates to whether a model of care is acceptable and sustainable for the stakeholders involved in providing the model or who may be impacted by it.

Midwives are the key resource in the midwifery continuity of care model. It is essential to consider their skills, confidence and the positive and negative impacts a midwifery continuity of care model may have both on the midwives and on other team members involved and those around them who are essential support networks. A variety of surveys and tools have been used to measure the acceptability of the program to service users and staff, and work-related stress, to help to ascertain the optimum caseload (number of women birthing per midwife per month) and to inform on program sustainability. Surveys may be anonymous and should always be voluntary and confidential.

A critical part of sustainability is whether the model of care is acceptable to the midwives working in it. Collecting data on unplanned sick leave may provide some information on whether the model of care is causing undue stress in the midwives. A number of tools may also be useful for assessing burnout and sustainability. These include the following:
- The **Copenhagen Burnout Inventory** (Kristensen et al., 2005) measures the degree of physical and psychological fatigue experience in three dimension of burnout: personal, work-related and client-related. All items use a 5-point scale and scores range from low through moderate and high to severe.
- The **Perceptions of Empowerment in Midwifery Scale** (Matthews et al., 2009) measures midwives' perceptions of their workplace and role across four subscales: autonomy, manager support, professional recognition, skills and resources. Higher scores indicate stronger feelings of empowerment.

- The **MBI Human Services Survey** (Maslach & Jackson, 2018) is universally recognised as a measure of burnout and has been validated across a number of studies and in a number of countries. Professional burnout may need to be considered when changing models of care and the Human Services Survey measures dimensions of burnout. The questionnaire includes 22 7-point Likert scales that explore three aspects of burnout syndrome.

In a survey, open-ended questions can ask midwives to consider what is working well in their roles and what is not working so well, with the option of suggesting improvements. Midwives are also asked to identify which of the issues that aren't working so well they would most like to change. Other ways of collecting data from midwives and other stakeholders would be in focus groups and interviews where the elements of sustainability care be exploded in depth including who it is working for, how is it working, whether it can continue into the future and what needs to change to ensure ongoing sustainability. Again, seeking advice from a researcher will be invaluable to ensure that you use the most appropriate tools and can analyse the data and report the findings.

CONCLUSION

Monitoring and evaluation of midwifery continuity of care is an essential component of implementation. Some of the key questions to ask in any monitoring and evaluation process include: What is the model?; What dimensions of continuity of care are being achieved?; Is it being implemented in the way it was intended; Is it working for the women, midwives and health system?; What does it cost?; and What needs to change to improve the model or build on its successes? It is essential to consider the context in which the model of care is being evaluated as each context will be specific and have its own challenges and benefits.

Monitoring and evaluation is a specialised field and this chapter has provided only an overview of some of the principles and tools that might be useful. Seeking advice and support from evaluators and researchers is important to enable you to design your evaluation to ensure that you will find the answers to the questions you are asking. Start thinking about the evaluation as you design your model of care, rather than along the way, as this will ultimately mean that you will ask the right questions and that the results you obtain can guide improvements and adaptations.

REFERENCES

Bauer M, Damschroder L, Hagedorn H, Smith J, Kilbourne A: An introduction to implementation science for the non-specialist, *BMC Psychol* 3:32, 2015.
Bougie E, Arim R, Kohen D, Findlay L: Validation of the 10-item Kessler Psychological Distress Scale (K10) in the 2012 Aboriginal peoples survey, *Health Rep* 27:3–10, 2016.

Care Quality Commission (CQC): *2017 survey of women's experiences of maternity care*. Statistical release, Newcastle upon Tyne, 2018, CQC. Online: https://www.cqc.org.uk/sites/default/files/20180130_mat17_statisticalrelease.pdf.

Cheyne H, Abhyankar P, McCourt C: Empowering change: realist evaluation of a Scottish government programme to support normal birth, *Midwifery* 29:1110–1121, 2013.

Cox JL, Holden JM, Sagovsky R: Detection of postnatal depression. Development of the ten point Edinburgh Postnatal Depression Scale, *Br J Psychiatry* 150:172–176, 1987.

Dencker A, Taft C, Bergqvist L, Lilja H, Berg M: Childbirth experience questionnaire (CEQ): development and evaluation of a multidimensional instrument, *BMC Pregnancy Childbirth* 10:81, 2010.

Donnolley N, Butler-Henderson K, Chapman M, Sullivan E: The development of a classification system for maternity models of care, *Health Inf Manag* 45:64–70, 2016.

Drummond M, Sculpher M, Torrance G, O'Brien B, Stoddart G: *Methods for the economic evaluation of health care programmes*, ed 3, Oxford, 2005, Oxford University Press.

EQUATOR Network: *Enhancing the quality and transparency of health research*, 2018. Online: https://www.equator-network.org.

Forster D, McLachlan H, Davey M, Biro M, Farrell T, Gold L, et al: Continuity of care by a primary midwife (caseload midwifery) increases women's satisfaction with antenatal, intrapartum and post-partum care: results from the COSMOS randomised controlled trial, *BMC Pregnancy Childbirth* 16:28, 2016.

Gao Y, Gold L, Josif C, Bar-Zeev S, Steenkamp M, Barclay L, et al: A cost-consequences analysis of a midwifery group practice for Aboriginal mothers and infants in the top end of the Northern Territory, Australia, *Midwifery* 30:447–455, 2014.

Haggerty JL, Reid RJ, Freeman GK, Starfield BH, Adair CE, McKendry R: Continuity of care: a multidisciplinary review, *BMJ* 327:1219–1221, 2003.

Harvey S, Rach D, Stainton M, Jarrell J, Brant R: Evaluation of satisfaction with midwifery care, *Midwifery* 18:260–267, 2002.

Homer C: Models of maternity care: evidence for midwifery continuity of care, *Med J Aust* 205:370–374, 2016.

Improvement Science Research Network: *What is improvement science?*, 2018. Online: https://isrn.net/about/improvement_science.asp.

Institute of Medicine (USA): *Committee on quality of health care in America. Crossing the quality chasm: a new health system for the 21st century*, Washington, 2001, National Academy Press. Online: https://www.ncbi.nlm.nih.gov/books/NBK222274/pdf/Bookshelf_NBK222274.pdf.

Jee S, Cabana M: Indices for continuity of care: a systematic review of the literature, *Med Care Res Rev* 63:158–188, 2006.

Kessler R, Andrews G, Colpe L, Hiripi E, Mroczek D, Normand S, et al: Short screening scales to monitor population prevalences and trends in non-specific psychological distress, *Psychol Med* 32:959–976, 2002.

Kildea S, Hickey S, Nelson C, Currie J, Carson A, Reynolds M, et al: Birthing on country (in our community): a case study of engaging stakeholders and developing a best-practice Indigenous maternity service in an urban setting, *Aust Health Rev* 42(2):230–238, 2018. doi:10.1071/AH16218.

Kristensen T, Borritz M, Villadsen E, Christensen K: The Copenhagen Burnout Inventory: a new tool for the assessment of burnout, *Work Stress* 19:192–207, 2005.

Loudon K, Treweek S, Sullivan F, Donnan P, Thorpe K, Zwarenstein M: The PRECIS-2 tool: designing trials that are fit for purpose, *BMJ* 350:h2147, 2015.

Lovibond P, Lovibond S: The structure of negative emotional states: comparison of the Depression Anxiety Stress Scales (DASS) with the Beck Depression and Anxiety Inventories, *Behav Res Ther* 33:335–343, 1995.

McCawley P: *Logic model for program planning and evaluation*, Moscow, Idaho, 2001, University of Idaho.

McNamara B, Banks E, Gubhaju L, Williamson A, Joshy G, Raphael B, et al: Measuring psychological distress in older Aboriginal and Torres Strait Islanders Australians: a comparison of the K-10 and K-5, *Aust N Z J Public Health* 38:567–573, 2014.

Maslach C, Jackson S: MBI: Human Services Survey, 2018. Online: https://www.mindgarden.com/314-mbi-human-services-survey.

Matthews A, Scott P, Gallagher P: The development and psychometric evaluation of the perceptions of empowerment in midwifery scale, *Midwifery* 25:327–335, 2009.

Molloy A, Martin S, Gardner T, Leatherman S: *A clear road ahead. Creating a coherent quality strategy for the English NHS*, London, 2016, The Health Foundation. Online: https://www.health.org.uk/sites/health/files/AClearRoadAhead.pdf.

National Health Service (NHS) Scotland: *Maternity care survey*. Edinburgh, 2015, Government of Scotland. Online: http://www.gov.scot/Resource/0048/00488961.pdf.

Nilsen P: Making sense of implementation theories, models and frameworks, *Implement Sci* 10:53, 2015. doi:10.1186/s13012-015-0242-0.

Pawson R: *The science of evaluation: a realist manifesto*, London, 2013, Sage.

Pawson R, Tilley N: *Realistic evaluation*, London, 2005, Sage.

Perriman N, Davis D: Measuring maternal satisfaction with maternity care: a systematic integrative review: What is the most appropriate, reliable and valid tool that can be used to measure maternal satisfaction with continuity of maternity care?, *Women Birth* 29:293–299, 2016.

Raine R, Fitzpatrick R, Barratt H, Bevan G, Black N, Boaden R: Challenges, solutions and future directions in the evaluation of service innovations in health care and public health, *Health Serv Res* 4:16, 2016.

RE-AIM: RE-AIM resources, 2018. Online: http://www.re-aim.org/.

Redshaw M, Martin C: Validation of a perceptions of care adjective checklist, *J Eval Clin Pract* 15:281–288, 2009.

Robert G, Fulop N: *The role of context in successful improvement. Perspectives on context. A selection of essays considering the role of context in successful quality improvement*, London, 2014, The Health Foundation.

Sandall J, Soltani H, Gates S, Shennan A, Devane D: Midwife-led continuity models versus other models of care for childbearing women, *Cochrane Database Syst Rev* (9):CD004667, 2016.

Saultz J: Defining and measuring interpersonal continuity of care, *Ann Fam Med* 1:134–143, 2003.

Saultz J, Lochner J: Interpersonal continuity of care and care outcomes: a critical review, *Ann Fam Med* 3:159–166, 2005.

Sawyer A, Ayers S, Abbott J, Gyte G, Rabe H, Duley L: Measures of satisfaction with care during labour and birth: a comparative review, *BMC Pregnancy Childbirth* 13:108, 2013.

Shiell A, Donaldson C, Mitton C, Currie G: Health economic evaluation, *J Epidemiol Community Health* 56:85–88, 2002.

The Health Foundation: *Evaluation: what to consider*, London, 2015, The Health Foundation. Online: https://www.health.org.uk/sites/health/files/EvaluationWhatToConsider.pdf.

The Health Foundation: *Improvement projects, tools and resources*, London, 2018, The Health Foundation. Online: http://www.health.org.uk/collection/improvement-projects-tools-and-resources?origin=lookingfor_topnav.

The World Café: *World Café method*, 2018. Online: http://www.theworldcafe.com/key-concepts-resources/world-cafe-method.

Uijen A, Schellevis F, van den Bosch W, Mokkink H, Van Weel C, Schers HJ: Nijmegen continuity questionnaire: development and testing of a questionnaire that measures continuity of care, *J Clin Epidemiol* 64:1391–1399, 2011.

Van der Waldt G: *Managing performance in the public sector: concepts, considerations and challenges*, Cape Town, 2004, Juta & Co.

Waldenström U, Hildingsson I, Rubertsson C, Radestad I: A negative birth experience: prevalence and risk factors in a national sample, *Birth* 31:17–26, 2004.

Walker K, Wilson P, Bugg G, Dencker A, Thornton J: Childbirth experience questionnaire: validating its use in the United Kingdom, *BMC Pregnancy Childbirth* 15:86, 2015.

Ware J, Snyder M, Wright R, Davies A: Defining and measuring patient satisfaction with medical care, *Eval Program Plann* 6:247–263, 1983.

Warwick Medical School: *Warwick–Edinburgh Mental Wellbeing Scale (WEMWBS)*, 2015. Online: https://warwick.ac.uk/fac/med/research/platform/wemwbs.

Wilde-Larsson B, Larsson G, Kvist L, Sandin-Bojo A: Womens' opinions on intrapartal care: development of a theory-based questionnaire, *J Clin Nurs* 19:1748–1760, 2010.

CHAPTER 9

Skilled, Motivated and Engaged: Do We Have the Midwifery Workforce to Deliver Continuity?

Suzanne Tyler, Ann Kinnear, Julie Simpson

Contents

INTRODUCTION

The most important aspect of providing any maternity service is the workforce. All maternity services need the right staff in the right place at the right time with the right skills and attitudes. In many high-income countries, maternity services face an immediate pressure to ensure that existing workforce numbers are sufficient to meet current demand. Many are also struggling with longer-term considerations of whether the composition of the current workforce will be able met the needs of women and families in future models of care, including those that provide midwifery continuity of care.

In designing and sustaining midwifery continuity of care models for today we have to be realistic about our starting points whilst being open, creative and innovative about the future. This is more than being just about sufficient numbers; it is also about the need to challenge and change the current situation, where much midwifery workforce planning and information is subsumed within nursing workforce planning and data. Long-term, strategic planning for models of midwifery continuity of care will require a clear and separate picture of the available midwifery clinical workforce, which is distinct from the information regarding the nursing workforce.

In addition, as we move forward to create new models of care for women, we need to recognise the tension that exists between midwives' loyalty and desire to be with the women they care for on the one hand and responsibilities to their employers or institutions on the other. Many working patterns and arrangements continue to be designed to meet the overall needs of the facility across a 24-hour period rather than putting resources into meeting the needs of the woman or midwives.

In this chapter, we will look at:

- the policy context of midwifery continuity of care in relation to maternity workforce development
- the issue of capacity and the number of midwives required to deliver models of midwifery continuity of care
- the development of competent midwives, focusing on skills and practice development in the provision of continuity of care
- the process of preparing confident midwives, focusing on attitudes, behaviours and cultures to enable the provision of midwifery continuity of care for the majority of women
- the employment conditions for all midwives that support models of midwifery continuity of care.

Professional context—midwifery workforce

From the outset, we acknowledge ongoing debate within the midwifery profession about whether working in continuity is achievable and sustainable for the entire midwifery workforce. It is clear that greater understanding about working in continuity is important if the models are to be attractive and enduring as a career choice for midwives.

Many midwives working in continuity of care feel passionate about their work and report higher professional satisfaction and lower burnout scores (Newton et al., 2014). In contrast, research reported by Goodwin et al. (2016) suggests that employment pressures associated with midwifery continuity of care models, such as working longer hours and isolation from other colleagues, are associated with significantly higher levels of emotional exhaustion and stress among the workforce (Yoshida & Sandall, 2013).

Goodwin et al. (2016) conjecture that it is possible that midwives who are reluctant to adopt this pattern of work from the outset, and did not choose to work in this way, were more likely to experience additional stress and job dissatisfaction. Drawing on data from focus groups with community and hospital midwives in one English region, they suggest that frontline or core midwives in current practice have concerns about providing midwifery continuity of care across the whole maternity continuum. Some of the reasons for this apprehension include an expectation that midwives will have to draw on clinical skills and abilities that they may no longer have. This work also highlights how productivity and retention may be further compounded if attention is not given to the individual circumstances and roster requirements of some midwives (Goodwin et al., 2016). Chapter 4 considers these matters along with the impact of midwifery continuity of care on the workforce.

Within the context of a growing body of evidence demonstrating greater satisfaction and less burnout for continuity of care midwives (Newton et al., 2016), it is clear that midwifery continuity of care models will, and indeed should, expand. Coupled with the weight of evidence of the real benefits for women and babies, including a Cochrane systematic review of midwife-led continuity of care (Sandall et al., 2016), we owe it to women to find a way for these models to work for all involved—from policy direction, service innovation and workforce development through to the organisation and provision of maternity services more broadly.

POLICY CONTEXT

Earlier chapters have demonstrated that the evidence base for midwifery continuity of care is strong in terms of its potential to improve outcomes for women and babies; hence policy has been developed to guide changes. Continuity of carer is a key requirement of England's 'Better Births' strategy (National Health Service (NHS) England, 2016) and of Scotland's 'best start' strategy (NHS Scotland, 2017). In Australia, the 2010 National Maternity Services Plan (Australian Health Ministers Conference, 2011) was built on the vision that all women should be able to access high-quality evidence-based care that is woman centred, by increasing and supporting a midwifery workforce that is able to provide care across the continuum:

> It will be necessary to ensure all maternity care professionals are utilised to their full scope of practice, and that new, smarter ways of working are introduced to maximise the use of their specialist knowledge and skills.
>
> **(Australian Health Ministers Conference, 2011, p. 17)**

The aspirations of Better Births, the English policy driver, clearly puts the workforce alongside women; its vision is not only: 'for maternity services to become safer, more personalised, kinder, professional and more family friendly' but also: 'for all staff to be supported to deliver care which is woman centred, working in high performing teams, in organisations which are well led and in cultures which promote innovation, continuous learning and break down organisational and professional boundaries' (NHS England, 2016, p. 8).

In its section on what health care professionals say, this report notes:

> Staff expressed concerns that providing continuity of carer would be difficult to deliver as the system is currently configured with particular fears being expressed about work/life balance. There was a concern that without additional resources it might not be possible.
>
> **(NHS England 2016, p. 40)**

As a health intervention, midwifery continuity of care is well demonstrated to be effective, in that it delivers improved outcomes. Determining the workforce implications and any efficiencies that might ensue are not yet well evidenced. Initiating or expanding models of continuity must begin with an assessment of both the number of staff required and the skills, competencies and behaviours which are necessary to minimise the number of different contacts a woman will have during her pregnancy, birth and early postnatal period and which ensure a positive working experience for midwives.

CALCULATING MIDWIFERY WORKFORCE NUMBERS

The most significant financial element of any maternity service is the cost of staff. Typically, in high-income countries up to 70% of health service expenditure goes on human resources; thus, staffing, budgets and financial pressures are all inextricably linked. In most high-income countries, the health service workforce has grown in recent years but this has, in most cases, been outstripped by demand—fuelled by population growth, a sharp rise in the number of people with long-term conditions and advances in health care. Health care workers are a precious resource and improvements in recruitment and retention are critical. In the maternity context increased numbers of births in many high-income countries, together with changes in the demographics of the childbearing population and advances in obstetrics and fetal medicine, have not only altered the volume of work but also shifted the balance between 'normal' and 'complex' maternity care provision. Continuing to deliver safe and appropriate maternity care in these circumstances raises new questions about the number of staff required, their skill expertise and models of care.

Determining the appropriate number of midwives in any given service has traditionally been a balance of professional judgement, empirical measurement and political will in terms of funding. It also depends on a number of different factors including buildings and facilities, as well as local geography and demographic factors, in addition to models of care, skill mix and the capacity and skills of individual midwives.

The very first step for any service considering how to implement greater continuity has got to be ensuring adequate staffing levels.

There are a number of tools designed to determine the nursing and midwifery workforce numbers based on activity, but only one has been specifically developed for use in midwifery services. It differs significantly from nursing workforce-modelling tools because it focuses on the needs of women rather than the activity of staff or the institution. The Birthrate Plus tool (Birthrate Plus, 2015) was founded in the UK, where it has been used for many years to capture and quantify the workload of midwives arising from women's care needs across the whole maternity pathway. This information is then translated into the number of full-time equivalent (FTE) midwives required to provide a high-quality service. Fundamental to this methodology is staffing that assures one-to-one care in labour for all women. Birthrate Plus is now being used to model and support the development of midwifery continuity of care group practices in New South Wales. It is also being used in the Australian Capital Territory and Tasmania.

The calculations in Birthrate Plus take into account the time needed for management, variability of workload, holiday, sickness and study leave. It can also account for activities that midwives perform and may include some that could, arguably, be delegated to other health care workers. Where Birthrate Plus is not used, many health services continue to plan their midwifery workforce using the same ratios and criteria that are applied in nursing. Where this happens, the ratios do not always reflect women's needs or the way maternity care is or could be delivered.

In the UK, Birthrate Plus has been used extensively for many years and has produced reliable and consistent data on the number of midwives (and more latterly additional maternity support workers) needed to safely provide the existing model of maternity care. It is currently the only maternity workforce tool accredited by the National Institute for Health and Care Excellence (NICE, 2015) and is currently being adapted to try to determine more accurately the workforce implications of delivering continuity of carer at scale.

Measuring workforce shortages

Although Birthrate Plus is widely used and accepted by individual maternity services, it has also highlighted workforce shortages. For example, in 2017 the Royal College of Midwives (RCM) used Birthrate Plus to estimate that the UK was at that time 3500 midwives short of the number required to provide safe care.[a] Maternity units in the UK are now routinely overworked and understaffed and many are struggling even to provide one-to-one care in labour (RCM, 2017a). Midwives in both the UK and Australia report that they have never felt so challenged in their ability to provide high-quality care and a worrying number do not feel confident in raising concerns about unsafe practice (Creedy et al., 2017; RCM, 2016). Services are now routinely reliant on midwives working through their breaks and well beyond their contracted hours to provide safe care for women. Research by the RCM in 2016 concluded that midwives are feeling stressed, burnt out and unable to give high-quality care. Whilst this research found a high level of camaraderie in midwifery, it also exposed many reports of bullying and undermining behaviours (RCM, 2017b).

In Australia, there are similar challenges in determining the right workforce numbers and then funding these positions. Health Workforce 2025 provided Australia's first long-term planning projections for midwives and concluded that demand will exceed supply in 2025 (Health Workforce Australia (HWA), 2012). This modelling, however, was based only on the ratio of projected number of births by population excluding antenatal and postnatal care and did not include new evidence-based contemporary ways of providing care, including midwifery continuity of care.

GETTING THE RIGHT WORKFORCE TO SUPPORT CONTINUITY OF CARER

The great unanswered question is whether it takes more, fewer or the same number of midwives to organise services along a continuity of carer model. In computer-simulated modelling, NHS England found that the two most significant factors affecting the success of continuity of care were having sufficient midwives and the design of protected time rosters (NHS England, 2017). Services that start with a shortage of midwives, particularly if that shortage prevents delivery of one-to-one care in labour, are unlikely to transfer successfully to models providing greater continuity.

Where staffing numbers are sufficient, getting the workforce right for midwifery continuity of care requires a different and more flexible approach to that required for traditional working patterns, deployment, ongoing training and professional development. Successful continuity models rely not just on the teams or group practices that provide continuity itself, but also on an appropriately resourced core of midwifery staff who provide support and backup if needed. Having this 'core' also provides the flexibility to move midwives in and out of continuity of care models should their circumstances change, or they need or want a break. This is discussed further in Chapter 4.

Identifying the needs of women and size of caseloads

The estimated workload for any continuity team or group practice should be determined by robust risk assessment of what women want in each group and the ability of the midwives to be flexible and adjust their workload to meet the changing health care needs of their clients. Continuity of carer, like traditional models of care, will involve a care package that spans around 40 weeks, crossing hospital and community settings and involving a series of scheduled appointments. Like women anywhere, those receiving midwifery continuity of care may need extra or unscheduled care, sometimes involving scans or other procedures or an unexpected admission to hospital. Continuity of care models need enough flexibility in their staffing to cope with risk escalation and referral or transfer of women to high-risk settings.

Within a continuity model, accommodating a part-time workforce means that a group of six FTE midwives could easily become eight or nine actual midwives (head count). This can potentially dissipate the benefits of continuity for women unless there can be some flexibility on the part of the midwives. For midwives too, all of the benefits of effective team working, a shared ethos and time to work, study and reflect together can become more challenging as the number of midwives in the group increases. Similarly, too high a caseload also undermines continuity of carer.

Each team or group of midwives will have a maximum number of women for whom they can realistically provide care. Given the unpredictability of labour and birth, at any one time the continuity of care midwife will rely on backup from another member of her group as well as support from a core midwife if the birth is planned to take place in the hospital. Core midwives are essential to the sustainability of continuity of care models because they provide interim care or specialist advice, antenatal monitoring and assessment, additional labour care for complex and high-risk women and inpatient postnatal care if any of these are required. In addition to ensuring sufficient staff to provide midwifery continuity of care, workforce numbers in all areas have to be sufficient to keep areas safe and ensure that quality care can be provided.

Skill mix and the midwifery workforce

Implementing any continuity of carer model challenges and changes the composition of the workforce as well as the overall numbers. In England, for example, 51% of midwives work part-time (Midwifery 2020, 2010). The characteristics of these midwives are not only those with childcare responsibilities but also, increasingly, midwives aged over 55 who have chosen flexible retirement. In Australia too there is an increasing trend to a part-time workforce that is not limited to those who are older or with childcare responsibilities. However, we should not think of this part-time workforce as a homogeneous group; some midwives will be very happy to work their hours in a flexible manner, matching hours worked to a reduced caseload, whereas for others fixed working days and shifts will best meet their out-of-work responsibilities.

Privately practising midwives

Some women may choose to pay to have their care with a privately practising midwife (PPM). In Australia, government subsidies known as Medicare rebates (public health insurance scheme) are provided to women who access private practitioners (midwives, GPs and obstetricians) on an activity-based funding model. The midwives self-determine the size of their caseloads and how their business is structured but the low subsidy has a tendency to drive up activity to ensure midwives can make a reasonable living. In New Zealand, midwives can choose to work in their own business as a lead maternity carer (LMC), which offers a successful model that can deliver both continuity and popular working arrangements. New Zealand midwives are an autonomous and distinct professional group—a position gained through years of planned political and professional activism. The central tenet in New Zealand is that midwifery is a partnership between midwives and women. It is asserted that New Zealand midwives most closely meet the International Definition of a Midwife by being able to practise across the full scope of practise (Pairman et al., 2015). Around the world, New Zealand midwifery is seen as a role model for what is possible in terms of midwifery continuity of carer. As in Australia, the New Zealand government provides a payment to the LMCs for care provided across the continuum, but until recently the payment for this has been low. This has the potential of actually undermining continuity, with some midwives taking caseloads as high as 60 women a year in order for their practice to be financially viable. A recent settlement between the government and New Zealand College of Midwives (NZCOM) will see the income of these midwives rise and presumably the need for such high caseloads will diminish (Meier, 2017). Private practice is one way for midwives to self-determine their caseload and their own preferred ways of working to increase continuity of carer, but this too is not without its challenges. For example, the Nursing and Midwifery Board of Australia (NMBA, 'the Board') regulates two professions but does not designate a place for a contemporary midwife on the Board.

Midwifery workforce regulation

In the current Australian context, private midwives are regulated differently to those who are employed in the public health system. The tight regulation and surveillance of privately practising midwives by the NMBA, the lack of professional indemnity insurance for homebirth and the subsequent scrutiny of the midwives' maintenance of knowledge and skills exceeds that which is required for all other midwives. This has the effect of causing significant distress and uncertainty amongst private midwives.

In the UK, the scope for private midwifery practice has also been limited by the legal requirement for all health professionals to carry adequate medical malpractice insurance, in a climate where no commercial insurer is willing to supply affordable cover for individuals. A small number of private midwifery organisations are emerging, often contracting back into the NHS. The value of these organisations in demonstrating a different way of working and a different way of organising services is probably greater than their reach in terms of the current number of women benefiting. Nevertheless, by demonstrating an alternative approach, these organisations might, over time, assist the NHS to consider what other models of care are possible.

Flexible ways of working

Back to our initial question—can we deliver midwifery continuity of care with our current workforce? The key to successful implementation in both the public and private systems is to design patterns of working that are flexible and also offer something which will benefit not only women as recipients of the improved model of care but also midwives, service managers and the organisation itself. This is described in detail in Chapter 4 of this book. Over the course of their careers, midwives in all settings should be supported to have the choice of where and how they wish to work, including the chance to 'dip in and out' of continuity models. The failure to achieve this flexibility, along with a dearth of leaders with a less rigid approach to workforce planning, is likely to be contributing to the growing attrition from the workforce. This is reinforced by the recent WHELM (Work, Health and Emotional Lives of Midwives) studies in Australia, New Zealand, Sweden, Canada, Norway and the UK (Hunter et al., 2017).

EMBEDDING MIDWIFERY AUTONOMY

Recognition of midwifery autonomy as one of the key factors in the provision of midwifery continuity of care has been slow. In Australia, there has been a generalised resistance to midwives' occupational autonomy. Historically this has mostly come from the medical profession, but in research conducted almost two decades ago it was also identified as a feature of the culture of dominance of midwifery by nursing (Brodie, 2002; Brodie & Barclay, 2001).

Until the early 2000s, fragmentation of the midwife's role, with subspecialisation into nursing and narrow areas of practice, was the norm in Australia (Tracy et al., 2000). Lack of professional recognition and the invisibility of midwifery within nursing became the catalyst for a landmark national review of midwifery—a 3-year research project known as the Australian Midwifery Action Project (AMAP). The Project examined issues relating to midwifery workforce, regulation, education, practice and service delivery (Barclay et al., 2003). This research identified a narrow scope of practice for midwives in Australia, most of whom were practising in one area of midwifery and subspecialising. This was associated with diminished opportunities to provide the full scope of midwifery practice, which reduced any capacity to build professional autonomy. The findings from AMAP provided useful guidance for many Australian midwifery leaders as they sought to build and enhance the profession, practice and education standards, working through and with the Australian College of Midwives to grow a workforce that could effectively implement midwifery continuity of care. The ensuing changes in the philosophy and organisational framework for midwifery led many midwives to shift their allegiances—away from the 'organisation' to individual 'women'—and this heralded a new era in the professionalisation of midwifery as an autonomous profession (Foureur et al., 2009).

In Australia, midwifery autonomy received some small recognition from recommendations in the National Maternity Services Plan (Australian Health Ministers Conference, 2011) for women to have greater access to midwifery care provided by PPMs with funding from Medicare (the public health insurance scheme). To be eligible, PPMs must undertake additional study and gain qualifications to prescribe medications for minor disorders and to order screening and diagnostics tests, also paid for by Medicare. Although the scope of practice of the PPM by definition is otherwise the same as all other midwives, this additional qualification gives them some formal recognition and goes some way towards recognising their professional autonomy.

Engaging students in continuity

Providing midwifery students with opportunities to learn about midwifery continuity of care is another way to build skills and a confident workforce for the future. For example, in Australia, there is a requirement in the Midwife Accreditation Standards (Australian Nursing and Midwifery Accreditation Council (ANMAC), 2014) that programs of study leading to initial registration as a midwife must support the students to attain at least 10 continuity of care experiences (Leap et al., 2017). These midwifery students are prepared for continuity of care, with many of them having their clinical placements in caseload or midwifery group practice (MGP) models. In one example of how to do this, a small district hospital in New South Wales provided interested third-year midwifery students with a buddy in a caseload group. The students participated in team meetings, case note review and medical officer appointments with the midwife and the woman, mirroring working in midwifery continuity of care. Since 2007, UK midwifery students have also had the opportunity to explore continuity of carer as part of their education.

SUPPORTIVE TRANSITION AND ROLE DEVELOPMENT

There are many midwives in Australia and the UK who report that they lack confidence or competence to work autonomously and provide midwifery continuity of care (Harris et al., 2011). This is mainly due to their experience in providing care that is specialised in one area of practice. These midwives may require some additional support and training, such as refresher courses, or shadowing opportunities as part of their professional development and to build their confidence.

Midwives providing continuity of carer must be able to coordinate care across various professional and organisational boundaries in order to address each woman's needs. She therefore needs not just sound clinical and interpersonal skills, but also the ability to facilitate connections with other professional colleagues including building collegial networks with those who may be outside of maternity services. This requires a flexible and adaptable workforce that is confident and competent to meet increasingly complex needs while working across different care settings and with multidisciplinary teams. Building the confidence to work in this way may require additional support for those more used to traditional hospital-only or community-only models. As discussed in Chapter 4, recruitment practices should include the early identification of midwives with the propensity for working in this way, including newly qualified midwives (Cummins et al., 2015, 2016).

Such support of midwives may be provided in a number of ways including buddy systems, shadowing and mentoring. These provide opportunities for midwives to reflect on the challenges and opportunities and share with others as they begin to adapt to new roles and new ways of working. Another supportive and potentially powerful strategy to encourage and motivate midwives as they transition and grow in their role is 'supportive clinical supervision'. In some professions, such as mental health nursing, psychology and social work, clinical supervision is recognised as crucial to safety and practice. This allows free and open discussion of, and reflection upon, challenges that emerge from practice whilst giving midwives the opportunity to acknowledge their weaknesses, and vent their distress and concerns, which in turn can contribute positively towards retention.

For maternity services managers the first challenge is to have protected time for staff learning and professional development and to secure funds to invest in sharpening not just clinical skills but also the attitudes and ways of working that make continuity a success. The second challenge is for managers to adopt both a supportive and a flexible style with their teams, trusting self-management and self-rostering and respecting professional autonomy. Styles of leadership and ways of supporting and developing staff have been further described in Chapter 4.

EFFECTIVE WORKING WITH OTHERS

Whilst every woman needs a midwife and midwifery care, some women will in addition require clinical (medical) interventions and support from others. Midwives can be seen as the conductors of the maternity orchestra and, even when they are the sole caregiver, they must be able to recognise that they work within multiprofessional teams. Midwifery continuity of care is not about working in professional isolation. Even though midwives working from community settings are more isolated that those working shifts in hospital settings, they must understand and be clear about the importance of collaboration, working in partnership with the woman and her family and having strong advocacy skills. Key skills for midwives working in midwifery continuity of care must include working in a collaborative manner—whether it be understanding partnerships with women or forging relationships with health professionals or with others who form part of the health and social care environment. Chapter 5 considers the issues of collaboration in more depth.

Skill mix that supports continuity of care

When considering the wider parameters of an effective maternity service, skill mix is as important as numbers. Other staff roles should be employed in the context of supporting midwifery continuity of care where this leads to greater efficiency. Clearly, this requires that support staff members are appropriately trained and that any delegated roles do not undermine the principle of women receiving the bulk of their care from a midwife they know and trust.

Effective skill mix is dependent on clarity of roles and efficient maternity care depends on a suitable balance of midwives, doctors, allied health and other care providers including maternity care assistants and support workers. In the UK, the role of the maternity support worker (MSW) and their contribution to high-quality care is now widely recognised. This unregulated but skilled group of staff works alongside midwives in both hospital and community settings, often undertaking tasks that would otherwise take midwifery time, thus releasing more time for the important midwife-to-woman relationship building, advice and support (Griffin et al., 2013). In one recent study, for example, an initiative involving MSWs supporting midwives in homebirths was implemented successfully, with emergencies well managed. This study concluded that MSWs have the potential for task shifting to release midwife capacity and provide reliable homebirth care to low-risk women (Taylor et al., 2018a).

THE IMPORTANCE OF THE WORKPLACE CULTURE

Much is made of whether or not midwives want to work in midwifery continuity of care in a climate where staff retention is a huge challenge. This is an important consideration for maternity managers. In England, recent data indicate that more than 7% of nursing and midwifery staff leaves the NHS each year for reasons other than retirement. The underlying factors causing this have been identified as pressure of work, lack of flexibility, pay and lack of career development (NHS, 2017). In a 2010 Australian study, the elements that kept midwives in their jobs were variety and normalising maternity care (Sullivan et al., 2011), whereas in another study the factors that prompted them to leave included working hours and schedules, poor remuneration, limited advancement opportunities and heavy workloads (Bogossian et al., 2011). Creedy et al. (2017) cite a number of different international studies demonstrating that workplace stress is consistently experienced by hospital-based midwives, with those working conventional shift patterns more likely to report harassment, abuse or bullying and burnout (Creedy et al., 2017). Research by the RCM (2016) indicates that the commonest reasons midwives give for leaving the profession are staffing, workload and not having enough time to spend giving women high-quality care.

Current models of care are leaving many midwives feeling unsupported and lacking control over their working lives (Hildingsson et al., 2016), whilst a number of services which have tried to introduce caseloading teams have reported friction between caseloading midwives and core staff (NHS, 2017).

JOB SATISFACTION AND WORK–LIFE BALANCE

The most recent evidence we have on midwives' attitude to their working lives has been captured in the WHELM studies, which have been undertaken in the UK, Australia, New Zealand, Sweden, Canada and Norway (Hildingsson et al., 2016). In the UK, 2000 midwives participated in an online survey in 2016 for this study. This found that 83% of participants were suffering from personal burnout and 67% from work-related burnout. At the time of this research very few English midwives were working in continuity of carer teams, which is a good indication that the way midwives are currently working is not good for their wellbeing. Over one-third scored in the moderate / severe / extreme range for stress and depression. Both scores put UK midwives in a far more vulnerable place than colleagues completing the study in other countries. Sixty-six percent of the midwives in the study reported that they had considered leaving the profession within the last 6 months; the top two reasons were dissatisfaction with staffing levels at work and dissatisfaction with the quality of care able to be provided. This highlights earlier work by Hunter (2004), which showed that midwives needed to manage their emotions, particularly during interactions with their colleagues with different ideologies and views about midwifery practice.

In contrast, Box 9.1 profiles the positive impact on the emotional wellbeing of midwives who are working in continuity of care.

BOX 9.1 Midwifery Continuity of Care Can Be Good for Midwives Too
Jenny Fenwick and Mary Sidebotham, Gold Coast University Hospital and Griffin University, Queensland, Australia
Wide-scale implementation of midwifery continuity of care has been slow and in some places is non-existent. When questioned about this, midwifery managers commonly respond: 'midwives don't want to work that way', 'the on-call is too intrusive and stressful', 'there is no work–life balance' and 'the model is not sustainable and causes burnout'. Faced with these perceptions many managers just do not believe that they can staff continuity models. The

Continued

BOX 9.1 Midwifery Continuity of Care Can Be Good for Midwives Too—cont'd

Work, Health and Emotional Lives of Midwives (WHELM) study has been designed to explore workforce sustainability and, in particular, the factors that impact onto midwives' emotional health and wellbeing. It provides an opportunity to test the correlation between continuity of care models and burnout (Creedy et al., 2017).

Our work began in one large Queensland hospital. At the time, the health service was planning to move to a new site and was committed to increasing the availability of continuity of midwifery care for local women. Part of the transition process was understanding the impact of the working environment on midwives' emotional wellbeing. We developed a survey using a number of validated tools including measures of burnout, stress, anxiety and depression, empowerment and the practice environment. We asked specific questions that enabled us to identify the employment model that midwives worked in as well as to understand the demographics of the midwifery workforce. One of the encouraging findings was that the midwives who provided caseload care for women were less likely to experience stress, anxiety, depression and burnout. We looked at this more closely and discovered that, unlike their colleagues working in a shift-based standard care model, they experienced greater control over their working life and enjoyed and valued the longitudinal relationship they were able to establish with women. These factors, they said, sustained them. We discussed these preliminary findings within our international networks and realised there was genuine interest in replicating this work more widely with larger cohorts. The WHELM consortium emerged from these early discussions alongside a decision to look more closely at the emotional wellbeing of the midwifery workforce at a national level in the contributing countries. The results from the New Zealand and Australian arms now provide the midwifery community with the largest body of evidence to date clearly showing that, although midwives do experience significant emotional pressure within their work, their ability to provide woman-centred care, the organisation of their work and how they are supported within the practice environment all significantly impact the risk of burnout. The clear message is that midwives providing continuity of care are less likely to experience anxiety, depression and burnout. Indeed, once adjusted to working in a flexible way, most consider that their ability to positively manage work and family life improves.

Conversely, midwives who are not working in caseload models consistently report feeling a growing sense of distress and disempowerment in the workplace. Many midwives are highly dissatisfied with their excessive workloads and their subsequent inability to provide woman-centred care. In addition, midwives consistently report feeling unsupported by their line managers and/or employers. Very worrying is the fact that in some countries participating in the WHELM study over 50% of those surveyed were seriously considering leaving the profession. This has significant implications for workforce planning. Currently the WHELM consortium are looking at solutions to this impending workforce crisis. It is becoming increasingly evident, however, that resourcing and supporting midwives to work across their full scope of practice within a caseload model that facilitates relational-based maternity care is the solution for many midwives.

Meeting the needs of different generations of midwives

A new challenge for managers, educators and policy makers is to ensure that the whole workforce is willing and able to shift to either providing midwifery continuity of care or supporting it in a variety of ways. Amongst long-serving midwives used to years of working in traditional patterns of either a community or hospital setting, there will undoubtedly be concerns and fears of change. For example, in a 2018 survey of midwives in Birmingham, UK only 35% said they would be willing to work in continuity teams which included intrapartum care, with 41% saying they were unable to change their shift patterns or current working arrangements (Taylor et al., 2018b). At the same time, it is too easy to assume that younger or more recently qualified midwives can more easily fit into new models just because their education included continuity of care. Between 2014 and 2016 in England, a large-scale project was undertaken to try to understand why so many early-career nurses and midwives who, in spite of high-cost education, were quitting the professions (Jones et al., 2015). This work certainly gives some hope, but also contains some warnings. It confirms other findings about profound intergenerational differences in the way that job satisfaction, professional autonomy and organisational loyalty is felt (Kings Fund, 2013).

For the first time in our health services' history we have four different generations working together. These generations have been labelled as: Baby Boomers (born between 1946 and 1964), who currently dominate much of the profession's upper echelons but are also likely to be retiring in the foreseeable future, Generation X (born between 1965 and 1980) and Generation Y or Millennials (born between 1981 and 2000). Although these three generations make up the bulk of the existing workforce, those newly qualified and currently in training are more likely to belong to the group known as Generation Z or post-Millennials (born since 2000). What motivated and suited yesterday's midwives does not necessarily suit today's or tomorrow's. There are clear differences in values, expectations, perceptions and motivations across those both in the current workforce and, more significantly, those currently still in education. At the same time the world of work is changing everywhere: the demands for highly skilled, particularly IT-confident, individuals are growing; pension affordability means future generations will work longer and the redesign of existing roles foreshadows greater integration across health and social care. Being ready to adapt workplaces to meet the needs of the Generation Y and Z midwives is going to be crucial to ensuring their retention and loyalty (Jamieson, 2012; Lavoie-Tremblay et al., 2010).

The study by Jones et al. (2015) identified a number of key factors to enhance retention of recently qualified nurses and midwives:

- clear, structured career development and progression pathways
- care and support (personally and professionally) from leaders and teams
- team spiritedness—to meet the need to be accepted, valued and appreciated

- feedback, guidance and developmental support
- flexibility to achieve work–life balance
- support and being enabled to meet the expectations of the patients and the public
- engagement in meaningful work—to make a difference.

Much of what Gen Y early-career midwives want seems closely aligned to the most positive conditions found in midwifery continuity of care: they will get to form relationships with women, provide holistic care, organise work around the woman not the system, work within small self-supporting and supportive teams, be supported by flexible bureaucracy and management and get the chance to practice autonomously using all their skills. The question remains, though, whether continuity models can meet Gen Y's other big motivational factor: an acceptable work–life balance. For maternity services, the challenge is how to match the expectations of midwives and the growing expectations of women with delivering efficient services. From the research available here it is clear that, although nurses and midwives enter the profession fully committed to working hard, even over shifts, they expect flexibility, professional respect, supportive development and the ability to enjoy a good balance in their working and home lives. Health service employers need to get much better at creating working environments that are diverse and recognise and accommodate differences if they are going to improve recruitment and retention.

Employment conditions and staff wellbeing

Most midwives reading this chapter will be working for a health service employer and most midwifery continuity of care models are likely to be introduced in the context of employed midwives. There is a wealth of evidence to demonstrate a strong link between the health and wellbeing of staff and the safety and quality of care being provided (Bryson et al., 2014). Given the unprecedented challenges facing many health services in terms of finances, staffing shortages, dissatisfaction with pay and mounting work pressures, it is crucial that any new models of care have staff wellbeing at their heart.

Maternity is a 24-hour, 7 days a week service; therefore unsocial hours come with the territory of being a midwife. That said, in most services routine antenatal and postnatal care has typically been provided within consistent core hours, with staff rostered into shift patterns that match scheduled appointments and predicted unscheduled and urgent care. Midwifery continuity of care models usually require midwives to be available not just at these fixed times for routine booked appointments but also on-call to manage urgent and unscheduled appointments and, importantly, to provide intrapartum care.

National legislation as well as employment policies are designed to protect workers whilst maintaining efficient and responsive services. In the UK, midwives' working conditions must be compliant with the EU Working Time Directive,[b] NHS Agenda for Change and safe staffing legislation, as well as the NMC Code. These set out very clearly the number of hours a midwife can work in any given stretch and in any week and the length of compensatory rest and off-duty to which she is entitled. They also restrict the number and manner of on-call working arrangements. Very often midwives require 'saving from themselves' as their commitment to women may lead them to disregard these employment safeguards. The principle of continuity must be that hours to provide care to a caseload align with contractual hours without the need to work any extra time.

Employment terms and conditions must reward the nature of the work as well as protect midwives from the risks associated with providing a high-pressured service that is available on demand at any hour, day and night. However, a necessary element of continuity of care models is a move away from traditional shift working to a greater reliance on on-call working. With this comes a trade-off between increased continuity for women and potentially enhanced job satisfaction for midwives, and certain terms and conditions of employment that both reward and incentivise flexibility whilst also protecting midwives' work–life balance.

In most states and territories in Australia, midwives working in continuity of care models are governed by an industrial framework that sets out their caseload, working hours, on-call arrangements and remuneration for working in this way, with specific working arrangements such as rosters left to local determination. The industrial frameworks can differ from state to state and from hospital to hospital. As a general rule, salaries are annualised (base plus a percentage) with guidelines around the number of hours that can be worked in any stretch of time.

Research from the UK's British Medical Association has focused on the risk of fatigue caused through long working hours and exposure to high-intensity working (British Medical Association (BMA), 2018). The risks of shift working are compounded by working practices that include short recovery times between shifts, rapidly rotating schedules and working full shifts in succession. Its key messages are that this comes with a personal cost to practitioners and a safety risk to patients, and has a direct link to midwifery, where shift working is the norm.

The intergenerational studies already cited (Jones et al., 2015) suggest that ways of working that come at this type of personal cost are now less likely to be tolerated by those entering the profession. Building a sustainable and resilient midwifery workforce for the future and rolling out continuity of carer can be mutually compatible goals. For this to be achieved, however, health services must be willing to embrace innovative approaches that give midwives autonomy and flexibility and to design working models around the needs of women rather than the needs of an organisation.

> **BOX 9.2 Sustaining a Rural Midwifery Caseload Program in Outback Australia**
>
> *Alison Isaacs, Midwifery Unit Manager, Danielle Toigo, Midwifery Group Practice Team Leader, Broken Hill Health Service Maternity Unit, NSW, Australia*
>
> Broken Hill is a small rural town situated about 1100 km west from Sydney and 500 km north of Adelaide.
>
> Rural maternity services have a unique opportunity to be able to provide gold-standard maternity care, meeting the needs of the community, and to be flexible and innovative to accommodate and support the needs of their local workforce in order to ensure the sustainability of a midwifery-led caseload program. It is possible for rural maternity services to be unique, innovative and flexible and thus sustain caseload midwifery programs. Once the value of this model of care can be demonstrated there is the potential for an amazing woman-centred, holistic service to be sustained and to overcome common challenges faced by rural maternity services.
>
> The Broken Hill Midwifery Group Practice (BHMGP) is an all-risk, no-exit caseload midwifery program which also offers shared care with the local Aboriginal Maternal and Infant Health Service, the Royal Flying Doctor Service and out-of-area private obstetricians. The BHMGP also launched a midwifery-led Early Pregnancy Assessment Service in early 2017, which is run by midwives within the MGP.
>
> The BHMGP was launched during a period of workforce stability and positions were offered to midwives on a permanent full-time basis only in order to maximise continuity of carer for women. Since then, a third of the midwifery workforce (three MGP midwives and two core midwives) went on maternity leave within a 3-month period and are planning to return to work on a part-time basis later this year. As such, job sharing within the MGP has been introduced in order to meet the needs of the workforce and sustain the current model of care.
>
> Two years after its launch it has evolved and there are plans to sustain it for the future for midwives working in this rural MGP, with relevant implications for similar models in other rural facilities.
>
> Broken Hill Maternity also supports the inclusion of new graduate midwives within the MGP in order to grow and sustain its own local workforce for the future; however, this relies on ongoing financial investment.

MAKING CHANGE A REALITY: EXAMPLES FROM PRACTICE

Boxes 9.2 and 9.3 contain two case studies from very different parts of the world that highlight the potential for making changes that suit both the workforce and women equally.

BOX 9.3 A Step-by-Step Approach in Scotland

Maureen McSherry, Consultant Midwife NHS Lanarkshire,
University Hospital Wishaw, Scotland

NHS Lanarkshire provides continuity of carer for scheduled antenatal and postnatal care within the community. Statistics provided by our electronic maternity system indicate an average of 74% of all women booked in Lanarkshire (approx. 4500 births per annum) have care provided by no more than three midwives, with over 50% of care provided by the named midwife. We have a homebirth rate <2% of all births.

We have midwives with contracts of employment based in community, rotational and hospital setting. We currently have an obstetric-led labour ward and a developing alongside midwifery unit (AMU) with no free-standing midwifery unit (FMU) in our area. Our ambition is to provide a midwife caseload model for the majority of our workforce with a core midwife staff to support, mentor and provide acute care skills to meet the level of complexity of women entering our care systems.

We believe if staff are unhappy then any change will not be received well, and will fail. So, in an attempt to be successful with the change, we want to understand how our staff feel, address their concerns and shape our model of working in a way which is acceptable to all. We also want the change to belong to all staff and are actively encouraging involvement in change areas.

We have participated in and hosted events with the Royal College of Midwives (RCM) to provide information to the workforce on continuity of carer. This also provides opportunities for our staff to ask questions or raise concerns. We have been holding 'buzz' sessions within the acute and community settings to inform staff since November 2017. We know staff are anxious and fearful that the new way of providing care will impact on their work–life balance, so we want to have the opportunity to listen to their concerns but also provide the evidence on why caring for women differently will improve outcomes.

We have also sent a staff experience survey to all our midwives to have an understanding of what currently works well, what frustrates them and how they would like to work. This will also provide baseline measures, which will be re-evaluated after implementation of the new way of working. Analysis of initial feedback is still awaited.

We have involved staff side representation from the outset and have set up a maternity strategy group involving all key players. This group meets on a monthly basis.

CONCLUSION

Returning to our opening intentions in this chapter, we conclude firstly that establishing and sustaining midwifery continuity of care schemes cannot be viewed in isolation from the wider workforce challenges facing health systems. The small and large 'p' political environment has got to be right, with a recognition of the true costs associated with moving from one service model to another. Health systems that find themselves unable to invest in and support improvements in maternity care have an obligation to be honest with women and with their workforce about what is possible within the resources available.

Furthermore, we still cannot say with any certainty whether, in the long term, sustainable continuity of carer models require more, fewer or the same number of midwives when compared with more traditional models. What we can say with certainty is that a maternity service already struggling to staff existing models that guarantee one-to-one care in labour for all women is unlikely, with the same resources, to be able to move to properly functioning midwifery continuity of care models. In relation to the skills and competence required to work effectively in a continuity model, we face an immediate paradox: throughout the developed world, midwifery education is focused on the full role of the midwife across antenatal, intrapartum and postnatal care; however, too many existing service models have fragmented midwifery care to such a degree that some midwives are deskilled and no longer feel confident to work across the entire pathway. Helping these midwives regain the skills will require a supportive transition. Continuity of care should be and could be synonymous with what we mean when we say 'midwifery'.

Finally, our combined experiences and understanding of the literature and emerging evidence has led to us to suggest a number of principles for getting the workforce right whilst at the same time aspiring to introduce the midwifery continuity of care schemes that women want. Our suggested principles for getting the workforce right include:

- Use an evidence-based midwifery workforce planning tool to review staffing and workload.
- Introduce an appropriate skill mix to create flexibility.
- Promote and enable occupational autonomy.
- Provide support for those moving to a new way of working.
- Commit to finding a place for everyone within your model of care.
- Facilitate multiprofessional education and continuing professional development.
- Ensure today's education prepares midwives for the models of care we want tomorrow.
- Pay attention to factors that maximise recruitment and retention.
- Introduce productive working to eliminate waste time.
- Limit working patterns that are known to disrupt circadian rhythms.
- Provide inbuilt rest breaks whilst on duty to allow adequate recovery time.
- Encourage team-based approaches to care that allow staff to take breaks without interruptions.
- Build plans for developing continuity with full staff engagement.

This chapter has identified the significant effort required to reorganise the midwifery workforce to incorporate midwifery continuity of care and carer throughout the continuum of pregnancy, birth and the postnatal period, in both community and hospital settings. Evidence-based tools for effective workforce planning that help determine the number and mix of midwifery staff needed in each birthplace have been described. Importantly, these will further assist in the important task of making the planning of midwifery workforce visible and distinct from nursing.

The workforce of today and tomorrow is changing, with many midwives wanting to work more flexibly and with greater autonomy and professional recognition than previous generations. If we can achieve a successful reorganisation of midwifery services and improved models of care through continuity, women will be cared for in the right place and at the right time, by the right people with the right skills, values and self-belief to deliver high-quality midwifery care.

Notes

a. In April 2018 the then Secretary of State for Health, Jeremy Hunt, acknowledged this shortage and committed to a 25% increase in midwifery training places over a 4-year period.

b. The Working Time Directive (WTD) is EU legislation designed to protect the health and safety of workers by establishing minimum requirements for working hours, rest periods and annual leave. It was enacted into UK law in the form of Working Time Regulations in 1998.

REFERENCES

Australian Health Ministers Conference: *National maternity services plan*, Canberra, 2011, Commonwealth of Australia.

Australian Nursing and Midwifery Accreditation Council (ANMAC): *Midwife accreditation standards 2014*, Canberra, 2014, ANMAC. Online: https://www.anmac.org.au/sites/default/files/documents/ANMAC_Midwife_Accreditation_Standards_2014.pdf.

Barclay L, Brodie P, Lane K, Leap N, Reiger K, Tracy S: *The AMAP report*, Volumes 1 and 2. Australian Midwifery Action Project. Sydney, 2003, Centre for Family Health and Midwifery, University of Technology.

Birthrate Plus: *Birthrate Plus: safe staffing for maternity services*, 2015. Online: https://www.birthrateplus.co.uk/.

Bogossian F, Long MH, Benefer C, et al: A workforce profile comparison of practising and non-practising midwives in Australia: baseline data from the midwives and nurses e-cohort study, *Midwifery* 27:342–349, 2011.

British Medical Association (BMA): *Fatigue and sleep deprivation—the impact of different working patterns on doctors*, London, 2018, BMA.

Brodie P: Addressing the barriers to midwifery—Australian midwives speaking out, *Aust J Midwifery* 15:5–14, 2002.

Brodie P, Barclay L: Contemporary issues in Australian midwifery regulation, *Aust Health Rev* 24(4): 103–118, 2001.

Bryson A, Forth J, Stokes L: *Does worker wellbeing affect workplace performance?* London, 2014, Department of Business Innovation and Skills. Online: https://assets.publishing.service.gov.uk/government/uploads/system/uploads/attachment_data/file/366637/bis-14-1120-does-worker-wellbeing-affect-workplace-performance-final.pdf.

Creedy D, Sidebotham M, Gamble J, Pallant J, Fenwick J: Prevalence of burn out, depression, anxiety and stress in Australian midwives: a cross-sectional survey, *BMC Pregnancy Childbirth* 17:13, 2017.

Cummins A, Denney-Wilson E, Homer C: The experiences of new graduate midwives working in midwifery continuity of care models in Australia, *Midwifery* 31:438–444, 2015.

Cummins A, Denney-Wilson E, Homer C: The challenge of employing and managing new graduate midwives in midwifery group practices in hospitals, *J Nurs Manag* 24:614–623, 2016.

Foureur M, Brodie P, Homer C: Midwife-centered versus woman-centered care: a developmental phase?, *Women Birth* 22:47–49, 2009.

Goodwin I, Taylor B, Kenyon S, McArthur C: *Continuity of carer in midwifery practice—a briefing paper*, Maternity Theme of the Collaboration for Leadership in Applied Health Research and Care (CLAHRC), West Midlands, 2016, Institute of Applied Health Research, College of Medical and Dental Sciences, University of Birmingham.

Griffin R, Richardson M, Morris-Thompson T: An evaluation of the impact of maternity support workers, *Br J Midwifery* 20:884–889, 2013.

Harris F, Teijlingen E, Hundley V, Farmer J, Bryers H, Caldow J, et al: The buck stops here: midwives and maternity care in rural Scotland, *Midwifery* 27:301–307, 2011.

Health Workforce Australia: *Health workforce 2025—doctors, nurses and midwives*, Volume 1. Canberra, 2012, Commonwealth of Australia. Online: https://submissions.education.gov.au/forms/archive/2015_16_sol/documents/Attachments/Australian%20Nursing%20and%20Midwifery%20Accreditation%20Council%20(ANMAC).pdf.

Hildingsson I, Gamble J, Sidebotham M, Creedy D, Guilliland K, Dixon L, et al: Midwifery empowerment: national surveys of midwives from Australia, New Zealand and Sweden, *Midwifery* 40:62–69, 2016.

Hunter B: Conflicting ideologies as a source of emotion work in midwifery, *Midwifery* 20(3):261–272, 2004.

Hunter B, Henley J, Fenwick J, Sidebotham M: *Work, health and emotional lives of midwives in the UK: The UK WHELM Study*, Cardiff, 2017, School of Healthcare Sciences, Cardiff University. Online: https://www.rcm.org.uk/sites/default/files/UK%20WHELM%20REPORT%20final%20180418-May.pdf.

Jamieson I: *What are the views of generation Y New Zealand registered nurses towards nursing work and career? A descriptive exploratory study*, PhD thesis. Canterbury, NZ, 2012, University of Canterbury.

Jones K, Warren A, Davies A: *Mind the gap: exploring the needs of early career nurses and midwives in the workplace*, London, 2015, Health Education England, National Health Service. Online: http://www.nhsemployers.org/-/media/Employers/Documents/Plan/Mind-the-Gap-Smaller.pdf.

King's Fund: *Time to Deliver Differently project*, London, 2013, King's Fund. Online: https://www.kingsfund.org.uk/projects/time-tothink-differently.

Lavoie-Tremblay M, Leclerc E, Marchionni C, Drevniok U: The needs and expectations of generation Y nurses in the workplace, *J Nurses Staff Dev* 26:2–10, 2010.

Leap N, Brodie P, Tracy S: Collective action for the development of national standards for midwifery education in Australia, *Women Birth* 30:169–176, 2017.

Meier C: *Midwives settle pay equity fight and get $8 million pay rise*, 2017. Online: https://www.stuff.co.nz/national/health/93079280/Midwives-settle-pay-equity-fight-and-get-8-million-pay-rise.

Midwifery 2020: *Workforce and workload workstream: final report*, Edinburgh, 2010, Midwifery 2020 Programme.

National Health Service (NHS): *Facing the facts, shaping the future: a draft workforce strategy for England to 2027*, London, 2017, NHS. Online: https://www.hee.nhs.uk/sites/default/files/documents/Facing%20the%20Facts%2C%20Shaping%20the%20Future%20-%20a%20draft%20health%20and%20care%20workforce%20strategy%20for%20England%20to%202027.pdf.

National Health Service (NHS) England: *Better Births: improving outcomes of maternity services in England, a Five Year Forward View for maternity care*. National Maternity Review. London, 2016, NHS England. Online: https://www.england.nhs.uk/wp-content/uploads/2016/02/national-maternity-review-report.pdf.

National Health Service (NHS) England: Maternity system modelling, London, 2017, NHS England.

National Health Service (NHS) Scotland: *The best start: a five-year forward plan for maternity and neonatal care in Scotland*, Edinburgh, 2017, NHS Scotland. Online: https://www.gov.scot/Resource/0051/00513178.pdf.

National Institute for Health and Care Excellence (NICE): *Safe midwifery staffing for maternity services*, London, 2015, NICE. Online: https://www.nice.org.uk/guidance/ng4.

Newton M, McLachlan H, Forster D, Willis K: Understanding the 'work' of caseload midwives: a mixed-methods exploration of two caseload midwifery models in Victoria, Australia, *Women Birth* 29:223–233, 2016.

Newton M, McLachlan H, Willis K, Forster D: Comparing satisfaction and burnout between caseload and standard care midwives: findings from two cross-sectional surveys conducted in Victoria, Australia, *BMC Pregnancy Childbirth* 14:426, 2014.

Pairman S, Tracy SK, Dahlen HG, Dixon L: *Midwifery: preparation for practice*, ed 3, Chatswood, NSW, 2015, Churchill Livingstone.

Royal College of Midwives (RCM): *Why midwives leave—revisited*, London, 2016, RCM. Online: https://www.rcm.org.uk/sites/default/files/Why%20Midwives%20Leave%20Revisted%20-%20October%202016.pdf.

Royal College of Midwives (RCM): *Evidence to the NHS Pay Review Body*, London, 2017a, RCM. Online: https://www.rcm.org.uk/sites/default/files/Evidence%20to%20the%20NHS%20Pay%20Review%20Body%202017%20A4%2056pp_2FINAL.pdf.

Royal College of Midwives (RCM): *RCM campaign for healthy workplaces delivering high quality care*, London, 2017b, RCM. Online: https://www.rcm.org.uk/sites/default/files/Caring%20for%20You%20-%20Working%20in%20Partnership%20Guide%202016%20A5%2024pp_9%20spd.pdf.

Sandall J, Soltani H, Gates S, Shennan A, Devane D: Midwife-led continuity models versus other models of care for childbearing women, *Cochrane Database Syst Rev* (9):CD004667, 2016.

Sullivan K, Lock L, Homer C: Factors that contribute to midwives staying in midwifery: a study in one area health service in New South Wales, Australia, *Midwifery* 27:331–335, 2011.

Tracy S, Barclay L, Brodie P: Contemporary issues in the workforce and education of Australian midwives, *Aust Health Rev* 23(4):78–88, 2000.

Taylor B, Croos-Sudworth F, MacArthur C: *Better Births and continuity: midwife survey results*, West Midlands, 2018b, University of Birmingham. Online: https://www.birmingham.ac.uk/Documents/college-mds/applied-health/better-birth-and-continuity.pdf.

Taylor B, Henshall C, Goodwin L, Kenyon S: Task shifting maternity support workers as the second health worker at a home birth in the UK: a qualitative study, *Midwifery* 62:109–115, 2018a. doi:10.1016/j.midw.2018.03.003.

Yoshida Y, Sandall J: Occupational burnout and work factors in community and hospital midwives: a survey analysis, *Midwifery* 29:921–926, 2013.

CHAPTER 10

Midwifery Continuity of Care for Specific Groups

Jyai Allen

Contents

INTRODUCTION

The evidence presented so far in this book demonstrates that women and babies benefit from midwifery continuity of care, including those with identified risk factors. The benefits of continuity of care are largely social, psychological and emotional; these in turn contribute to the physical benefits women experience. Part of the midwife's role is to identify, plan, provide and evaluate care for specific groups to ensure equity and access (National Health Service (NHS) England, 2017; Nursing and Midwifery Board of Australia (NMBA), 2006). Women who are from vulnerable or marginalised communities gain significant benefit from individualised care (Rayment-Jones et al., 2015).

This chapter provides several short stories as examples of how midwifery continuity of care can be designed to meet the needs of specific groups: women who are socially disadvantaged; women from a refugee background; women at risk of having their baby removed by a child protection / safeguarding agency; lesbian, gay, bisexual or transgender (LGBT) families; and young women. It also provides a focus on working, in Australia, with Aboriginal and Torres Strait Islander (herein referred to as 'Aboriginal') families in a variety of contexts.

We invited several people who are involved in providing care to specific groups to contribute to this chapter. The authors come from Australia, Canada and the

United Kingdom (UK). We asked them to talk about their highlights, challenges and strategies for success by providing a brief example from practice (all names have been changed using pseudonyms to protect confidentiality of the women and their families). Some of the stories you may find challenging and even disturbing. We acknowledge this and trust you will use this reflection to gain an understanding of the different issues facing midwives in these ways of working. The next sections will explore how midwifery continuity of care embeds a primary health care approach and can be used as a public health strategy.

PRIMARY HEALTH CARE

Social determinants of health (e.g. housing, education, employment, social support, discrimination) strongly influence the health of individuals and their access to health services (Marmot & Wilkinson, 2005). By addressing these social determinants of health, primary health care aims to:

- improve health care for all, particularly those who experience inequitable health outcomes
- keep people healthy
- prevent illness
- reduce the need for unnecessary hospital presentations
- improve the management of complex and chronic conditions (Department of Health, 2013).

A primary health care approach that addresses the social determinants of health for mothers and babies is an essential component of woman–centred care (Kaufmann, 2002). Therefore, it has long been suggested that midwifery continuity of care should be underpinned by primary health care principles (Brodie, 2003; Leap & Edwards, 2006).

MIDWIFERY AS PRIMARY HEALTH CARE

In Australia, the national competency standards for the midwife (NMBA, 2006) have primary health care as one of the four essential domains. This document states that, in their role as primary health care providers, midwives:

- understand that health is influenced by sociocultural, spiritual and politico-economic environments
- have an ability to develop relationships with the women for whom they care as well as others with whom they interact in their professional lives
- have an important advocacy role in protecting the rights of women, families and communities whilst respecting and supporting their right to self-determination
- are committed to cultural safety within all aspects of practice and act in ways that enhance the dignity and integrity of others

- work collaboratively with health care providers and other professionals referring women to appropriate community agencies and support networks
- promote wellness for the woman, her family and the community (NMBA, 2006). Although this is an Australian document, it will have resonance in many other countries. The midwife's primary health care role is crucial to optimise outcomes during pre-conception, pregnancy, birth and the postnatal period, particularly for women with complex social factors (McNeill et al., 2012).

MIDWIFERY AS A PUBLIC HEALTH STRATEGY

In the UK, the Nursing and Midwifery Council's standards of competence for registered midwives similarly refer to midwifery as part of a public health strategy which encourages women to optimise the health and wellbeing of themselves and their babies (Nursing and Midwifery Council (NMC), 2009). In low-, medium- and high-income countries, interventions involving midwives are the most potent way to address health inequalities (Bick, 2006). However, the potential for midwifery as a public health strategy to improve the lives of women and their families continues to be underrecognised (Biro, 2011; McNeill et al., 2012). It is important for midwives to explicitly acknowledge the public health benefits of their practice (Biro, 2011). In Box 10.1, we provide an example of how midwifery is being articulated as a public health strategy in the UK (Chief Nursing Officers of England, Northern Ireland, Scotland and Wales, 2010); the principles are relevant to midwives working in any setting or context across the world.

When you read the stories highlighted in this chapter, we encourage you to consider the ways in which the midwife uses a primary health care approach to address the social determinants of health and to improve public health outcomes within the community.

Midwifery continuity for women from vulnerable groups

Socioeconomic inequalities continue to widen in resource-rich countries like Australia and the UK with detrimental consequences for women and children in disadvantaged circumstances (Wilkinson & Pickett, 2006). This includes women who are black, Asian or from a minority ethnic group (BAME), migrants and those from a refugee background. Women who are vulnerable because of their 'social class' or 'ethnicity' are at a higher risk of maternal and perinatal morbidity and mortality (Marmot, 2010; Raleigh et al., 2010).

Women who have socially complex lives often struggle to engage effectively with maternity services (Ebert et al., 2011; National Insitute of Clinical Excellence (NICE), 2010; Rayment-Jones et al., 2015). This equates with 'late' booking for antenatal care, irregular attendance for antenatal visits or no antenatal care at all (Raatikainen

> ## BOX 10.1 The Midwife's Role in Reducing Inequalities
> - By 2020, 'midwives will embrace a greater public health role. Individual midwives and the midwifery workforce will expect support from those who plan and commission to enable them to meet the challenges of reducing inequalities and improving maternal and family health' (p. 5).
> - 'Midwives' unique contribution to public health is that they work with women and their partners and families throughout pregnancy, birth and the postnatal period to provide safe, holistic care. For optimum effect, midwifery needs to be firmly rooted in the community where women and their partners live their lives. Midwives should have a good knowledge of the health and social care needs of the local community; be well networked into the local health and social care system; and be proactive in identifying women at risk, and engaging with the woman, her family and other services as appropriate' (p. 6).
> - 'Seamless maternity services which work effectively between community and hospital settings should continue to be developed. These will support families to achieve improvements in early childcare and development and will facilitate access to parenting programmes and good quality early years' education' (p. 7).
> - 'Midwives should use their advocacy role for influencing and improving the health and wellbeing of women, children and families. This will include making the economic case for committing resources so that the midwife can deliver public health messages in the antenatal and postnatal periods and ensuring that there is a midwifery contribution at policy, strategic, political and international level' (p. 7).
>
> *(Chief Nursing Officers of England Northern Ireland Scotland and Wales 2010* Midwifery 2020. Delivering expectations. *Department of Health UK. Online: https://www.gov.uk/government/publications/midwifery-2020-delivering-expectations)*

et al., 2007). Underattending antenatal care is independently associated with adverse perinatal outcomes because abnormal processes that are potentially life threatening (e.g. pre-eclampsia or intrauterine growth restriction) are less able to be detected and managed (Raatikainen et al., 2007). Improving access to maternity care in a way that is acceptable to women with social complexity is therefore of paramount importance (NICE, 2010).

Midwifery continuity of care addresses the needs of women from vulnerable groups through the opportunity to build trusting relationships and enable access to safe, supportive services (Homer et al., 2017; Rayment-Jones et al., 2015). Continuity of carer enhances the social and emotional support women receive, which helps them confide their problems to a trusted midwife (Beake et al., 2013). For this to occur, the midwife must 'be available' and have sufficient time and attention to focus on the woman's individual needs to enable her to feel valued and safe (Ebert, 2012; Ebert et al., 2011). Ideally, midwives working in continuity of care have specific personal attributes that enable them to work with women in way that facilitates them to feel empowered and in control during pregnancy, birth and the postnatal period (Allen

---

BOX 10.2 A Reflection on Working in a Caseload Practice for Women With Socially Complex Lives

Hannah Rayment-Jones, Midwife, United Kingdom

Looking after women who live socially complex lives meant our working days were erratic and often unplanned. I would spend a lot of time trying to get in touch with women who were hard to reach, and distrusting of health care professionals. A significant amount of time was put into developing a relationship with each woman to be able to understand her individual needs. This might have been through reaching out via home visits, phone calls or text messages depending on what the woman was most comfortable with. Having the time to start conversations, often from home in the evening, is particularly important when trying to build relationships with women whose first priority may not be their maternity care.

One woman, Amena, a recent asylum seeker from Syria, was expecting her first baby and living alone; she spoke very little English. She had sparse knowledge of the maternity services in the UK and did not access any health care until late in her pregnancy. Getting in touch with Amena was difficult; understandably she did not want to answer her door to people she did not know. I started leaving short letters, translated into Arabic, explaining what the role of a midwife is, what would happen during an appointment and the reasons why; also, how we could prepare her to have her baby. Amena eventually agreed to a home visit, and then attended appointments after being shown how to use the bus to get to the hospital. She went on to attend an Arabic women's group in the area where she made friends with other mothers. Her care was based around her individual needs, and she always had an interpreter present for appointments. Amena was discharged from maternity care with a support network, a social worker and health visitor she knew and trusted.

It is vulnerable women like Amena who benefit so much from the more flexible continuity model of care, especially in improving their access and engagement with services and, in turn, clinical outcomes and the longer-term health and emotional wellbeing of the woman and her family.

---

et al., 2017; Leap, 2010). 'Endorphic' midwives promote feelings of safety, relaxation and reassurance so that women move through pregnancy and into birth feeling confident and unafraid (Allen et al., 2017).

Our first story (Box 10.2) is from Hannah Rayment-Jones, who worked for 4 years as a caseload midwife in a specialised service for women from a vulnerable community in London, UK. This work is also outlined in Chapter 2 by Vicki Cochrane. Every year, Hannah had a caseload of approximately 35 women living socially complex lives. The caseload team was made up of six experienced, compassionate midwives. Hannah is confident the sustainability and success of the service was in part due to the relationships between the midwives and their willingness to support each other. The midwives were flexible with their time, and met regularly to debrief about particularly difficult experiences or very complex cases.

Women from a refugee or asylum seeker background experience poorer perinatal outcomes including an increased instance of stillbirth; this can partly be explained by obstetric risk factors, lack of access to or engagement with maternity care (Biro & East, 2017) and / or communication barriers with care providers (Yelland et al., 2016). Women from a refugee background describe experiences of extreme suffering, abuse and loss, going 'literally through hell and back' (Balaam et al., 2016, p. 133). This means their emotional and mental health and wellbeing may be particularly challenged during the childbearing year. Standard 'fragmented' maternity care, for women from a refugee background, results in traditional birthing and recuperative practices being interrupted by the imposition of high-resourced, biomedical notions of appropriate care (Stapleton et al., 2013).

Providing quality, culturally responsive and accessible care is fundamental to addressing maternal and perinatal health inequalities in women who are refugees (Biro & East, 2017). Caseload midwifery for women from a refugee background has been associated with greater levels of advocacy, individualised care and improved outcomes (Bulman & McCourt, 2002). Midwifery continuity of care is particularly valued by newly arrived women as it offers security and support to negotiate an unfamiliar maternity system (Stapleton et al., 2013).

Our second story (Box 10.3) is from Michelle Steel, a midwife who established continuity of antenatal care for women from a refugee background in 2008 in Australia. This model was supported by a clinical (senior) midwife, a named social worker and a named obstetrician. Together they provided continuity of antenatal care for approximately 240 women each year. After 5 years, and following evaluation of the service, Michelle began providing midwifery continuity of postnatal care to women at home. In 2016, the service transformed into a midwifery continuity of care model: a midwifery group practice (MGP) specialising in maternity care for women from a refugee background. This is a perfect example of how continuity of care can evolve to address the needs of women from vulnerable communities.

Midwives providing continuity of care have an important role when pregnant women are at risk of having their babies removed by a child protection / safeguarding agency. Midwives need to share information, work collaboratively with a multidisciplinary team and develop pathways that best support the vulnerable woman and her baby (Everitt et al., 2017; Leap et al., 2010). Developing positive relationships with women and keeping them engaged within a maternity service are integral to providing quality care (Everitt et al., 2015). Midwifery continuity of care is an ideal model because a midwife who knows and cares about the woman's social circumstances can act as an advocate and support the woman to remain engaged in maternity care (Marsh et al., 2015).

Our third story in this section (Box 10.4), from Louise Everitt, explores how midwifery continuity of care can strengthen and protect families at risk. Louise is a

---

BOX 10.3 Working With Women From a Refugee Background in a Midwifery Group Practice

Michelle Steel, Midwife, Australia

Women from a refugee background prefer to come to our service because there is a greater understanding of their cultural needs. Women trust us not to treat them differently or 'otherly' when they describe female genital mutilation (FGM), preferences for perineal care, previous pregnancy and child losses, or their experiences in refugee camps. Women in general prefer not to have to explain their circumstances to multiple health care providers; and we strive to ensure women have the same known and trusted midwife with each pregnancy.

There is a large family from an African country who continue to come back to our service with each subsequent pregnancy. Everyone from the family—the matriarch, all her daughters and daughters-in-law—have had babies with us. Understanding the family dynamics has helped identify family violence, social isolation, homelessness, a woman with decreased mental capacity as a young mum, immigration issues and so forth. Because I am known and trusted by the family, I can bring up these topics in such a way that it can be openly discussed.

Another family I have cared for includes three sisters and their mother (who is a midwife); eleven babies so far. Knowing and being part of the birthing story for this family means there is no need for the woman to re-live difficult experiences through giving her 'history' and it is easier to identify potential risks in subsequent pregnancies. Building greater trust and acceptance in the midwife–family relationship results in higher levels of disclosure, which means her needs can be identified and met.

The Refugee MGP has seen a reduction in 'late' bookings and an increase in antenatal attendance and acceptance of maternity care. Women from a refugee background have a maternity service that 'belongs' to them; they take ownership of it. They have an easy route into the somewhat scary tertiary hospital system. They have someone on their side to walk by their side as they journey through pregnancy, birth and new motherhood and deal with all the trauma and challenges faced by refugees in our culture.

Clinical Midwifery Consultant at St George Public Hospital in Sydney, Australia. Her role is to provide direct clinical care or assist the midwives and doctors to care for women with complex pregnancies, specifically those who are very young and those whose lives involve social / emotional pressures (e.g. mental health, domestic violence, homelessness, sexual assault). Louise emphasises that working collaboratively with a great multidisciplinary team means not just providing, the clinical care, but also creating the ongoing support to enable situations in which women can feel empowered to make significant changes.

BOX 10.4 Working to Strengthen Families at Risk of Having Their Babies Removed

Louise Everitt, Midwife, Australia

When I first met Jade, she was 16 years old; she lived in a group home under the care of workers and community services. The workers from the home came with her for all her antenatal appointments. At 16 she had no family to support her and a history of serious sexual abuse in her past. She had no significant health problems but her fear of birth and her ability to parent were overwhelming to her. From a midwifery perspective she was cared for by a team of three midwives in the birth centre providing continuity of care and a homelike environment.

Jade's pregnancy, birth and postnatal stay were uncomplicated except that, after a long labour, she required transfer to the delivery suite. Her known midwives accompanied her, and she gave birth to her son with the assistance of a vacuum extractor. Sadly, whilst both were under the care of community services, at 16 weeks old her son died of sudden infant death syndrome (SIDS). As midwives we were asked to attend the funeral. A tiny white coffin, a grief-stricken young women surrounded by her only supports: the house mates and workers and her midwives. What words can help at such a distressing time? Our presence, however, was important to her.

Two years later, at 18, Jade was pregnant again. She had a choice to go to another hospital, but she chose to return to the midwives she knew and trusted. We knew her story, which meant recounting the memories with people previously involved made her feel comfortable. This time her history was different. She had had significant depression following her son's death and now had a story involving the use of illegal drugs and domestic violence. Without knowing her past history, this story could easily have evoked judgemental attitudes from staff. Knowing the extent of the trauma already experienced in her short 18 years, and her lack of support and role models, we understood that the way she chose to deal with her pain was perhaps not unexpected.

Immediately following the birth of her son, we received a phone call from community services that we were not predicting. They had decided to remove Jade's newborn baby from her care; he would be placed in foster care after discharge from hospital. Jade would be able to have contact with her baby in hospital and then only limited access a few times a week at the community services offices. This was distressing for all of us but we understood that the protection of a baby is always paramount. The alternative options we tried to organise were not considered a viable possibility.

At 21 Jade returned pregnant for the third time, choosing again to return to her trusted midwives, this time with a new partner and supportive extended family. Her second son remained in the care of community services and she still had some supervised access visits. Significant depression still accompanied her life, but she had worked hard to remain off illegal drugs; this new relationship was safe and supportive. Her pregnancy remained overshadowed by the involvement of community services and their questioning of her parenting abilities. The conversations at the antenatal visits always touched on fears of the past and fears for the future.

> ### BOX 10.4 Working to Strengthen Families at Risk of Having Their Babies Removed—cont'd
>
> Jade gave birth to a healthy baby girl without complication following a long labour. It was the first birth experience where she had a supportive partner and family around her. On the day of her discharge we took some happy family photos. She said to me, "I finally get to leave hospital and go home with my baby". This was the first steps in the next chapter of two new lives. I am glad I was able to share her journey and see her achieve something she had worked harder than most: to be, a new mum, baby in arms leaving hospital like everyone else.

Midwifery continuity of care for lesbian, gay, bisexual and transgender families

A shortage of heath care providers with knowledge of LGBT health issues and relevant competence in care provision impacts negatively on people within these communities (United States Department of Health and Human Services, 2013; Walker et al., 2016). For example, lesbians experience covert and overt homophobia and prejudice (Dahl et al., 2013). Conversely, when staff members demonstrate a positive and informed attitude, combined with small gestures of support, this positively impacts on lesbian mothers' experience of maternity care (Dahl et al., 2013). Developing cultural competence in this area, like any area, starts with identifying one's own beliefs and biases about people who are perceived as different from oneself (Jesse & Kirkpatrick, 2013). Case studies, reflective journaling and group work can help midwives to: examine personal bias, learn how to take a respectful and competent sexual health history, provide comprehensive health education, initiate appropriate referrals (Walker et al., 2016) and respond in appropriate ways when colleagues identify as belonging to the LGBT community (Mander, 2012). To work in a culturally safe way with lesbian families means to acknowledge that lesbian sexuality is normal and healthy, and that the 'co-mother' is an equal parent in the family who should be included as such (Dahl et al., 2013). Further, midwives should be able to consider how the co-mother's role and needs may be different from those of fathers (Spidsberg & Sørlie, 2012); for example, both mothers may wish to breastfeed.

Our first story in this section (Box 10.5) is from Karen Hollidale, who has been a midwife for over 17 years in a variety of contexts. She has worked in public hospital systems and team care models, and now is a privately practising midwife who enjoys working closely with families in a continuity of care model. Karen has worked with several families in the LGBT community and values all the relationships she has formed over the years.

Many LGBT families do not conform to a model of two parents of two genders (Greenfield, 2017). There may be more than two parents, different parents may have

BOX 10.5 Community-Based Private Midwifery Care for Lesbian Families
Karen Hollindale, Midwife, Australia

Getting to know couples during their pregnancy journey and supporting them through their birth and postnatal time is a privilege. Working in a continuity model, a relationship grows during those months of visits during pregnancy, and comes to fruition during the labour and birth, and the postnatal period.

Melina and Maree came to me seeking a connection. They had been to see a few different midwives and just could not find the right match. As a lesbian couple, Melina and Maree had sought out a model that would be supportive, and where they did not need to tell their story over again to new people. They wanted someone they could trust and walk with them on their journey. They had previously experienced a continuity of care relationship with their first baby, Kieran, and knew the benefits this offered their family.

Melina was a reserved but engaging person during the pregnancy. We had many in-depth discussions around her pregnancy questions, her concerns with her wider family unit, and her life in general. I got to know Melina and Maree well, and had a wonderful time involving and preparing Kieran for his sister's arrival. Kieran was going through the process of spectrum assessment and would become upset easily if things were out of routine—so working with him during the pregnancy was a wonderful growing relationship for us all—and we watched a big brother grow.

We all prepared for Melina's birth at home, processed and discussed her last birth, vocalised her hopes and dreams for this birth, wiped away tears, discussed books to read with Kieran and waited patiently.

Five days past Melina's estimated due date, Maree called me in the middle of the night when Melina's contractions started. She had a small fluid leak and was crampy: 'but you don't need to come yet Karen—they are too short'. My midwife's intuition told me her birth journey had begun and I decided to drive to their place—despite being told differently. I walked in to find Melina on the floor rocking through a strong contraction lasting for well over a minute—I knew her baby was well on her way. She reached around to grab my hand and said,

'I'm glad you're here Karen.'

'I'm glad I'm here too!'

Less than 30 minutes later we all welcomed a sweet little girl into her mummy's arms. Just Maree and I were there, as the rest of the team hadn't made it yet, and Kieran had slept on. His sweet little face came sleepily out to greet his new little sister about 30 minutes after she was born. The rest of Melina's team arrived—and Melina looked proudly up to all and said:

'I'd like introduce you to Ella.'

Our journey continued with more smiles, tears and teaching. We reminisced about Kieran's birth, and the wonderment of Ella's birth—and I got to share the joy of seeing confidence grow for Melina and Maree in their new parenting journey. During the postnatal period, I saw healing, confidence and wonder at each special milestone. I got to see the special relationship that the 'Mummy' and 'Mumma' shared with their new baby girl, and of course to watch a big brother blossom in his new role. I will never forget the picture Kieran drew for me of his family: Melina, Maree, Kieran, Ella *and Karen*. I was teary to think I was such a special part of their journey, especially for him.

BOX 10.5 Community-Based Private Midwifery Care for Lesbian Families—cont'd

I'm still in touch with Melina and Maree more than 12 months later and they say Kieran still remembers me at weird little times—brushing his teeth at the sink saying *'Karen has nice teeth too Mummy'.* However a family is made up, it is always such a pleasure to be part of their journey. Treating families with the care and understanding they all deserve makes each journey so special. Some birth journeys, however, stay with you forever!

different roles and levels of involvement, and a parent's gender may not necessarily denote their role (Greenfield, 2017). Transmasculine individuals or 'transmen' are people who were assigned as female at birth, but their inner sense of gender identity is on the male side of the gender spectrum; they may have the physical capacity to become pregnant, give birth and lactate (MacDonald et al., 2016). 'Transwomen' are individuals who identify as female, yet may have the physical capacity to supply sperm, owing to their anatomical sex (Greenfield, 2017). It can be problematic for transmen when midwives use terms with them such as 'mother' and female pronouns like 'she'; similarly, it can be problematic for transwomen when midwives use terms with them like 'man' and 'father' (Greenfield, 2017). Non-binary or agender people prefer to avoid the use of 'male' and 'female' and instead use pronouns like 'them' and 'theirs' (MacDonald et al., 2016). For some trans people the use of gendered terms for body parts can reinforce underlying gender dysphoria (Greenfield, 2017). For example, research shows that some transmen preferred to use the term 'chest feeding' instead of 'breastfeeding' because 'breast' denotes gender (MacDonald et al., 2016). Box 10.6 has been adapted from Greenfield's (2017) guide to inclusive language when working with these families.

Our final story in this section (Box 10.7) is from Canadian midwife Cora Beitel. In 2013, Cora co-founded The Strathcona Midwifery Collective, a community midwifery practice in Vancouver. In Canada, midwives are primary care providers offering: continuity of carer, antenatal care in free-standing clinics, birth at home or in hospitals, and postnatal care for clients for about 2 months after the birth. Cora, who is non-binary, has had the privilege of caring for many queer, trans and non-binary clients and their families, and in recent years has teamed up with a local doula to facilitate the Queer and Trans Pregnancy and Parenting Group (QTPP) out of the clinic. This group offers trans and queer families a space to share ideas and build community and support as they move along the parenting journey. Cora is committed to building better inclusivity practices in medical spaces for pregnant trans people and their families.

BOX 10.6 Inclusive Language When Working With LGBT Families

1. If you're not sure what pronoun a person wants to use, simply ask.
2. Use names instead of roles (*e.g.* 'mother' implies there is only one and that the person who is pregnant identifies as female).
3. Be aware of your assumptions and be open to alternative possibilities (e.g. there may be one mother, two mothers or no mother; or one father, two fathers or no father).
4. Don't be afraid to ask questions, but first think about whether they're necessary.
5. Ask open questions (e.g. 'Who are the baby's parents?' 'Who gave birth?').
6. Avoid questions about why and how parents decided to conceive, who was to carry the child and non-medically relevant details of transition.
7. Think about what it is you actually want to find out and then phrase your question accordingly.
8. Avoid repeated questions (i.e. record the answers to your questions).

(Adapted from: Greenfield, M 2017 He's not the mother. AIMS J 29(2): 7-9)

BOX 10.7 Working With Transgender and Non-Binary People
Cora Beitel, Midwife, Canada

As midwives, our responsibility is to provide client-centred care, and to me this means getting to know each family, honouring each person's knowledge about their body and tailoring my care as best I can to meet their needs. Within our model there is an opportunity to slow down the antenatal care, taking the time that's needed to provide respectful, informed-choice conversations, while creating a space that is both physically and emotionally safe for our clients. This kind of care benefits everyone and is particularly important when caring for trans and non-binary persons. When your gender identity does not match the expected gender of a pregnant person, discrimination is an everyday possibility and there is a heightened potential for vulnerability stemming from being misgendered, physical dysphoria and mistreatment from the health care system. Midwifery care rooted in advocacy allows time to delve more into each client's needs regarding their care, focusing on safety and support along with the routine clinical care.

Most of the trans or non-binary clients that I have cared for have planned homebirths. People have chosen to give birth at home usually for reasons of comfort, peacefulness and reduced interventions. However, this choice is also made because of fearing being misgendered, mistreated or disrespected by hospital staff who may not be sensitive to the care needs of a transgender pregnant patient. When caring for trans clients planning to birth at home, special considerations need to be put in place in the event of a transfer to hospital in labour.

One person I was caring for, who was having his first baby, started early labour with his water breaking at 38 weeks. I spent the night at his house with his partner and doula, trying to get labour to move forward with natural remedies. By morning, it was clear that labour wasn't progressing and he was getting exhausted. We decided a transfer to hospital was best. My focus in this moment became about creating as much emotional safety as possible at the

BOX 10.7 Working With Transgender and Non-Binary People—cont'd

hospital. I called ahead, spoke to the charge nurse and discussed the need for a caring and sensitive team. I wanted my client to walk into the hospital and feel seen and respected, with the focus being on his medical needs and not unnecessarily on his gender identity. We were in luck! We had the best team of fabulous nurses at the hospital and my client was surrounded with an excellent care team. Every time someone new entered the room, I would catch them in the hallway first and discuss what my client needed—proper use of his pronouns, thoughtful use of language, slowing down with exams. Over all, the care was very appropriate. The birth was challenging, as births can be, but the care in the room felt very respectful and client centred. This allowed my client and his partner the space to focus on their needs and their baby and not on educating hospital staff.

We can't control whether someone has a homebirth, or how a birth will unfold, but we can take steps to change the spaces our clients walk into in the hospital. Birth is a vulnerable and intense time for our clients and their partners and family, and how they are treated in hospital can make a significant difference to their experience. Change is slow in large institutions, but it is happening. With feedback from families and care providers we are seeing more education on inclusivity happening in our institutions and it is making a difference to client care.

Midwifery continuity of care for young women

Working with young women to identify and modify the risk and protective factors in their daily lives improves health outcomes (Viner et al., 2012). Young pregnant women are more likely to have challenges including emotional and mental health issues (Siegel & Brandon, 2014) related to psychosocial stressors such as low income, exposure to violence and intense loneliness (Bloom et al., 2013). These vulnerabilities can be associated with smoking, alcohol and illicit drug use during pregnancy (Bottorff et al., 2014).

The relationship between the midwife and woman facilitated by continuity of care promotes health engagement: turning up for care and 'buying in' to care (Allen, 2015). As a public health strategy, midwifery continuity of care works by promoting earlier maternity booking, enabling access to quality antenatal care, supporting greater emotional resilience, promoting good nutrition and ideal gestational weight gain, encouraging reduction in smoking/drug use and diagnosing/treating genitourinary infections (Allen et al., 2016). Health engagement is the mechanism behind the better outcomes experienced by young women and their babies who received caseload midwifery compared with other models—namely lower rates of pre-term birth and separate neonatal nursery admission, and higher rates of breastfeeding (Allen et al., 2015).

The story in Box 10.8 focuses on providing care within a midwifery group practice designed for young women in Australia. The author of this chapter, Jyai Allen,

BOX 10.8 Working With Young Women in a Specialised Midwifery Group Practice

Jyai Allen, Australia

I remember doing a booking home visit for 14-year-old Lianna at her mother's home on the outskirts of Brisbane. Lianna was softly spoken, avoided eye contact, and did not ask any questions. Through obtaining her history, I learnt that she had been raped on the school grounds by a peer and was not in any contact with the boy who raped her. Lianna was having her baby alone with the support of her mother.

Lianna and her mother came regularly to the group antenatal care sessions. She was painfully shy and didn't interact with the other young women, who were older teenagers. Towards the end of her pregnancy, we spent larger amounts of time one-on-one talking about labour and active birth strategies. I was never sure how much Lianna was engaging in the discussion because she always kept her head down, with her eyes focused on the table in front of us.

At about 39 weeks gestation, Lianna telephoned me, in early labour. When I met her in birth suite she was managing well. She sat on a birth ball, rolling her hips during contractions and doing Sudoku between them! Her mother was present, quietly supportive in an armchair. With Lianna's permission, I invited a young final-year medical student into the room.

Lianna progressed quickly and within a few hours she moved spontaneously into a hands-and-knees position for birth. The room was dim and quiet as Lianna pushed her baby out instinctively, without direction. I quietly supported the medical student to pass the baby through her legs onto the bed. Lianna picked her baby up and within 15 minutes she was breastfeeding, and the placenta was born physiologically.

I visited Lianna and her baby at home for 6 weeks. Everything about Lianna's demeanour had changed. She made eye contact, she asked questions, she kept detailed records of the baby's output and she wrote down any concerns to discuss at the visits. She breastfed confidently and without the usual adolescent embarrassment. She was clearly bonded to her baby and thriving as a mother.

When the final visit came she handed me a handmade 'thank you' card with my name cut out and pasted on, along with a photo of her and her baby. I'll never forget Lianna—and how being informed and supported during her whole experience by a midwife she knew and trusted enabled her to step into her power and transform through birth to become the strong and confident mother she needs to be. All young women should have that opportunity as they transition into motherhood.

I talked to the medical student as we were walking to the car park after the birth. He told me this had been his last rotation on birth suite, but his first normal birth. He was ecstatic and effusive about what an incredible experience that had been. He said he wanted to pursue a speciality in obstetrics.

was a caseload midwife involved in establishing and working within the practice prior to conducting a 5-year evaluation of the service as part of her PhD (Allen, 2015). The practice provides community-based pregnancy and postnatal care, with labour and birth care in a tertiary birth suite. Young women have a booking visit in their home, followed by group antenatal care with other young women of similar gestation at a suburban clinic. There is access to an obstetrician and a social worker either on site or via telecommunication technologies (e.g. telemedicine). The midwives facilitate a social postnatal group for young women to reconnect with each other after their babies are born. Postnatal care is provided in the home until 4–6 weeks after birth.

Midwifery continuity of care for Aboriginal women

In this next section, we focus on Aboriginal and Torres Strait Islander peoples, who share a similar colonised history to Indigenous peoples in Canada and New Zealand. Aboriginal health is holistic—it 'means not just the physical wellbeing of an individual but refers to the social, emotional and cultural wellbeing of the whole Community in which each individual is able to achieve their full potential as a human being thereby bringing about the total wellbeing of their community' (National Aboriginal Community Controlled Health Organisation (NACCHO), 2018). For Indigenous peoples across the world, the impact of European invasion (often referred to as 'colonisation') has resulted in dispossession, racism, marginalisation, poverty and intergenerational disadvantage which profoundly affects Aboriginal health and wellbeing (Congress of Aboriginal and Torres Strait Islander Nurses and Midwives (CATSINaM), 2017).

Australian Aboriginal maternal and infant mortality rates are double the non-Aboriginal rate (Australian Government, 2011, 2013, 2018), and Aboriginal babies are more likely to be born pre-term and with low birth weight (Australian Institute for Health and Welfare (AIHW), 2017; Hoy & Nicol, 2010; Singh & Hoy, 2003). Aboriginal women are less willing and able to engage in maternity care owing to a lack of culturally appropriate services, institutional racism within health services, the absence of local services, and the lack of Aboriginal health care workers, transport and childcare (Arnold et al., 2009). Conversely, Aboriginal peoples are more likely to access and engage with health services that are respectful and culturally safe (CATSINaM, 2017), holistic and integrated (Kildea et al., 2013).

First nations women across the world have requested the return of birthing services to their lands, their communities and their control for many years; this is known as 'Birthing on Country' (Australian College of Midwives (ACM), Congress of Aboriginal and Torres Strait Islander Nurses and Midwives (CATSINaM), Council of Remote Area Nurses of Australia, 2016; Kildea & Van Wagner, 2012). Birthing on Country has been defined as:

… maternity services designed and delivered for Indigenous women that encompass some or all of the following elements: are community based and governed; allow for incorporation of traditional practice; involve a connection with land and country; incorporate a holistic definition of health; value Indigenous and non-Indigenous ways of knowing and learning, risk assessment and service delivery; are culturally competent and are developed by, or with, Indigenous people.

(Kildea & Van Wagner, 2012, p. 5)

In Northern Quebec (Canada) the Inuit model, involving three Birthing on Country services that operate in places which are many hours by plane from access to caesarean section facilities, provides the most robust evidence of an 'exemplar model' (Kildea et al., 2016a). Such models have improved maternal and infant health outcomes because they meet community expectations, address clinical / medical, social / cultural, spiritual and emotional risks, and support Indigenous midwifery training (Van Wagner et al., 2012). Since the first remote maternity service opened in the mid eighties there has been a slow return of birthing services to remote communities, with 16 now open across Canada. In Chapter 11, Vicki Van Wagner, Brenda Epoo, Aileen Inukpuk Moorhouse and Kim Moorhouse provide a story exemplifying how, for the Inuit, Birthing on Country means continuity, not only of your caregiver but also with your family, your language, the land and Inuit history.

The Australian Birthing on Country model combines:

- Aboriginal knowledge, ownership and governance
- continuity of midwifery carer
- choice of place of birth
- culturally safe care
- development of the Aboriginal maternal and infant workforce; and
- programs to strengthen the capacity of families (Kildea et al., 2016b).

A staged approach to the introduction of Birthing on Country models is occurring in a number of areas in Australia.

Our next story (Box 10.9) was contributed by Lise Robertson, a Danish-born, Australian-trained and experienced caseload midwife. For the last 4 years, she has

---

BOX 10.9 A Partnership Model Between Aboriginal Community Controlled Health Organisations and a Tertiary Maternity Hospital

Lise Robertson, Midwife, Australia

This is the story of my professional partnership with an Aboriginal woman, through the pregnancies and births of her two children, and beyond. Her name is Bell and I cared for her through the Birthing in Our Community (BiOC) MGP. Bell's story is unique, as is the childbearing journey of every woman I have worked with in this diverse community—a community with common strengths such as: straightforward honesty, 'this is how it is, and how I tell it', a proud sense of belonging to family and place and an ability to live in the moment much more

BOX 10.9 A Partnership Model Between Aboriginal Community Controlled Health Organisations and a Tertiary Maternity Hospital—cont'd

than people in my Western culture. Working in this community, I have learned to be a more flexible and patient midwife, enjoying days where little runs to plan, yet so much is achieved.

I first met Bell during a BiOC yarning session 4 years ago. She was 20 years old, a little shy and carrying her first baby Ben with great anticipation. I was not her caseload midwife, but through the group antenatal sessions I knew Bell was with her boyfriend David and that Ben was not planned but welcomed. Bell trusted her own ability to grow and birth a healthy baby so much that she declined ultrasound scans, routine blood tests and fetal heart rate auscultation during pregnancy.

I cared for Bell and David during her first labour, which lasted over 12 hours and was uncomplicated. She stuck to her plan of no analgesia. She agreed to intermittent fetal heart rate auscultation and the only other intervention was an artificial rupture of membranes (ARM) when her contractions slowed during transition. Bell was active throughout labour, she gave birth on her hands and knees and she had a physiological third stage.

Two years later Bell asked me to be the midwife for her second child: 'you were with me through Ben's birth and I'd like you to be there this time too please'. It was a very different journey for both of us, as the BiOC model had changed, and I now saw Bell for individual home visits during her pregnancy (instead of group antenatal care sessions). We simply called each other when a visit was due, or she wanted me to come, and I would swing by her place on my route home. Again, she chose to have no ultrasound scans or fetal heart rate monitoring during pregnancy. I came to know Bell much better during her second pregnancy: a beautiful woman and a confident mother. Bell still breastfed Ben until she decided to stop in late pregnancy, she made excellent choices for her family with David by her side and she dreamt of a career in midwifery in the future for herself.

Bell's second birth was the waterbirth she had hoped for. She and David came in mid morning, and by dinnertime she had given birth to her daughter Anna in the warm water with grace and calmness. Again, the only intervention was an ARM she requested during active first stage, when contractions had slowed. I remember watching David holding Bell as she lifted her baby out of the water and onto her chest. Ten minutes later, I watched as she put Anna to the breast still in the water, and noticed David was no longer in the room. Laughingly she explained he had gone to help his mate in their fish and chip shop with the dinner rush. Four hours later David was back, and they left for home with their newborn daughter. We had 6 weeks of mostly social postnatal home visits; Bell really did not need much guidance from me this time.

But the story does not end there. Last year Bell, with a little encouragement from me, successfully applied for and became one of our Aboriginal family support workers in BiOC. For 6 months, I had the pleasure of working alongside Bell, who connected with and supported the women in my caseload with great professionalism and kindness. Bell is starting her midwifery education program this semester with some funding support and she will have some clinical placements with BiOC MGP. I feel so lucky to have been a part of Bell's journey. When I retire soon, I am looking forward to handing over the baton to Bell—Aboriginal midwives are best placed to do this job!

worked as a caseload midwife in an urban model known as 'Birthing in Our Community' which aims for equity in birth outcomes, health status and life expectancy for Aboriginal and Torres Strait Islander families. The model is governed by a partnership between two Aboriginal community-controlled health organisations and a tertiary maternity hospital. Over the last 4 years, Lise has seen the model evolve from four midwives and two Aboriginal health care workers operating from the hospital into a community-based and -controlled 'Mums and Bubs Hub', where each woman has her own midwife and family support worker. At the Hub, families can access culturally appropriate services including a social worker, psychologist, paediatrician, woman's health general practitioner and a Stop Smoking Program.

The final story in this chapter (Box 10.10) is from Melanie Briggs, an Aboriginal midwife working with an Aboriginal community-controlled health organisation in a

---

BOX 10.10 Aboriginal Midwives Providing Midwifery Continuity for Aboriginal Women

Melanie Briggs, Midwife, Australia

As a child I remember living on the mission, in a four-bedroom house with my older sister and two older brothers. We shared the house with my Nan, aunty and two uncles, who also had two little boys and a girl. The floors were simple unpolished timber floorboards, the kitchen was a single bench top with curtains to cover the shelves and one huge timber dining table where everyone would sit and yarn about life, laugh and tell stories of the old people. This is where I felt safe, being surrounded by family and empowered to be myself, knowing that there is no judgement and the stories were the creation of our people and our journeys. In 2018, this type of living arrangement has been referred to as overcrowding. However, we grew to learn and respect our Elders, listen and be grateful for what we have been given. Growing up, we learnt how all things were created by the mother earth and how creations are returned in a cultural and spiritual way.

Recently I cared for my 25-year-old cousin Leslie, who was pregnant with her first baby. Leslie is a direct descendant of one of the original tribes from the area and has been handed down many stories relating to birth and the rituals that were performed prior to invasion. Throughout our yarns about her birth expectations, Leslie said that she wanted her five sisters involved in the birth experience. I understood Leslie's request to have her sisters with her because having family surround you with stories, comfort and safety makes you feel empowered.

Leslie was around 36 weeks pregnant when we conducted a hospital tour. As we walked into the hospital we were greeted by the ward clerk, who acknowledged Leslie and me. A midwife then politely said hello and walked us through the labour and postnatal wards. As we walked into the hospital ward with 'white walls and polished vinyl floors', we inspected what seemed to be a small 3.5 metre × 3.5 metre room that had a single bed where women were expected to labour and birth, one reclining chair for the support person and a neonatal resuscitation table.

BOX 10.10 Aboriginal Midwives Providing Midwifery Continuity for Aboriginal Women—cont'd

Leslie advised that she had been to the labour ward before to support her sister when she was giving birth. Leslie described this experience as 'lonely and sad', as both Leslie and her sister felt they needed more people in the room to support them during the labour. Leslie then asked me if she was going to be able to be supported by her sisters during her birth. The midwife from the hospital interrupted abruptly and responded to Leslie by saying 'we only allow two family members to be in the room with you at one time, for safety reasons'. The abrupt response caused significant distress for Leslie, and I could see her automatic disengagement from the hospital midwife.

I asked the hospital midwife if I could speak with her outside of the room to explain Leslie's situation. The midwife followed me outside of the room and before I could explain Leslie's situation the midwife stated that the rooms do not facilitate large families and that she is not allowed to have more than two people in the room with her at one time. I continued the discussion around the importance of family and the rituals that her family follow that relate to birth, and how not having all her sisters present at the birth would impact her negatively and may cause her to disengage and not be present when in labour. We continued to discuss other ways her family could all be present and how the hospital could manage this. The midwife was unable to make decisions and the situation had to be escalated to the midwifery unit manager (MUM).

I had a meeting with the MUM and explained Leslie's situation, and the MUM was very understanding. The MUM was very knowledgeable of the local Aboriginal community and the importance of family during birth. The MUM and I planned for Leslie's family to alternate times during labour and birth as well as have all sisters there at the time of the birth but the most significant issue for the MUM was to ensure the carer was not impacted during the routine checks. I communicated this plan to Leslie and she felt relieved knowing that she would be able to have her family present during labour and birth.

At term, Leslie went into spontaneous labour; her family attended the labour ward and the maternity staff seemed to be welcoming. Leslie progressed to full dilation in approximately 12 hours and gave birth to a live female bubba (baby) with immediate skin-to-skin contact. Her sisters surrounded her and welcomed the new bubba with songs, yarning and laughing.

Immediately following the birth, you could sense Leslie's pride, strength and the joy of having her family with her during labour and birth. The moment the bubba was born, the sisters surrounded her and protected her. Leslie felt safe and knew that she was protected by her family and her midwife.

---

rural town in New South Wales, the same place where she grew up. Melanie provides antenatal and postnatal continuity of care in the community for Aboriginal women or women who are having an Aboriginal baby. In addition, she provides intrapartum *support* (not clinical care) in the local hospital. Melanie provides vital advocacy and support for mothers specifically relating to cultural practices that women request.

CONCLUSION

This chapter has highlighted real-life experiences and the learning of midwives engaged in practice with specific groups across a range of different settings. Through reflection on these stories we hope you can appreciate how best you can work with women who are isolated, marginalised or vulnerable—for whatever reasons. The themes in the stories have included how:

- the midwife identifies and helps address the social determinants of health in each woman's life
- the midwife–woman relationship enables responsive midwifery focused on the woman's individual needs and advocacy for these
- the midwife promotes the normalcy of pregnancy while keeping a close eye on potential risks and acting in a timely way
- the midwife appreciates the value of professional relationships and allied health services to support the woman in a holistic way
- the midwife is part of the community—she is known and trusted by the community
- the midwife is reflective, and aware of her personal bias and privilege, which makes her more able to respond in culturally safe ways with clients who are culturally different from the midwife
- the midwife focuses on developing the woman's strengths and resilience so that she starts life with a new baby in the best possible circumstances.

We hope these themes will help guide you when providing midwifery continuity of care to women from specific groups.

REFERENCES

Australian College of Midwives (ACM), Congress of Aboriginal and Torres Strait Islander Nurses and Midwives (CATSINaM), Council of Remote Area Nurses of Australia: Birthing on Country position statement, 2016. Online: http://catsinam.org.au/static/uploads/files/birthing-on-country-position-statement-endorsed-march-2016-wfaxpyhvmxrw.pdf.

Australian Government: *National Aboriginal and Torres Strait Islander health plan 2013–2023*, 2013. Online: http://www.health.gov.au/internet/main/publishing.nsf/content/B92E980680486C3BCA257BF0001BAF01/$File/health-plan.pdf.

Australian Government Department of Health: *National maternity services plan*, 2011. Online: http://www.health.gov.au/internet/publications/publishing.nsf/Content/pacd-maternityservicesplan-toc.

Australian Government Department of the Prime Minister and Cabinet: Closing the Gap: Prime Minister's report, 2018. Online: http://closingthegap.pmc.gov.au/sites/default/files/ctg-report-2018.pdf?a=1.

Australian Institute for Health and Welfare (AIHW): *Aboriginal and Torres Strait Islander Health Performance Framework (HPF)*, 2017. Online: https://www.aihw.gov.au/reports/indigenous-health-welfare/health-performance-framework/contents/summary.

Allen J: (How) does the way maternity care is provided affect the health and well-being of young women and their babies? PhD thesis, Australian Catholic University, 2015. Online: http://researchbank.acu.edu.au/theses/546.

Allen J, Gibbons K, Beckmann M, Tracy M, Stapleton H, Kildea S: Does model of maternity care make a difference to birth outcomes for young women? A retrospective cohort study, *Int J Nurs Stud* 52(8):1332–1342, 2015.

Allen J, Kildea S, Stapleton H: How optimal caseload midwifery can modify predictors for preterm birth in young women: integrated findings from a mixed methods study, *Midwifery* 41:30–38, 2016.

Allen J, Kildea S, Hartz DL, Tracy M, Tracy S: The motivation and capacity to go 'above and beyond': qualitative analysis of free-text survey responses in the M@NGO randomised controlled trial of caseload midwifery, *Midwifery* 50:148–156, 2017.

Arnold JL, Costa CM, Howat PW: Timing of transfer for pregnant women from Queensland Cape York communities to Cairns for birthing, *Med J Aust* 190(10):594–596, 2009.

Balaam MC, Kingdon C, Thomson G, Finalyson K, Downe S: 'We make them feel special': the experiences of voluntary sector workers supporting asylum seeking and refugee women during pregnancy and early motherhood, *Midwifery* 34:133–140, 2016.

Beake S, Acosta L, Cooke P, McCourt C: Caseload midwifery in a multi-ethnic community: the women's experiences, *Midwifery* 29:996–1002, 2013.

Bick D: The importance of public health: let history speak for itself, *Midwifery* 22:287–289, 2006.

Biro MA: What has public health got to do with midwifery? Midwives' role in securing better health outcomes for mothers and babies, *Women Birth* 24:17–23, 2011.

Biro MA, East C: Poorer detection rates of severe fetal growth restriction in women of likely refugee background: a case for re-focusing pregnancy care, *Aust N Z J Obstet Gynaecol* 57(2):186–192, 2017.

Bloom T, Glass N, Curry MA, Hernandez R, Houck G: Maternal stress exposures, reactions, and priorities for stress reduction among low-income, urban women, *J Midwifery Womens Health* 58(2): 167–174, 2013.

Bottorff JL, Poole N, Kelly MT, Greaves L, Marcellus L, Jung M: Tobacco and alcohol use in the context of adolescent pregnancy and postpartum: a scoping review of the literature, *Health Soc Care Community* 22(6):561–574, 2014.

Brodie P: The invisibility of midwifery: will developing professional capital make a difference?, D Mid thesis, Sydney, 2003, UTS. Online: http://epress.lib.uts.edu.au/dspace/handle/2100/339.

Bulman K, McCourt C: Somali refugee women's experiences of maternity care in west London: a case study, *Crit Public Health* 12:365–380, 2002.

Chief Nursing Officers of England, Northern Ireland, Scotland and Wales: *Midwifery 2020: delivering expectations*, 2010. Online: https://www.gov.uk/government/publications/midwifery-2020-delivering-expectations.

Congress of Aboriginal and Torres Strait Islander Nurses and Midwives (CATSINaM): Position statement: embedding cultural safety across Australian nursing and midwifery, 2017. Online: https://www.catsinam.org.au/static/uploads/files/embedding-cultural-safety-accross-australian-nursing-and-midwifery-may-2017-wfca.pdf.

Dahl B, Fylkesnes AM, Sørlie V, Malterud K: Lesbian women's experiences with healthcare providers in the birthing context: a meta-ethnography, *Midwifery* 29(6):674–681, 2013.

Department of Health: National Primary Health Strategic Framework, 2013. Online: http://www.health.gov.au/internet/publications/publishing.nsf/Content/NPHC-Strategic-Framework.

Ebert L: Woman-centred care and the socially disadvantaged woman: an interpretative phenomenological analysis, PhD thesis, University of Newcastle, 2012. Online: http://hdl.handle.net/1959.13/936189.

Ebert L, Ferguson A, Bellchambers H: Working for socially disadvantaged women, *Women Birth* 24: 85–91, 2011.

Everitt L, Fenwick J, Homer CS: Midwives experiences of removal of a newborn baby in New South Wales, Australia: being in the 'head' and 'heart' space, *Women Birth* 28(2):95–100, 2015.

Everitt L, Homer CS, Fenwick J: Working with vulnerable pregnant women who are at risk of having their babies removed by the child protection agency in New South Wales, Australia, *Child Abuse Rev* 26:351–363, 2017.

Greenfield M: He's not the mother, *AIMS J* 29(2):7–9, 2017.

Homer C, Leap N, Edwards N, Sandall J: Midwifery continuity of care in an area of high socio-economic disadvantage in London: a retrospective analysis of albany midwifery practice outcomes using routine data (1997–2009), *Midwifery* 48:1–10, 2017.

Hoy W, Nicol J: Birthweight and natural deaths in a remote Australian aboriginal community, *Med J Aust* 192(1):14–19, 2010.

Jesse DE, Kirkpatrick MK: Catching the spirit of cultural care: a midwifery exemplar, *J Midwifery Womens Health* 58:49–56, 2013.

Kaufmann T: Midwifery and public health, *MIDIRS Midwifery Digest* 12(Suppl 1):S23–S26, 2002.

Kildea S, van Wagner V: *'Birthing on Country,' maternity service delivery models: a rapid review*. An evidence check rapid review brokered by the Sax Institute. Canberra, 2012, Maternity Services Inter-Jurisdictional Committee for the Australian Health Minister's Advisory Council. Online: https://www.saxinstitute.org.au/wp-content/uploads/Birthing-on-Country1.pdf.

Kildea S, Magick Dennis F, Stapleton H: Birthing on Country workshop report. Alice Springs, Brisbane, 2013, Australian Catholic University and Mater Medical Research Institute on behalf of the Maternity Services Inter-Jurisdictional Committee for the Australian Health Minister's Advisory Council.

Kildea S, Tracy S, Sherwood J, Magick-Dennis F, Barclay L: Improving maternity services for Indigenous women in Australia: moving from policy to practice, *Med J Aust* 205(8):374–379, 2016a.

Kildea S, Lockey R, Roberts J, Magick Dennis F: *Guiding principles for developing a Birthing on Country service model and evaluation framework, phase 1*. Maternity Services Inter-Jurisdictional Committee for the Australian Health Ministers' Advisory Council. Brisbane, 2016b, Mater Medical Research Unit and the University of Queensland.

Leap N: The less we do the more we give. In Kirkham M, editor: *The midwife–mother relationship*, ed 2, Basingstoke, Hants, 2010, Palgrave Macmillan, Ch. 2, pp 17–35.

Leap N, Edwards N: The politics of involving women in decision making. In Page LA, Campbell R, editors: *The new midwifery: science and sensitivity in practice*, ed 2, London, 2006, Churchill Livingstone, pp 97–123. Ch. 5.

Leap N, Fowler C, Homer C, for Australian Centre for Child Protection: *Nurturing and protecting children: a public health approach. A learning resource for midwives and child and family health nurses*, 2010. Online: https://www.unisa.edu.au/PageFiles/90644/ppcn_mcurriculummaterials.pdf.

MacDonald T, Noel-Weiss J, West D, Walks M, Biener M, Kibbe A, et al: Transmasculine individuals' experiences with lactation, chestfeeding, and gender identity: a qualitative study, *BMC Pregnancy Childbirth* 16:106, 2016.

McNeill J, Lynn F, Alderice F: Public health interventions in midwifery: a systematic review of systematic reviews, *BMC Public Health* 12:955, 2012.

Mander R: Midwifery and the LGBT midwife, *Midwifery* 28(1):9–13, 2012.

Marmot M: *Fair society, healthy lives*. The Marmot Review executive summary. The Marmot Review, 2010. Online: http://www.ucl.ac.uk/gheg/marmotreview/FairSocietyHealthyLivesExecSummary.

Marmot M, Wilkinson R: *Social determinants of health*, ed 2, Oxford, 2005, Oxford University Press.

Marsh CA, Browne J, Taylor J, Davis D: Guilty until proven innocent? The assumption of care of a baby at birth, *Women Birth* 28(1):65–70, 2015.

National Aboriginal Community Controlled Health Organisation (NACCHO): Aboriginal health definitions, 2018. Online: http://www.naccho.org.au/about/aboriginal-health/definitions/.

National Health Service (NHS) England: *Implementing Better Births: continuity of carer. A Five Year Forward View for maternity care*, London, 2017, NHS. Online: https://www.england.nhs.uk/mat-transformation/implementing-better-births/.

National Insitute of Clinical Excellence (NICE): *Pregnancy and complex social factors: a model for service provision for pregnant women with complex social factors*, London, 2010, NICE.

Nursing and Midwifery Board of Australia (NMBA): National competency standards for the midwife, 2006. Online: https://www.nursingmidwiferyboard.gov.au/search.aspx?q=national%20competency%20standards%20for%20the%20midwife.

Nursing and Midwifery Council (NMC): Standards for competence for registered midwives, 2009. Online: https://www.nmc.org.uk/globalassets/sitedocuments/standards/nmc-standards-for-competence-for-registered-midwives.pdf.

Raatikainen K, Heiskanen N, Heinonen S: Under-attending free antenatal care is associated with adverse pregnancy outcomes, *BMC Public Health* 27(7):268, 2007.

Raleigh VS, Hussey D, Seccombe I, Halt K: Ethnic and social inequalities in women's experience of maternity care in England: results of a national survey, *J R Soc Med* 103:188–198, 2010.

Rayment-Jones H, Murrells T, Sandall J: An investigation of the relationship between the case load model of midwifery for socially disadvantaged women and childbirth outcomes using routine data—a retrospective observational study, *Midwifery* 31(4):409–417, 2015.

Siegel RS, Brandon AR: Adolescents, pregnancy and mental health, *J Pediatr Adolesc Gynecol* 27(3):138–150, 2014.

Singh G, Hoy W: The association between birthweight and current blood pressure: a cross-sectional study in an Australian Aboriginal community, *Med J Aust* 179(10):532–535, 2003.

Spidsberg BD, Sørlie V: An expression of love—midwives' experiences in the encounter with lesbian women and their partners, *J Adv Nurs* 68(4):796–805, 2012.

Stapleton H, Murphy R, Correa-Velez I, Steel M, Kildea S: Women from refugee backgrounds and their experiences of attending a specialist antenatal clinic. Narratives from an Australian setting, *Women Birth* 26(4):260–266, 2013.

United States Department of Health and Human Services: Healthy people 2020, 2013. Online: http://www.healthypeople.gov/2020/default.aspx.

Van Wagner V, Osepchook C, Harney E, Crosbie C, Tulugak M: Remote midwifery in Nunavik, Quebec, Canada: outcomes of perinatal care for the Inuulitsivik Health Centre, 2000–2007, *Birth* 39:230–237, 2012.

Viner RM, Ozer EM, Denny S, Marmot M, Resnick M, Fatusi A, et al: Adolescence and the social determinants of health, *Lancet* 379(9826):1641–1652, 2012.

Walker K, Arbour M, Waryold J: Educational strategies to help students provide respectful sexual and reproductive health care for lesbian, gay, bisexual, and transgender persons, *J Midwifery Womens Health* 61(6):737–743, 2016.

Wilkinson RG, Pickett KE: Income inequality and population health: a review and explanation of the evidence, *Soc Sci Med* 62:1768–1784, 2006.

Yelland J, Riggs E, Szwarc J, Casey S, Duell-Piening P, Chesters D, et al: Compromised communication: a qualitative study exploring Afghan families and health professionals' experience of interpreting support in Australian maternity care, *BMJ Qual Saf* 25(4):e1, 2016.

CHAPTER 11

Midwifery Continuity of Care: Theorising Towards Sustainability

Lorna Davies, Susan Crowther, Billie Hunter

Contents

INTRODUCTION

The term 'sustainability' currently has a seemingly ubiquitous presence in academia, popular culture and everyday conversation. In health care it could be seen to translate as the potential for the 'long-term maintenance of health and wellbeing of the human population' (Davies, 2017, p. x). Our health is dependent on the health of the environment that we inhabit, the social structures that we create and function within and the frameworks that regulate our economic models.

An interest in the concept of sustainability in relation to midwifery care and practice has increased exponentially in recent years (Crowther et al., 2016; Davies, 2017; Donald, 2012; Hunter & Warren, 2014; McAra-Couper et al., 2014; Sandall et al., 2016; Tracy et al., 2013; Wakelin & Skinner, 2007; Young, 2011). Researchers have explored the sustainability of models of midwifery care, sustainable workforce requirements, burnout and the emotional wellbeing of midwives, the resilience of midwives, and how midwives view the concept of sustainability within their professional lives. Interestingly, much of the available research on sustainable midwifery practice has been carried out within a continuity of care setting. The findings of these studies have provided insight into how midwifery continuity of care models may sustain both midwives and the women whom they serve, revealing factors that may facilitate sustainable approaches within practice as well as those that militate against it.

In this chapter we delve into some theoretical depths to discuss the notion of sustainability in relation to midwifery continuity of care. We unpack its conceptual and theoretical origin and meaning, consider how it is challenged by neoliberalism and the associated concept of individualism, and explore how it relates to professional practice in midwifery models of care that facilitate relational continuity.

SUSTAINABILITY: THEORETICAL AND CONCEPTUAL FRAMEWORK

Before exploring further the phenomenon of sustainability and its effects within midwifery care, it may be useful to consider the meaning of the concept of 'sustainability' in order to bring some context to its use in practice. The word has evolved from the Latin word '*sustinere*', which means 'the capacity to endure' (World Commission on Environment and Development, 1987). It appeared in a dictionary as a word as recently as 1972, emerging from the field of ecology. The comprehensive nature of the concept means that it is not easy to pin it down to a 'one size fits all' definition (Vos, 2007). The only consensus on sustainability seems to be that, although there is a huge potential for interface between aspects of the concept and the entities that use it, a shared universal understanding of what sustainability means has not been forthcoming (Ratner & Blake, 2004). The term is, however, generally recognised as representing the three tenets of environmental/ecological, economic and social equity (Bromley & Paavola, 2008). These tenets have been depicted in a variety of ways, including 'pillars' supporting a roof (Fig. 11.1a) and as overlapping circles (Fig. 11.1b).

Within a balanced situation framework where all tenets are considered to be of equal importance, they should theoretically achieve the outcomes of social equity and justice, economic welfare and ecological health (Littig & Grießler, 2005, p. 67). However, critics of the tripartite models have argued that the use of pillars or concentric circles have led to a compartmentalised approach that fails to acknowledge the integrative nature of a sustainable approach.

It has also been proposed that there is an urgent need for greater inclusion of spiritual and cultural tenets, particularly by Indigenous groups (Morgan, 2004). This line of argument suggests that an economy will not flourish without the holistic wellbeing of the community and this wellbeing is reliant on cultural identity (Davies, 2017). Additionally, beyond the social context there is a relationship with the earth's

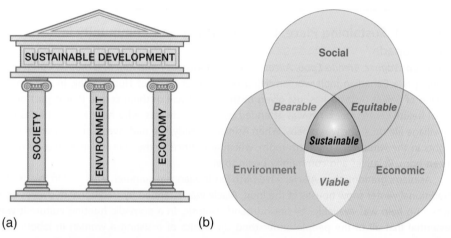

Figure 11.1 *Different ways to consider the concept of sustainability:* (a) 'pillars' supporting a roof; (b) overlapping circles *(Source: (a) http://www.sustainability-ed.org/pages/what3-1.htm; (b) adapted from http://humanhealthimpact.org).*

resources. As explored by Crowther & Hall (2017) in relation to childbirth, 'spiritual' can be construed as a shared and individual sense of purpose and finding meaning in the activities we engage with; it may or may not be related to religion and connection to a sense of 'other' and is associated with holism and wellbeing.

In Box 11.1 midwife Vicki van Wagner and her Inuit colleagues illustrate the concept of sustainability from the experience of midwifery continuity of care in remote Inuit regions of Canada. They highlight the holistic nature of midwifery care and how it can be used as a way of culturally, spiritually and environmentally reclaiming childbirth, thus sustaining the life of communities.

The story in Box 11.1 clearly shows how the values of a community help to integrate and inform the provision of midwifery care in a community: an approach that is based on values rather than being economically based (Morgan, 2004). Indigenous models often depict a more holistic perspective. The concentric model in Fig. 11.2 integrates these values and principles in a New Zealand Māori cosmological worldview—one that offers a philosophical representation of human relationships with the earth, based upon a perspective that is participative and equitable.

Aspects of the Māori worldview have been incorporated into mainstream New Zealand culture and this is apparent in maternity care. The three mainstays of Māori culture—partnership, participation and protection—are explicitly woven into the midwifery model of care, which is embedded in continuity of care. Although this is a model specific to New Zealand, there are resonances for midwifery in other Indigenous cultures, as identified in Box 11.2 where Deanna Stuart-Butler describes a service for Aboriginal women in South Australia that has grown from strength to strength. She highlights the importance of non-Indigenous people embracing 'cultural

BOX 11.1 Sustaining Place, Culture, History and Community in Inuit Canada

Vicki Van Wagner, Brenda Epoo, Aileen Inukpuk Moorhouse and Kim Moorhouse, Canada

Asiniaq is a Canadian Inuit woman living on the east coast of Hudson Bay, in the remote village of Salluit. Asiniaq has just given birth in the small birthing centre that is part of the local health centre. Her birth was attended by local midwives, who have known her as part of village life since she was a baby. When Asiniaq is ready, the midwives turn on a set of small lights in the window of the birth room, which announce to the community that a baby has been born. Relatives and community begin to visit.

Asiniaq's grandmother, Alacie, gave birth 'on the land' in summer tents and in igloos, the traditional winter snow houses of the Inuit. Alacie was attended by traditional midwives and, when no help was available, by her husband Paulosie. In a nomadic hunting culture it was essential that all of the people understood the basics of assisting a woman in labour and helping at a birth.

When Asiniaq's mother, Elisapee, gave birth the people had moved into villages and local priests and teachers had forbidden traditional healing. Midwifery and traditional healing had gone underground and people feared the power of the authorities. Elisapee's first birth was in the nursing station, staffed by nurses with midwifery training. She was also attended by her Aunt Minnie, the local midwife. Despite the lack of respect for her skills, Minnie continued to go with women in labour and provide suggestions and support in Inuit, which the nurses could not speak. When Elisapee gave birth to Asiniaq several years later she was flown 'south' to a hospital staffed with physicians, where none of the caregivers spoke her language. According to the authorities, babies were no longer to be born in the village. Elisapee waited weeks for labour to begin, worried about her children and her husband back in the village. She was disoriented being away from home and community, her language and traditional foods and was frightened in the big city. She cried with loneliness and called out for her mother and aunt as she laboured alone in the hospital.

For her next child, Elisapee refused to leave the village. The nurse in the nursing station had no experience with birth and threatened her and told her that the baby might die. She quietly but strongly refused to leave and trusted in her body and the advice of the elders. When talk of bringing birth back to the communities began in the villages of the Hudson Coast, Elisapee joined the local women's group and the work to reclaim Inuit midwifery and local birth. Minnie began to teach traditional ways to the young women who wanted to learn. The young midwives learned both traditional and southern ways to help at births.

Now Asiniaq has given birth in the birth centre that her mother fought to establish, with her mother and her great aunt beside her. The midwives who attend her not only know her, but also know her language and her culture.

In the remote communities of the Inuit regions of Canada, where local activism has returned birth and midwifery to the communities, continuity of care also means continuity of place, culture, language and tradition. Continuity of carer flows from reclaiming birth as part of the life of the community. For the Inuit, local birth means continuity not only of your caregiver but also continuity with your family, your language, the land and Inuit history.

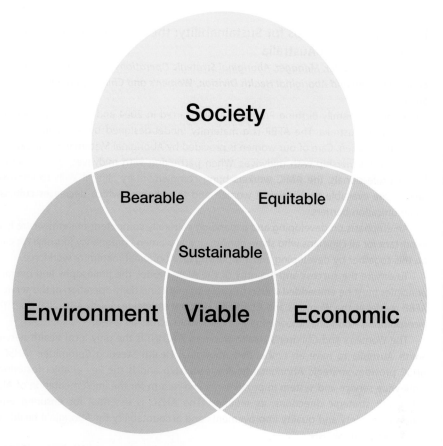

Figure 11.2 *Mauri model of sustainability* (Mauri refers to 'life force' or essence in Te Reo Māori) *(Source: Morgan, 2004* A Tangata Whenua perspective on sustainability using the Mauri model *p. 7).*

humility' as an ongoing tenet of partnerships that promote sustainability and wellbeing for Aboriginal women, their babies and their communities.

MIDWIFERY AND SUSTAINABILITY

It could be inferred that the midwifery profession has many features that affiliate it with sustainability. The endurance and resilience of midwives suggest that midwifery is the ultimate sustainable health care role, having survived as an entity regardless of the oppression and persecution that has been endured over the centuries (Borsay & Hunter, 2012). When mapped against the tenets of sustainability—environmental, economic and social—midwifery continuity of care appears to hold a strong position, as we will explore in the following sections.

BOX 11.2 Partnerships for Sustainability: the Aboriginal Family Birthing Program in South Australia

Deanna Stuart-Butler, Manager, Aboriginal Strategic Operations (Hospital) Women's and Babies' Division and Aboriginal Health Division, Women's and Children's Health Network, South Australia

The Aboriginal Family Birthing Program (AFBP) started in 2004 and is located in seven sites across South Australia. The AFBP is a maternity model designed by Aboriginal women for Aboriginal women. Care of our women is provided by Aboriginal Maternal Infant Care (AMIC) workers in partnership with midwives. When partnering with midwives, doctors and other health professionals, the AMIC workers bring complementary clinical skills to improve the health care available to Aboriginal women and their babies, which decreases cultural and communication barriers.

An emphasis on developing and expanding culturally competent maternity care is vitally important for all clinicians who share our Aboriginal women's pregnancy journey. We can also do this together by developing and supporting an Aboriginal maternity workforce.

To ensure the success and integrity of the AFBP model, the philosophy and overarching principles must be embedded within the development and daily operation of the service. The AFBP model at the Women's and Children's Hospital (Adelaide, South Australia) does this by incorporating Aboriginal knowledge and leadership across all levels.

The Women's and Children's Health Network (WCHN) is the only local health network in South Australia to have an embedded Aboriginal Health Steering Committee (AHSC). The AHSC provides strategic Aboriginal health leadership and is the key enabler fostering network-wide service and system improvements and reform for the implementation of Aboriginal health strategic directions, as required. The AHSC is essential for ensuring effective continuous safety and quality improvements and accountability for Aboriginal health across the whole of the WCHN.

The AFBP is recognised as the evidence-based best-practice model of maternity care for Aboriginal women. It certainly has not been easy to influence change, particularly in addressing the cultural considerations of our women and their families. I'm grateful that I have the opportunity here at the Women's and Children's Hospital as part of my role in partnership with Centre for Education and Training (CET) to facilitate cultural training. In attendance we have 1st, 2nd and 3rd year students from our local universities in Adelaide.

We greatly appreciate the dedication of our non-Aboriginal clinicians—particularly our midwives, as we know they chose this profession because they truly care for women. I have seen first-hand how these midwives always put the women at the centre of their care. All we ask as Aboriginal women is that all midwives reflect on the cultural needs, social complexities and emotional wellbeing of the Aboriginal women at the centre of your care. Please put yourself in her shoes. This is what we like to call 'cultural humility' and we know that cultural humility is a lifelong journey of learning about and being sensitive to cultural differences. We are only too happy to walk with midwives, if they let us.

Environmental

In promoting physiological birth, the midwifery model supports a low resource and minimal intervention approach (Davies, 2017), which reduces consumption and therefore supports the principles of environmental sustainability. Davis (1987) speaks of midwifery as being aligned with natural forces and of midwives being ecologically attuned. She surmises that this should foster an imperative to explore how we can reduce environmental impact by sourcing appropriate assessment tools and by carrying out interventions only when they are required (Davies, 2017). Furthermore, the introduction of sustainability literacy within programs of midwifery education has the potential to promote judicious use of materials in practice, such as replacing disposable materials with more durable and reusable items wherever possible and promoting the importance of low-impact materials for parenting use, such as reusable over disposable nappies (Davies et al., 2011).

Economic

As discussed in Chapter 7 of this book, from an economic perspective midwifery continuity of care potentially offers a less expensive alternative to other forms of care within maternity services and it can be seen as a viable economic model (Tracy et al., 2013). Improved outcomes for mothers and babies related to midwifery-led care are consistent in a range of studies (Dixon et al., 2014; Homer, 2016; Sandall et al., 2016) including where care for low-risk women is provided in homebirth or midwifery-led units (Grigg et al., 2014; Homer et al., 2014; Monk et al., 2014). Conversely, for low-risk women, birth in a tertiary hospital is linked with an increase in a broad spectrum of costly interventions including augmentation of labour, emergency caesarean section and admission to neonatal units (Birthplace in England Collaborative Group, 2011; Davis et al., 2011; Tew, 1995; Tracy et al., 2007). These outcomes are all likely to be less common with midwifery continuity of care.

Social

An approach that embraces a midwifery philosophy of pregnancy and birth as a normal event aligns well with the concept of social sustainability (Davies, 2017), which is commonly described in relation to community, communication and relationships (Barron & Gauntlett, 2002; Leap, 2010; McKenzie, 2004). Within a social model of childbirth, the midwife is expected to support the physical, psychosocial, cultural and spiritual wellbeing of the woman (Davies, 2017); she concerns herself with the social conditions and stresses that might affect the woman and she facilitates relationships in the family and wider community (Kitzinger, 2012). This potentially enables women to resolve fears and concerns (Dahlberg & Aune, 2013; Forster et al., 2016; Huber & Sandall, 2009) in a way that assists them to develop autonomy and a sense of empowerment (Davies, 2017; Leap & Hunter, 2016; Niven, 2013).

Midwives working in midwifery continuity of care could be described as 'social connectors' (Gladwell, 2006)—people who take on a networking role within a community (Leap, 2010). They engage within a broad spectrum of social, cultural, professional and economic circles and facilitate connection within these communities, involving other health professionals and agencies where appropriate, thus building social capital or capacity (Crowther et al., 2018). The term 'social capital' refers to the effective functioning of the networks of relationships among people who live and work together in communities. This is a familiar role in midwifery that has been played out globally and across time and space. By negotiating care with women, encouraging active involvement of other family members and 'facilitating the eco-niche of the mother/baby dyad' (Davies, 2017, p. 190), the midwife acts as a catalyst for social connection.

PROTECTING, PRESERVING AND PROMOTING THE 'ECO-NICHE'

Within sustainable midwifery continuity of care, the midwife is able to support the development of the mother–baby dyad by protecting, preserving and promoting the 'eco-niche' (Davies et al., 2011). An eco-niche is defined as an area within a habitat that is occupied by an organism (Vandemeer, 1972). The mother–baby dyad delivers an ecosystem that meets the baby's needs within a feedback loop system. A midwifery continuity of care model that enables a midwife to foster a holistic and relational approach with a woman is likely to provide emotional sustenance for the mother in a way that transcends the monitoring and surveillance role of contemporary technocratic maternity care (Kitzinger, 2012). When a woman feels safe and nurtured emotionally during pregnancy, her baby is more likely to flourish (Leclère et al., 2014; Odent, 1999).

Studies have demonstrated that early attachment with her/his mother offers the baby a strong foundation for forming relationships for the rest of its life (Grossmann et al., 2006). The ability to form strong social bonds and relationships is viewed as being highly significant in the context of achieving wellbeing and it would seem that people who readily form relationships are, broadly speaking, healthier and happier (Layard, 2011; Wood et al., 2013; Youngson, 2014). This in turn should encourage the development of a more balanced and less individualistically focused society. It is likely that the relationality fostered within a midwifery continuity of care framework will mean that both midwives and the women for whom they are caring will be more likely to thrive emotionally. These relationships in turn help those within them to feel safe (physically and emotionally), feel seen, feel understood and feel loved. In other words, how we birth and how we are born matters.

A key element in protecting, preserving and promoting the 'eco-niche' is holism. The concept of 'holistic' is characterised by the 'belief that the parts of something are intimately interconnected and explicable only by reference to the whole' (Oxford Dictionary, 2018). Where there is relational continuity of care, midwives can potentially work with women to address their individual psychological, social, cultural and spiritual needs within a holistic framework that incorporates awareness of the wider contributing issues associated with ecological health, social equity and economic welfare.

MIDWIFERY CONTINUITY OF CARE AND THE CHALLENGES OF NEOLIBERALISM

At this point it is important to acknowledge the significant challenge presented to providing sustainable midwifery continuity of care within the current complexity of the social and political realities in which midwives practise and women give birth. Like all areas of health care, midwifery is influenced and embedded with the sociopolitical constructs of the day. We argue that midwifery has been significantly impacted by the ideological concept of neoliberalism and the values of the free market, and that this militates against a sustainable framework for practice (Cervantes, 2013; Klein, 2014; Kumi et al., 2013; Sandall et al., 2009).

Neoliberalism

Neoliberalism is based on the belief that wellbeing is most likely to be achieved by encouraging free markets, free trade, strong private property rights and individual entrepreneurialism within an institutional framework (Harvey, 2005; Stegar & Roy, 2010). People are held to account for their own wellbeing and self-management, and welfare provision is considered inappropriate and too expensive (Beck & Beck-Gernsheim, 2002; Sandall et al., 2009). Neoliberal governments therefore work to establish streamlined health care systems based around a business model. Approaches such as strategic planning, risk management strategies, performance-based targets and cost–benefit analyses are borrowed from the worlds of industry and commerce and are designed to encourage market-based behaviour within publicly funded health care facilities. This invariably impacts on high-needs schemes and projects that do not aim for monetary success or attract a business focus—such as midwifery continuity of care projects for women in disadvantaged communities (Homer et al., 2017; Rayment-Jones et al., 2015).

Individualism

A significant constituent within the ideology of neoliberalism is individualism (Watts, 2014). Neoliberalism operates on the principle that most humans will safeguard their own interests before those of others and their environment and in many cases this has led to a societal focus on self. In terms of human development, this self-focus can be considered to be an emergent phenomenon associated with the breakdown of community and social unity (Heron, 2008). It has been argued that individualism has resulted in a separation from a sense of community and has led to what has been described as 'compulsive and obligatory self-determination' (Bauman, 2013, p. 32).

Is midwifery continuity of care sustainable in a culture driven by neoliberalism?

Although we have established that a midwifery continuity of care framework has the potential to provide a good fit for a sustainable model of care, if neoliberalism and the allied concept of individualism have such a strong hold on societal values, including those within health care, is sustainability a realistic aim within the broad sphere of midwifery practice? How can we guarantee endurance within a system that is essentially focused on economic considerations? Does the model of midwifery continuity of care really have the potential to foster the altruism, empathy and community-based values necessary to embed social justice and equity when it is placed within the shadow of neoliberalism? How do we ensure the sustainability of those who are working within the model? In the next section we will consider these challenging questions.

MIDWIFERY CONTINUITY OF CARE AND RESILIENCE

The answer to the questions posed above may lie to some degree in the form of resilience. The introduction of a sustainable approach in any area involves accepting the need for adaptability and change, and the concept of resilience can help us better understand and support this.

It is not unusual for sustainability and resilience theory to be considered synonymous, which has led to the terms being used interchangeably (Crowther et al., 2016). However, this tends to disguise the true nature of resilience, which, like sustainability, arose as an ecological term in the 1980s. Resilience is generally associated with the notion of adjusting to, and recovering from, change by 'bouncing' or 'springing' back into shape (American Psychological Association, 2018). Because the capacity to recover generates from resilience, it tends to be seen as a way of achieving a state of sustainability; in terms of ecology, resilience is embedded within ecosystems. However, in the neoliberal context, the expectation to find resilience tends to be placed in the hands of the individual citizen, who is expected to find reserves of personal strength in adversity; thus resilience is seen as an individual response rather than something being developed as part of a collective (Tainter, 2006).

Crowther et al. (2016) suggest that resilience-building initiatives are often hailed in midwifery as a panacea that can be used to resolve a multitude of difficulties in practice, by encouraging midwives to 'toughen up' in workplace settings that are 'socially, economically and culturally challenging' (p. 47). The concept of resilience may also be used to isolate individual winners and losers in a workplace setting. This is particularly pertinent in workplace settings that are characterised by dysfunctional and less than collegial relationships at the interface of care, staff shortages, power differentials, gender inequalities and unrealistic workloads (Catling et al., 2017). The

2016 publication by the World Health Organization (WHO) *Midwives voices, midwives realities* reported findings from a survey of 2500 midwives representing 93 countries; it concluded that social, economic and professional barriers were impacting on the delivery of safe and effective maternity services. In such circumstances, notions of resilience may be reduced to coping strategies aimed at surviving rather than thriving in the workplace.

Studies by Hunter & Warren (2014) and Crowther et al. (2016) suggest, however, that resilience can be experienced much more expansively and collectively, and can include the development of self-awareness and nurturing of self and others. Crowther et al. (2016) also reported that the cultivation of relationships with women and their families and a love for midwifery encourages a sense of self-determination and self-care that enables midwives to transcend the model they are working within in order to provide good-quality, personalised and holistic care.

This understanding of resilience suggests that, even within the context of neoliberalism, midwives are able to achieve ways of working that make their professional role more sustainable. As discussed in previous chapters, a substantial amount of literature available on midwifery continuity of care indicates that there are a number of factors that can be drawn upon to help midwives achieve this including: nurturing a strong sense of professional identity, ensuring self-care, fostering good interprofessional relationships, future proofing the profession within undergraduate and postgraduate education and providing strong models of preceptorship/mentorship for new practitioners. At a broader systems level, sustainability means ensuring that the models are built with a recognition of the importance of endurance and that they can be scaled up without losing the quintessence of sustainability that midwifery continuity of care has to offer (Davies, 2017; Hunter & Warren, 2014).

PROFESSIONAL IDENTITY AND INTERPROFESSIONAL RELATIONSHIPS

Midwives need to have a strong sense of professional identity, at both a personal and a collective level, in order to ensure sustainability. A profession with a strong self-identity is much more likely to build resilience amongst its members and is therefore more likely to be sustainable (Davies, 2017). A midwifery workforce that has a distinct a sense of identity can be expected to: experience greater job satisfaction (Caza & Creary, 2016), provide a better quality of midwifery care (Ferlie et al., 2005) and make fewer referrals and transfers in care, resulting in fewer interventions (Hunter & Segrott, 2014). These enhancements are likely to increase the confidence and improve the experiences of women accessing care (Lothian, 2008; Tracy et al., 2013); they are also likely to relieve pressure on obstetric and neonatal services, thus potentially improving interprofessional and interpersonal relationships. The resulting cost savings (Bartlett et al., 2014; Tracy, 2011, Tracy et al., 2013) might also mean less resource-intensive environments, conferring economic benefits (Martis, 2011). Such changes could also lead to a more sustainable midwifery 'ecosystem' in addition to a more sustainable broader maternity services network.

A caveat lies in the recognition that a strong professional identity can be achieved only when midwives feel empowered and experience real autonomy in their working lives (Davies, 2017). Autonomy is a concept that is central to the definition of a midwife (International Confederation of Midwives (ICM), 2017); however, the level of autonomy a midwife is able to demonstrate is variable and dependent on the practice setting where the midwife is situated; the authority granted by employers; the level and quality of educational preparation, professional regulation and professional association; and midwives' own willingness to accept autonomy. Reassuringly, as described in other chapters in this book, research carried out on midwifery continuity of care in a number of different countries and settings consistently reports an increasing sense of autonomy within the working lives of midwives (Crowther et al., 2016; Davies, 2017; Hunter & Warren, 2014; McAra-Couper et al., 2014; Newton et al., 2014).

The importance of respectful interprofessional working and collaboration has been discussed in Chapter 5. This may be easier to achieve within the framework of midwifery continuity of care than in a more fragmented model—for example, midwives in a New Zealand study spoke of respectful and equal relationships with obstetricians whilst acknowledging that this had taken many years to achieve (Davies, 2017). Through the lens of sustainability, a new egalitarianism based on partnership, not competition for occupational territory, could be used to replace the old vertical system of obstetric control (Gulliland & Pairman, 1995).

Sustainability and the wellbeing of midwives

As discussed in previous chapters, relational continuity would appear to be effective in maintaining emotional wellbeing for midwives, particularly when comparisons are made with midwives working hospital-based shifts (Dixon et al., 2017). Self-sustainability is a key factor in ameliorating potential stress and burnout (Donald, 2012; Wakelin & Skinner, 2007), with protective factors including occupational autonomy, collegial and social support, and the ability to develop meaningful relationships with women (Dixon et al., 2017; McAra-Couper et al., 2014; Sandall et al., 2016). It is becoming evident that, when these factors are present, midwives are able to pull upon their own reserves of resilience that allow them to cope better with stressful situations. According to Crowther (2017), in order to achieve sustainable healthy psychosocial resilience for midwives it is crucial that these factors are continually present. In Box 11.3, Jackie Kitschke, Midwifery Manager of Midwifery Group Practices at the Women's and Children's Hospital in South Australia, outlines strategies that illustrate how this is achieved in practice.

BOX 11.3 Sustaining Midwifery Group Practices

Jackie Kitschke, Midwifery Manager, Women's and Children's Hospital, Adelaide

Our midwifery group practice (MGP) was established in 2004 and has continued to develop over the last 14 years to meet the needs of the women accessing care and the midwives wanting to work in this way.

There was wide consultation across the division in the initial setup, which was vital to enable MGP to articulate into each area of the maternity service. We have developed documents with each area that describes how MGP works in that area. This provides clear communication about the roles of the MGP and ward midwives in relation to the care of women. These documents are revised regularly and updated when new procedures are introduced. This has proven very helpful when there is confusion or disagreement about the role and responsibility of the MGP midwife when women are in the hospital.

We have a detailed 'Ways of working' document that is a living document and updated as required. It is vital in outlining the group norms so everyone is clear what is expected of them and of each other. It covers areas including rosters, annual leave, how long to work, managing inductions of labour, etc. The number of hours midwives work and the considerations around how long to stay, etc., need to be clear with everyone. In my experience, when you have some midwives working harder than others, over time they become exhausted and overwhelmed and want to leave. We reinforce the importance of having your allocated days off to recuperate. One day a week is a non-call day, which is used to catch up on delayed appointments, education, follow up results or recuperate if they have been called in a lot that week.

The most important day of the week is our meeting day on Wednesday. Everyone who is on-call is expected to come unless looking after a woman in labour. We discuss the births from the week (an obstetrician and neonatologist are invited to attend for this), our statistics and any business arising and we have an hour for education including simulations. It is a great opportunity to catch up, have cake, share our learning and get energy from each other. Sometimes we have this meeting in a café for breakfast and schedule a meeting with other MGPs a couple of times a year.

Being visible in the division is important for the sustainability of MGP because even though MGP is in its 14th year it is often misunderstood. We achieve this by being involved in many initiatives, writing articles for the Health Network newsletter, celebrating successes, having representatives on committees and keeping the words 'woman' and 'midwife' on the agenda.

Future proofing the workforce

Education for sustainable professional practice recognises the importance of applying the principles of sustainability to a specific area of practice (Goodman, 2013). Ensuring that new midwives understand the importance of building a strong and resilient midwifery profession is crucial, and this is best achieved at the level of undergraduate education in programs that are fully aligned with midwifery continuity of care models (Sweet & Glover, 2013). Programs that embrace sustainability literacy and endeavour to offer student midwives the opportunity to work within models reflecting the principles of sustainability are best placed to achieve this. This means that the midwifery student is able to experience the joys and challenges of the midwifery continuity of care model at first hand under the guidance of experienced midwives, providing an opportunity to situate students' learning about what it is to be a midwife within a sustainable and holistic context (Gray et al., 2016).

A cultural ecosystem model for midwifery

Sustainability could ostensibly prove to be the missing link that provides a clear rationale for the more widescale implementation of midwifery continuity of care. A cultural ecosystem approach can be used to illustrate this. This approach explores the emotional and psychological wellbeing as well as the physical wellbeing of individuals within their specific cultural setting. It also acknowledges the relationship between the components.

To return to Morgan's Indigenous model of sustainability introduced earlier in the chapter (Morgan, 2004), Fig. 11.3 illustrates how a cultural ecosystems model based

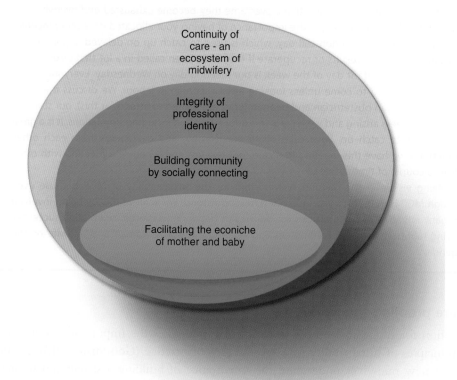

Figure 11.3 *A cultural ecosystem model (Adapted from Davies, 2017 Midwifery: a sustainable health-care profession? PhD thesis. University of Canterbury, Christchurch, NZ).*

on the Māori principles relating to sustainability could be used effectively to link the two spheres of sustainability and midwifery practice, within a context of midwifery continuity of care.

The layers of the model are intersecting yet interdependent. The holistic tenets of the environmental, sociocultural, economic and spiritual integrity coalesce in the ecosystem of midwifery practice provided by continuity of care. However, the ecosystem of midwifery practice will maintain its integrity only if all of these elements are supported. Likewise, 'the 'mother / baby dyad' will only flourish if midwives have a strong sense of their own identity and respectful collegial relationships within the larger network of maternity care' (Davies, 2017, p. 300).

CONCLUSION

Health care professionals are being entreated to recognise the links between sustainability and health and, as we have outlined in this chapter, midwives have a valuable part to play in such a drive for change. A midwifery continuity of care model works on the premise that the underlying philosophy of the midwifery profession supports a community-based primary health service that strengthens family relationships and promotes normal birth This model would appear to support the principles of social sustainability such as equity, social justice and community capacity, as well as addressing resource and economic issues and helping to meet the cultural and spiritual needs of women, their babies and families.

In this chapter we have suggested a cultural ecosystem model, which brings together midwifery (practised within a midwifery continuity of care model) with sustainability. We argue that midwifery continuity of care offers a natural abode for a sustainable approach to midwifery practice that could provide the potential for midwifery to lead the field in sustainable health care.

REFERENCES

American Psychological Association: *The road to resilience*, 2018. Online: http://www.apa.org/helpcenter/road-resilience.aspx.

Barron L, Gauntlett E: Housing and Sustainable Communities Indicators Project, 2002. Online: http://www.regional.org.au/au/soc/2002/4/barron_gauntlett.htm.

Bartlett L, Weissman E, Gubin R, Patton-Molitors R, Friberg IK: The impact and cost of scaling up midwifery and obstetrics in 58 low- and middle-income countries, *PLoS ONE* 9(6):e98550, 2014. doi:10.1371/journal.pone.0098550.

Bauman Z: *Liquid modernity*, Chichester, W. Sussex, 2013, John Wiley & Sons.

Beck U, Beck-Gernsheim E: *Individualization: institutionalized individualism and its social and political consequences*, Thousand Oaks, CA, 2002, Sage / Theory, Culture & Society.

Birthplace in England Collaborative Group: Perinatal and maternal outcomes by planned place of birth for healthy women with low risk pregnancies: the birthplace in England national prospective cohort study, *BMJ* 343:d7400, 2011.

Borsay A, Hunter B: *Nursing and midwifery in Britain since 1700*, London, 2012, Palgrave Macmillan.

Bromley D, Paavola J: *Economics, ethics, and environmental policy: contested choices*, Oxford, 2008, Blackwell.

Catling C, Reid F, Hunter B: The culture of birth in Australia, *Women Birth* 30:21–22, 2017.

Caza B, Creary SJ: The construction of professional identity. In Wilkinson A, Hislop D, Coupland C, editors: *Perspectives on contemporary professional work: challenges and experiences*, Cheltenham, Glos, 2016, Edward Edgar, pp 259–285. Online: https://scholarship.sha.cornell.edu/cgi/viewcontent.cgi?article=1875&context=article.

Cervantes J: Ideology, neoliberalism and sustainable development. human geographies, *J Stud Res Hum Geog* 7(2):25–34, 2013.

Crowther S: Resilience and sustainability amongst maternity care providers. In Thomson G, Schmied V, editors: *Psychosocial resilience and risk in the perinatal period: implications and guidance for professionals*, Abingdon, Oxon, 2017, Routledge, pp 185–200.

Crowther S, Hall J: *Spirituality and childbirth*, Abingdon, Oxon, 2017, Routledge.

Crowther S, Hunter B, McAra-Couper J, Warren L, Gilkison A, Hunter M, et al: Sustainability and resilience in midwifery: a discussion paper, *Midwifery* 40:40–48, 2016.

Crowther S, Deery R, Daellenbach R, Davies L, Gilkinson A, Kensington M, et al: Joys and challenges of relationships in Scotland and New Zealand rural midwifery: a multi-centre study, *Women Birth* 2018. pii: S1871-5192(17)30321-9. doi:10.1016/j.wombi.2018.04.004. [Epub ahead of print].

Dahlberg U, Aune I: The woman's birth experience—the effect of interpersonal relationships and continuity of care, *Midwifery* 29(4):407–415, 2013.

Davies L: Midwifery: a sustainable healthcare profession?, PhD thesis. Christchurch, NZ, 2017, University of Canterbury. Online: https://ir.canterbury.ac.nz/bitstream/handle/10092/14670/Davies%2C%20Lorna%20final%20PhD%20thesis.pdf?sequence=1&isAllowed=y.

Davies L, Daellenbach R, Kensington M: *Sustainability, midwifery and birth*, Abingdon, Oxon, 2011, Routledge.

Davis D, Baddock S, Pairman S, Hunter M, Benn C, Wilson D, et al: Planned place of birth in New Zealand: does it affect mode of birth and intervention rates among low-risk women?, *Birth* 38(2): 111–119, 2011.

Davis E: *Heart and hands*, ed 2, Berkeley, CA, 1987, Celestial Arts.

Dixon L, Prileszky G, Guilliland K, Millar S, Anderson J: Place of birth and outcomes for a cohort of low risk women in New Zealand: a comparison with birthplace England, *NZCOM J* 50:11–18, 2014.

Dixon L, Guilliland K, Pallant JF, Sidebotham M, Fenwick J, McAra-Couper J, et al: The emotional wellbeing of New Zealand midwives: comparing responses for midwives in caseloading and shift work settings, *NZCOM J* 53:5–14, 2017.

Donald H: The work–life balance of the case-loading midwife: a cooperative inquiry, DHSc thesis. Auckland, 2012, University of Technology. Online: http://aut.researchgateway.ac.nz/bitstream/handle/10292/4663/DonaldH.pdf?sequence=3.

Ferlie EL, Wood FM, Hawkins C: The nonspread of innovations: the mediating role of professionals, *Acad Manag J* 48(1):117–134, 2005.

Forster DA, McLachlan HL, Davey M-A, Biro MA, Farrell T, Gold L, et al: Continuity of care by a primary midwife (caseload midwifery) increases women's satisfaction with antenatal, intrapartum and postpartum care: results from the COSMOS randomised controlled trial, *BMC Pregnancy Childbirth* 16:28, 2016.

Gladwell M: *The tipping point: how little things can make a big difference*, New York, 2006, Little, Brown and Company.

Goodman B: Education for sustainability—principles for nursing curricula. Education briefing. Plymouth, 2013, Plymouth University. Online: https://www.academia.edu/3109351/Education_for_Sustainability__Principles_for_nursing_curricula.

Gray J, Taylor J, Newton M: Embedding continuity of care experiences: an innovation in midwifery education, *Midwifery* 33:40–42, 2016.

Grigg C, Tracy SK, Daellenbach R, Kensington M, Schmied V: An exploration of influences on women's birthplace decision-making in New Zealand: a mixed methods prospective cohort within the evaluating maternity units study, *BMC Pregnancy Childbirth* 14:210, 2014. doi:10.1186/1471-2393-14-210.

Grossmann KE, Grossmann K, Waters E: *Attachment from infancy to adulthood: the major longitudinal studies*, New York, 2006, Guilford Press.

Guilliland K, Pairman S: *The midwifery partnership: A model for practice*, Wellington, NZ, 1995, Dept of Nursing and Midwifery, Victoria University of Wellington.

Harvey D: *A brief history of neoliberalism*, Oxford, 2005, Oxford University Press.

Heron T: Globalization, neoliberalism and the exercise of human agency, *Int Int J Polit Cult Soc* 20(1–4): 85–101, 2008.

Homer CSE: Models of maternity care: evidence for midwifery continuity of care, *Med J Aust* 205(8): 370–374, 2016.

Homer CSE, Thornton C, Scarf V, Ellwood DA, Oates JJN, Foureur M, et al: Birthplace in New South Wales, Australia: an analysis of perinatal outcomes using routinely collected data, *BMC Pregnancy Childbirth* 14:206, 2014.

Homer CSE, Leap N, Edwards N, Sandall J: Midwifery continuity of carer in an area of high socio-economic disadvantage in London: a retrospective analysis of Albany midwifery practice outcomes using routine data (1997–2009), *Midwifery* 48:1–10, 2017.

Huber US, Sandall J: A qualitative exploration of the creation of calm in a continuity of carer model of maternity care in London, *Midwifery* 25(6):613–621, 2009.

Hunter B, Segrott J: Renegotiating inter-professional boundaries in maternity care: implementing a clinical pathway for normal labour, *Sociol Health Ill* 36(5):719–737, 2014.

Hunter B, Warren L: Midwives' experiences of workplace resilience, *Midwifery* 30(8):926–934, 2014.

International Confederation of Midwives (ICM): *International definition of the midwife*, 2017. Online: https://internationalmidwives.org/assets/uploads/documents/CoreDocuments/ENG%20Definition_of_the_Midwife%202017.pdf.

Kitzinger S: Rediscovering the social model of childbirth, *Birth* 39(4):301–304, 2012.

Klein N: *This changes everything: capitalism vs. the climate*, London, 2014, Allen Lane / Penguin.

Kumi E, Arhin AA, Yeboah T: Can post-2015 sustainable development goals survive neoliberalism? A critical examination of the sustainable development–neoliberalism nexus in developing countries, *Environ Devel Sustain* 16(3):539–554, 2013.

Layard R: *Happiness: lessons from a new science*, ed 2, London, 2011, Penguin.

Leap N: The less we do the more we give, Ch. 2. In Kirkham M, editor: *The Midwife–mother relationship*, ed 2, London, 2010, Palgrave Macmillan, pp 17–35.

Leap N, Hunter B: *Supporting women for labour and birth: a thoughtful guide*, Abingdon, Oxon, 2016, Routledge.

Leclère C, Viaux S, Avril M, Achard C, Chetouani M, Missonnier S, et al: Why synchrony matters during mother–child interactions: a systematic review, *PLoS ONE* 9(12):e113571, 2014.

Littig B, Grießler E: Social sustainability: a catchword between political pragmatism and social theory, *Int J Sustain Dev* 8(1 / 2):65–79, 2005. Online: https://www.ihs.ac.at/pdf/soz/test2.pdf.

Lothian JA: Choice, autonomy, and childbirth education, *J Perinat Educ* 17(1):35–38, 2008.

McAra-Couper J, Gilkison A, Crowther S, Hunter M, Hotchin C, Gunn J: Partnership and reciprocity with women sustain lead maternity carer midwives in practice, *NZCOM J* 49:29–33, 2014.

McKenzie S: *Social sustainability: towards some definitions*. Working paper no. 27. Magill, 2004, Hawkes Research Institute, University of South Australia. Online: http://naturalcapital.us/images/Social%20Sustainability%20-%20Towards%20Some%20Definitions_20100120_024059.pdf.

Martis R: Good housekeeping in midwifery practice. In Davies L, Daellenbach R, Kensington M, editors: *Sustainability, midwifery and birth*, Abingdon, Oxon, 2011, Routledge, pp 141–155.

Monk A, Tracy M, Foureur M, Grigg C, Tracy SK: Evaluating midwifery units (EMU): a prospective cohort study of freestanding midwifery units in New South Wales, Australia, *BMJ Open Access* 4: e006252, 2014.

Morgan B: *A Tangata Whenua perspective on sustainability using the Mauri model*, 2004. Online: http://www.thesustainabilitysociety.org.nz/conference/2004/Session5/36%20Morgan.pdf.

Newton M, McLachlan H, Willis K, Forster D: Comparing satisfaction and burnout between caseload and standard care midwives: findings from two cross-sectional surveys conducted in Victoria, Australia, *BMC Pregnancy Childbirth* 14:426, 2014.

Niven CA: *Psychological care for families: before, during and after birth*, Oxford, 2013, Butterworth-Heinemann.

Odent M: *The scientification of love*, London, 1999, Free Association Books.

Oxford Dictionary: Holistic definition, 2018. Online: https://en.oxforddictionaries.com/definition/holistic.

Ratner BD, Blake D: 'Sustainability' as a dialogue of values: challenges to the sociology of development, *Sociol Inq* 74(1):50–69, 2004.

Rayment-Jones H, Murrells T, Sandall J: An investigation of the relationship between the case load model of midwifery for socially disadvantaged women and childbirth outcomes using routine data—a retrospective observational study, *Midwifery* 31(4):409–417, 2015.

Sandall J, Benoit C, Wrede S, Murray SF, van Teijlingen ER, Westfall R: Social service professional or market expert? Maternity care relations under neoliberal healthcare reform, *Curr Sociol* 57(4): 529–553, 2009.

Sandall J, Soltani H, Gates S, Shennan A, Devane D: Midwife-led continuity models versus other models of care for childbearing women, *Cochrane Database Syst Rev* (4):CD004667, 2016. doi:10.1002/14651858. CD004667.pub5.

Steger MB, Roy RK: *Neoliberalism: a very short introduction*, Oxford, 2010, Oxford University Press.

Sweet LP, Glover P: An exploration of the midwifery continuity of care program at one Australian university as a symbiotic clinical education model, *Nurse Educ Today* 33(3):262–267, 2013.

Tainter JA: Social complexity and sustainability, *Ecol Complex* 3(2):91–103, 2006.

Tew M: *Safer childbirth? A critical history of maternity care*, ed 2, London, 1995, Chapman & Hall.

Tracy S: Costing birth as commodity or sustainable public good. In Davies L, Daellenbach R, Kensington M, editors: *Sustainability, midwifery and birth*, Abingdon, Oxon, 2011, Routledge, pp 32–44.

Tracy SK, Sullivan E, Wang YA, Black D, Tracy M: Birth outcomes associated with interventions in labour amongst low risk women: a population-based study, *Women Birth* 20(2):41–48, 2007.

Tracy SK, Hartz DL, Tracy MB, Allen J, Forti A, Hall B, et al: Caseload midwifery care versus standard maternity care for women of any risk: M@NGO, a randomised controlled trial, *Lancet* 382(9906): 1723–1732, 2013.

Vandermeer JH: Niche theory, *Annu Rev Ecol System* 3:107–132, 1972.

Vos RO: Defining sustainability: a conceptual orientation, *J Chem Technol Biotechnol* 82(4):334–339, 2007.

Wakelin K, Skinner J: Staying or leaving: a telephone survey of midwives, exploring the sustainability of practice as lead maternity carers in one urban region of New Zealand, *NZCOM J* 37:10–14, 2007.

Watts D: *Dictionary of American government and politics*, Edinburgh, 2014, Edinburgh University Press.

Wood V, Tesser A, Holmes JG: *The self and social relationships*, London, 2013, Psychology Press.

World Commission on Environment and Development: *Our common future*, Oxford, 1987, Oxford University Press.

World Health Organization (WHO): *Midwives voices, midwives realities*, Geneva, 2016, WHO. Online: http://apps.who.int/iris/bitstream/handle/10665/250376/9789241510547-eng.pdf;jsessionid=D2801 F5D2E7D31E23849D052C63E60E5?sequence=1.

Young CM: The experience of burnout in case loading midwives, PhD thesis. Auckland, 2011, University of Technology. Online: http://aut.researchgateway.ac.nz/handle/10292/244720.

Youngson R: Re-inspiring compassionate caring: the reawakening purpose workshop, *J Compassionate Health Care* 1(1):1, 2014. Online: https://jcompassionatehc.biomedcentral.com/track/pdf/10.1186/ s40639-014-0001-0.

CHAPTER 12

Midwifery Continuity of Care and Carer: The Future

Caroline Homer, Pat Brodie, Nicky Leap, Jane Sandall

Contents

INTRODUCTION

What lies ahead in developing and sustaining midwifery continuity of care and carer? The need for vision, creativity and strategic thinking is brought home to us when considering the diversity of: contexts, needs, choices, options, models, practitioners, opinions, beliefs, priorities, philosophies and uncertainties in modern maternity care. Clearly there is much to do, but there is an enormous amount of knowledge, skill and commitment out there as evidenced by many of the research studies, stories and experiences highlighted in this book. We hope you have found the chapters useful in helping you think through your specific context, issues and community while addressing your own opportunities and challenges.

Throughout this book we have shown compelling evidence that midwifery continuity of care can result in: improved outcomes; high levels of satisfaction for women, midwives and others; cost efficiencies; and in some cases savings. We have suggested various ways in which midwifery continuity of care can be provided and, in doing so, have explored definitions and accepted understandings of different organisational frameworks.

There are many ways to provide continuity of care and carer in order to enable women the opportunity to develop a relationship with a known midwife or small group of midwives. Several authors in this book have highlighted this, and have emphasised the need to include women who use maternity services in all phases of planning, implementation and evaluation.

The importance of building collaborative relationships with colleagues has been identified as a major factor when aiming for safe, supportive, sustainable services for women and their families. This particularly applies to developing trusting and respectful interprofessional relationships between midwives and medical colleagues and working in ways that are effective and rewarding. Partnerships with colleagues in community settings are also vital when applying primary health care principles to the development of midwifery continuity of care, especially when addressing issues related to equity and access to services. Some fine examples of how this can work have been provided in this book.

In the wealth of stories provided by contributors from a number of different settings, we hope that you will find ideas that can be adapted for your own context, whether you are practising in a small group practice or developing widespread changes in mainstream maternity service provision. The examples we have provided give an idea of the variety and diversity that exists in the provision of midwifery continuity of care and carer.

Several authors have addressed the challenges and complexity of evaluating midwifery continuity of care. Midwifery continuity of care is a complex intervention and, as such, simple evaluations may not always count the things that matter. Strategies and frameworks for addressing issues have been highlighted. The ultimate sustainability of midwifery continuity of care will be measured by how acceptable, appropriate and beneficial this way of providing care is for midwives and those who work to support safe and effective care; midwifery continuity of care needs to work well for midwives as well as for women.

REFLECTING ON YOUR OWN CONTEXT

Whether you are planning to establish a new service or are reviewing your current model, taking the time to reflect on your context is always helpful. The questions in Box 12.1 may be useful to reflect on what you already have or what you want to change. Working through this with women in your local community is critical to ensure that the service you develop is truly focused on what women want and need.

DEVELOPING FUTURE MIDWIVES

Midwifery continuity of care and carer requires more than just some rethinking of the various ways that care is provided. It also requires innovative approaches to the way in which we prepare future midwives for the challenges that they will no doubt face. We believe that it is now time for a fresh approach and greater creativity and innovation in the midwifery programs that prepare midwives for practice. We need curricula for undergraduate and postgraduate studies that promote and enable innovative thinking and approaches to midwifery practice. It is essential to ensure that students are exposed to midwifery continuity of care and carer from the outset. A

BOX 12.1 Questions to Reflect on Your Situation

- What are the current models or components of your service that are working well?
- What are the current models or components of your service that are not working well?
- Who benefits from the current models of care? Why?
- Who does not benefit from the current models of care? Why?
- What is your vision of an 'ideal' model of care for your setting?
- What are the obstacles in achieving this vision?
- Is there a midwifery continuity of care/carer model that will assist with this vision?
- How might you implement such a model?
- What are the strengths, weaknesses, opportunities and challenges?
- How do you plan to evaluate this model of care?
- How will you address the wider political and policy issues?

number of countries now have this as a requirement in their education standards—see, for example, the Australian Midwifery Accreditation Standards (Australian Nursing and Midwifery Accreditation Council (ANMAC), 2014). Another way to imprint this way of working on our future midwives is to employ students as assistants in midwifery or maternity support workers and place them to work alongside and support midwives providing continuity of carer services. In addition, also required are specific educational programs that address the needs of midwives already working in midwifery continuity of care or who wish to change the way they practise and work with women.

Revised educational and professional development programs will strengthen the foundations of midwifery and see many more midwives practising to their full scope of practice through:

- exploring the philosophy of woman-centred care and what it means for women and midwives
- developing specific skills that enable midwives to promote and protect the principles of 'normal' pregnancy and birth
- understanding primary health care as a system and framework for the organisation of maternity care and social change
- identifying the skills needed to work autonomously as part of a group or team providing continuity of care
- developing skills and structures for collegial support, peer review, critical thinking and interprofessional collaboration
- promoting and utilising evidence-based approaches to care
- strengthening skills that enable interprofessional collaboration and effective working with health system managers, commissioners of services, policy makers and professional leaders

- developing communication, self-care and personal management skills
- developing the political skills that enable midwives to advocate and lobby for adequate midwifery resources so they can fulfil their role.

Women need midwives who are competent and confident with clear vision, political consciousness, energy and passion. Having individual and collective self-confidence will see midwives through the labour of developing new systems and into being able to give birth to midwives, managers, organisations and health systems that are able to encourage and enable midwifery continuity of care and carer to flourish.

RECONCEPTUALISING MATERNITY CARE FOR THE FUTURE

Many countries are facing an imperative to redesign their services based on the evidence, safety and quality of care and to match the expectations of women and communities. The *Lancet* series on midwifery has highlighted the need to develop services based on what women and babies need and not just on what services or organisations are willing to provide (Renfrew et al., 2014; ten Hoope-Bender et al., 2014). It is time to act on this high-level guidance.

The big-picture issues that need to be addressed include workforce shortages, changed working hours and a new working ethic, fiscal challenges of needing to do more with less funding and increased interventions in labour and birth. The workforce of today and tomorrow is changing, with many midwives choosing to work part-time and wanting more flexibility and autonomy than did previous generations.

We need to reconceptualise maternity services and how they are provided. This 'rethink' of systems of health care delivery needs to:

- address priorities for quality care and safety through interdisciplinary collaboration
- be guided by evidence and the importance of translating that into reality
- meet the needs of consumers
- demonstrate cost–benefit, effectiveness and sustainability
- be based on primary health care principles regardless of location
- be mindful of the need to prepare the next generation of a skilled health workforce.

The process requires service providers to engage in strategies that incorporate the needs of those who use maternity services rather than work just from a basis of professional or provider's preferences. Although it is recognised that this is not necessarily easy, given the history of medical and managerial influences in health systems and organisations, it is important if services are to be of the highest quality and to meet the needs of the community. For example, the introduction of community-based maternity services developed as an outreach service attached to a hospital or health service that also provides more specialised obstetric and paediatric care is likely to achieve the goal of improved maternity care outcomes while improving continuity and satisfaction with care (Walsh, 2006).

As shown in this book, the way that midwifery continuity of care and carer is developed will vary according to the specific country and health system; the geographical location of services; the particular population characteristics of the women who use the service; the availability of midwives, general practitioners and obstetricians; and the range of current services already available. The common characteristics of the services in the future are likely to include:

- most women receiving continuity of care and carer from midwives across the antenatal, intrapartum and postnatal periods
- increased provision of maternity care in community settings, including postnatal care in the woman's home
- preparation for parenting and birth in community-based settings where women share ideas, information and experiences in groups facilitated by a midwife, often in collaboration with other health care providers (Department of Health / NCT / One Plus One / Fatherhood Institute, 2011)
- midwives taking responsibility for coordinating care and liaising with other service providers and organisations across hospital and community settings.

How these major characteristics might be applied across a region, city, state or country will require careful thought, detailed planning and extensive consultation before service redesign and implementation. Considerable time should be invested in the development of these planning processes, which should *precede* any change.

We are keen to see mainstream, widespread, 'mass' changes and reform in maternity services. It is essential that midwifery continuity of care and carer should not be seen as 'boutique' or 'exclusive' as this will restrict the potential for it to make a difference to most women. We need to be committed to the scaling up of midwifery continuity of care so that all women, regardless of risk profile, location or health insurance status, have their maternity care provided in this way.

The challenge for all of us interested in improving maternity services is how to achieve change within our current systems. We know that not all midwives want to practise in models of continuity of care, and sometimes their individual circumstances make this impossible. These midwives can be supportive of those who do want to work in new ways by providing effective core services, thus being an important part of the widespread changes that are required and that women are asking for (Gilkison et al., 2017).

Overall, it is worth remembering three overarching factors that will enhance the sustainability of midwifery continuity of care. First described by Jane Sandall in 1997, and equally relevant today, midwives working in successful continuity of care models are able to enjoy the following crucial factors:

- **meaningful relationships with women**—enough continuity through pregnancy, labour and birth and the postnatal period for a two-way, meaningful relationship to evolve

- **occupational autonomy**—the opportunity for midwives to have flexible arrangements regarding how they organise their working lives, including working out on-call arrangements with the colleagues in their MGP or team
- **social support: at home and at work**—this means that midwives meet at least once a week with other midwives in their team or MGP for collegial support to plan work and discuss pressing issues, but also to support each other around any potential uncertainty, overload of work or emotional difficulties that may be affecting their working lives.

CONCLUSION

We hope that this book has given you much to think about as you reflect on the way maternity care is provided in your setting, in particular how you can establish new models of continuity of midwifery care and 'reconceptualise' your own maternity service. Change is an ongoing process and requires energy, commitment and vision. We wish you well in all your endeavours.

REFERENCES

Australian Nursing and Midwifery Accreditation Council (ANMAC): *Midwife accreditation standards*, 2014. Online: https://www.anmac.org.au/sites/default/files/documents/ANMAC_Midwife_Accreditation_ Standards_2014.pdf.

Department of Health/NCT/One Plus One/Fatherhood Institute (Producer): Preparation for birth and beyond. A resource pack for leaders of community groups and activities, 2011. Online: https:// assets.publishing.service.gov.uk/government/uploads/system/uploads/attachment_data/file/215386/ dh_134728.pdf.

Gilkison A, McAra-Couper J, Fielder A, Hunter M, Austin D: The core of the core: what is at the heart of hospital core midwifery practice in New Zealand? *NZCOM J* 53:30–37, 2017.

Renfrew M, McFadden A, Bastos H, Campbell J, Channon A, Cheung N, et al.: Midwifery and quality care: findings from a new evidence-informed framework for maternal and newborn care. *Lancet* 384:1129–1145, 2014.

Sandall J: Midwives' burnout and continuity of care. *Br J Midwifery* 5(2):106–111, 1997.

ten Hoope-Bender P, de Bernis L, Campbell J, Downe S, Fauveau V, Fogstad H, et al.: Improving maternal and newborn health through midwifery. *Lancet* 384:1226–1235, 2014.

Walsh D: Birth centres, community and social capital. *MIDIRS Midwifery Dig* 16(1):7–15, 2006.

Epilogue: Why Midwifery Continuity of Care Matters to Women

Mary Newburn, Maternity Activist, UK

I am delighted to write the Epilogue for this important book, highlighting why mid-wifery continuity of care matters to women, their families and their communities. While it is impossible to do justice to the diversity of women's experiences of birth, there are common threads in women's stories about the difference it can make to their lives when they have a midwife who 'goes on the journey' alongside them through pregnancy, labour and birth, and into new motherhood. I shall include some stories from women I know well to illustrate the profound importance of that relationship, starting with my own story.

In the late 1970s, aged 18, I gave birth to my first child. It was a traumatic experi-ence, one that left me feeling isolated and vulnerable. It was, however, life changing in several positive ways. A kind midwife, whom I had never met before, 'delivered' me from the pain and terror I had been experiencing when she spoke the words that I have never forgotten: 'Come on, we can do this'. By connecting with me and talking about the two of us solving the problem together, I found new reserves. The psychological power of partnership is huge.

When I was pregnant with my second child, I attended antenatal classes with the National Childbirth Trust (NCT). This meant that, for my second birth, I had lots of practical labour preparation skills to draw on. My experience of this birth was transformative and, within a year or so, I started training to be an antenatal teacher for the NCT.

By the time I had my third child, I was a different woman in many ways. I was in a different relationship and I had been to college and to university. I had taken modules in the Sociology of Health and Women's Studies and been employed by the NCT at its national office in London for several years. I knew quite a lot about midwifery care and different options for birth. I had heard Caroline Flint, the celebrated author of *Sensitive Midwifery,* speak at study days. She was a pioneering midwifery leader, articulating the value of midwifery continuity of care and leading a randomised controlled trial of a project called 'Know Your Midwife'.

With my third child, I wanted a homebirth—I came from a family of home-birthers—but my GP didn't like the sound of that at all. I was determined to organise care from someone I wouldn't need to educate, persuade, argue with, put up with or defend myself against. I wanted to have care from someone who had read the evidence that I had read and who would share, or at least respect, my values and beliefs—someone who would understand what this was all about for me, and who would feel confident and comfortable in supporting me.

I needed continuity of care from a midwife who would be a constant, going on the journey with me, and sharing my delight in how the baby would grow and snuggle in for birth. I wanted a midwife who would get to know my passions and wishes—for example, my strong feeling that it should be my prerogative to be the first to touch and cradle my baby. Midwifery continuity of care was not available on the NHS where I lived and so I decided to find an independent midwife.

I subsequently gave birth at home and it was a profoundly special experience for me and Tim, and a family event for my mum and other children. Everything was on our terms. We were at the centre of the experience. The beauty of observing and enjoying the physiological process unfold was extraordinary. Like a flower bud waiting to bloom, my pregnancy continued to 10 days beyond 40 weeks. Labour was slow at first and then came on rapidly. I thought I wouldn't be able to cope at one point, but my midwife knew me and believed in me, and I trusted her. Everything was normalised and I never once felt my autonomy was compromised in this joyous experience.

In different ways, the births of each of my children motivated me to become a childbirth activist, coming together with other equally passionate women to try to improve and shape the way maternity services are delivered. Childbirth advocacy also became the focus of my working life as I continued to work for the NCT at national level in a role that spanned 27 years.

Over the years, my work has included: leading the development of evidence-based maternity policy and position statements, editing the NCT professional development journal, commissioning reviews of evidence, facilitating service user involvement in research, and speaking at professional conferences and on TV and radio. More recently, I was a co-investigator on the Birthplace in England cohort study and I have worked with NHS England to develop new guidance for 'patient and public involvement' in NHS maternity services by means of multidisciplinary bodies called Maternity Voices Partnerships (MVPs).

Having worked with women and families around the time of birth for close to 40 years, I know the importance of midwifery continuity of carer. My thinking has been shaped by all of my work over these four decades as well as my personal experiences of maternity care and my study of relevant literature. I know that being able to get to know your midwife and having the same person facilitate your care over time is profoundly important and can make us feel less like small cogs in grossly impersonal machines.

Apart from the growing evidence about improved outcomes associated with midwifery continuity of care—evidence that has been thoroughly discussed in this book—there is a wealth of evidence from individual women's stories to show how a relationship of ongoing care from a midwife matters to women and their families. As examples, three women have agreed for me to share their stories here.

Leigh's Story

Leigh and Robin were living in an Australian city and were very excited about having their first baby. At about 9–10 weeks they booked into a midwifery group practice (MGP) at their local maternity unit for a first visit with one of the two caseload midwives who would be providing their maternity care. Just a week later, Leigh had some vaginal bleeding and was referred to the early pregnancy assessment service (EPAS). She had a nuchal scan and several visits to the EPAS before the bleeding decreased. At 19–20 weeks gestation a subsequent scan identified that there were major problems with restricted growth and a lack of amniotic fluid around the baby; Leigh and Robin were referred to the maternal fetal medicine unit (MFMU) on the same day. The caseload midwife whom they had previously met was with them for this initial consultation as well as all subsequent hospital appointments. Likewise, the same consultant obstetrician saw them several times over the next 2 weeks. The pregnancy did not go well and it became clear that there was never going to be a living baby and that Leigh's own health was at risk from a possible infection.

Leigh and Robin had important decisions to make, which culminated in Leigh being induced. After a long labour, Leigh gave birth to their tiny, lifeless baby, who they named 'Jesse'.

Leigh was cared for throughout most of her labour by her caseload midwives, with other midwives in the midwifery group practice stepping in to relieve them after very long periods. Leigh remembers this as being really important:

'Both of our midwive made every effort to be present for the majority of our time in hospital. I often got the impression that they were doing additional hours beyond their rostered hours / days, such was their dedication to our care. This made the whole ordeal far less impersonal and scary.'

In her second pregnancy, Leigh was not eligible to book with the midwifery group practice because of her history of pregnancy problems and second trimester loss. Instead she had care from staff in the MFMU. When it became clear that her pregnancy was developing normally and that the medical team could step down, Leigh was told that the caseloading team was already fully booked. However, with a bit of help from a senior midwife who knew about Leigh and Robin's previous loss, a caseload midwife was assigned. This was a huge relief.

The weeks passed and Leigh and Robin got to know their caseload midwife, who called on them at home for appointments. They started attending birth preparation classes. The only concern was that their baby was persistently in a transverse position. Weeks passed and the baby did not change position. Leigh and Robin's midwife arranged for them to see an obstetrician who, responding to their wishes, referred them to a specialist in vaginal breech births at another hospital, and an attempt was made to turn the baby. This didn't work. The baby wasn't

Continued

Leigh's Story—cont'd

having any of it. An early planned caesarean birth was arranged (to avoid the risk of cord prolapse if Leigh went into labour).

It wasn't the birth that Leigh or Robin had hoped and planned for, but they took it in their stride. After losing their first baby, they had learned the hard way that the best-laid plans have to be flexible ones, adapting to circumstances. In all of this, their caseload midwife helped them through. She was there for each twist and turn of late pregnancy and planning for the birth, answering questions and alongside them. She was also there to help Leigh establish breastfeeding, daily at first when there were some difficulties and then less often as Leigh became confident and the baby thrived; in the first 6 weeks she was always at the end of the phone.

Both the less common parts of their journey (a transverse baby) and the very common (the highs and lows of getting breastfeeding established) were made safe by having a known midwife quietly working with them, not alarmed, not fussing, showing that all was well and passing on a sense of calm and confidence. They didn't have to keep explaining about their previous loss, or why they'd had an 'elective' caesarean, or later putting on a brave face when the feeding was feeling like a mountain to climb. Very soon, they were finding their feet, enjoying having an extra little person in the family, with breastfeeding now the new normal.

Leigh remembers the difference her midwife made to her experience of pregnancy and new motherhood:

'My caseload midwife became invaluable in supporting us through some difficult decisions in pregnancy, and with the breastfeeding she really came into her own—she was the very best support in the world. She helped every single day for weeks with the breastfeeding and made me feel more relaxed when I was anxious and more confident when I really felt I was struggling. The whole beginning of our journey would have been so much more difficult without her experience, confidence and support.'

Michelle's Story

Michelle was pregnant with her third baby, living in a city in the UK. She had had two caesareans and wanted to have a vaginal birth for her third baby. She knew, from her research online, that NICE guidelines and the Royal College of Obstetricians and Gynaecologists (RCOG) supported this as long as the pregnancy was going well and there were no underlying medical problems. Michelle needed a midwife who would advocate for her and help her make plans. She most definitely did not need a succession of different midwives and obstetricians to whom she had to explain her plans and situation repeatedly. She knew what she wanted, and she soon found out that this was at odds with what her local hospital doctors felt comfortable with. They rejected the NICE and RCOG guidance ('That's not what we do round here … we're not happy with the risks') and attempted to wear her down by repeatedly asking her to come back for extra appointments to discuss plans for the birth.

Michelle's Story—cont'd

Michelle felt that the doctors were always on the lookout for some deviation from normal that would strengthen their negotiating hand and put pressure on her to agree to a third caesarean. Emotionally, this was very difficult for Michelle. She felt that she had to resist the very people she was looking to for care and support. Her husband was wavering. She felt alone and vulnerable, on the brink of defeat.

Late in her pregnancy, Michelle was introduced to a consultant midwife who listened to her and said that what she wanted was perfectly reasonable; she offered to help Michelle to make arrangements for this to happen. The relief Michelle felt was immense. She'd had to contend with the implied suggestion that maybe she wasn't a caring mother who wanted the best for her baby. She stopped thinking she was going mad and that the whole world seemed to be against her.

The consultant midwife established a continuing interest, meeting with her regularly and sharing in the delight that Michelle and her husband felt after Michelle had a normal birth with no complications. This midwife's knowledge, support and continuing personal interest helped to validate Michelle's profound choice that so many had attempted to undermine and criticise. Where others had cast doubt, the consultant midwife stepped forward and acted as an advocate and reinforcer of Michelle's wishes.

Michelle felt empowered and transformed as a woman by her birth experience. She became a childbirth activist and blogger and has organised two 'Women's Voices' conferences, one hosted and funded in part by the RCOG. Michelle is acutely aware that for thousands of other women a supportive relationship with a midwife is not possible. She is passionate about coming together with others to change that: #continuitymatters.

Marie's Story

Marie has had two homebirths with the NHS in England. In her first pregnancy she had great continuity from the homebirth team, which operated a hybrid arrangement of modified caseload midwifery. This meant that Marie had her own named midwife—someone she really connected with who provided most of her antenatal care. Marie felt that this midwife was really positive about homebirth for first-time mothers and that she really believed in her, which built her confidence.

The whole experience was empowering and enjoyable. When Marie went into labour and called the homebirth team, the midwife on-call said that she could come out now or, if Marie was comfortable to wait a short while, her own midwife would be on duty in an hour and could come then. Marie was happy to wait and delighted to have her familiar, trusted midwife with her. The birth was straightforward and very special. However, there was one disappointment: the baby came a bit early while Marie's husband was out of the country. Through the use of Skype he was there to see the birth but it wasn't the same as if Marie could have nestled into his arms, and for him to hold their little one straight away. Marie emphasises that, while

Continued

Marie's Story—cont'd

the philosophy and friendly approach of her midwife seemed to be shared by all the other midwives in the homebirth team, it was lovely to have the midwife she knew best to be helping her to birth her baby.

In her second pregnancy, although she had not moved house, an NHS reconfiguration of community services meant Marie had to arrange for care with a different NHS trust. This time there was no midwifery continuity of care. Marie's second labour was going well until the midwife arrived. She wasn't the easiest person for Marie to work with. She wasn't encouraging and didn't seem relaxed or confident. Marie had hardly met her before and she seemed a bit jumpy. In the second stage the midwife said there were decelerations and Marie needed to push for all she was worth, whereas the first time she had breathed the baby out easily and serenely. The baby was born in robust health, breathing immediately, but because an ambulance had been called there were paramedics in the doorway. It wasn't the peaceful family birth she'd anticipated. Marie accepted Syntocinon, on the midwife's advice, but soon had a retained placenta, requiring transfer to hospital for a manual removal.

Marie is very sure that it made a real difference in her first pregnancy and labour having a midwife whom she knew well, someone who had belief in her and confidence in the physiological process of labour. This took away any anxiety of the unknown and allowed her to relax and give birth with ease. She feels the difference was tangible and now believes she must make her voice heard so that other women in the UK are able to have really high-quality midwifery continuity of carer within the NHS.

Each of these stories is an example of how connections are built over time and through developing conversations: situations where a woman and her midwife can get to know one another better, forging a trusting relationship. Gradually, they will formulate and revise plans, making adjustments along the way to respond to the woman's history and values, the midwife's professional responsibilities and the changing circumstances and needs of the woman, her baby and family. It should be said, though, that if it doesn't feel like the right fit there should always be an opportunity to ask for another midwife.

A midwife who believes that a woman is making sensible choices gives a woman a precious gift. This is an especially valued gift if the woman has previously experienced pregnancy complications and may have struggled against an impersonal or rigid maternity care system. Feeling understood and validated can be life changing for many women.

I finish with an appreciation of midwives. A wise and kind midwife will listen well, provide evidence-based information and offer gentle guidance if and when it is needed. She will advocate for a woman even if she would not make the same choices herself; this can facilitate profound positive changes in a woman's life. I want to acknowledge that this can happen in situations where midwives are not able to provide continuity of care.

Midwifery continuity of carer, however, offers the ideal situation for the building of a relationship with a focus on: intelligent listening, developing empathy and positive regard, and providing respectful, competent, woman-centred care. Having some accumulated knowledge of the woman and her pregnancy, her family and her history facilitates the midwife's understanding. Appreciation of this nuanced knowledge enables her to provide individualised care, tailored by a unique combination of understanding who the woman is, how her pregnancy is developing and what she and her family value.

We need more midwifery continuity of carer, for more women, in more countries. Please do what you can to be the change that many of us want to see in the world.

GLOSSARY

Collaboration A dynamic, active process that leads to a purposeful relationship based on the need to either solve a problem or create something. Health care collaborators in maternity care include midwives, doctors, students, allied health workers and students.

Consumers Users of maternity services.

Core midwives Midwives within a maternity unit who are not working in midwifery continuity of care. Core midwives are usually based in one clinical area (antenatal, labour and birth, or postnatal).

GP shared care When a woman's pregnancy care is shared between a hospital maternity unit and a GP.

Independent midwife A person authorised to practise midwifery in their country, who works privately and independently of a hospital or health service. See also Midwife in private practice.

Lead maternity carer 'Lead maternity carer (LMC)' is a term used in New Zealand. It refers to the person who has overall responsibility for ensuring that the care provided to the woman throughout her pregnancy, labour and birth, and early postnatal period is appropriate, safe and effective, based on her identified needs and individual situation. The LMC ensures that care of the woman and her baby is seamless across the interface between community-based health services and acute care, as well as other agencies and the general practitioner.

Mainstream maternity services Maternity services provided for the majority of women in publicly funded facilities.

Medicare The Australian system of universal health insurance, which is funded by revenue raised through a compulsory levy and taxes. Medicare provides access to public hospital services for all Australians through a negotiated payment to state governments. Medicare also supports access to general practitioners and specialist services including pathology, X-ray and ultrasound.

Midwife The International Confederation of Midwives (2017) defined a midwife as 'A person who has successfully completed a midwifery education program that is based on the ICM Essential Competencies for Basic Midwifery Practice and the framework of the ICM Global Standards for Midwifery Education, and is recognised in the country where it is located, who has acquired the requisite qualifications to be registered and/or legally licensed to practice midwifery and use the title 'midwife', and who demonstrates competency in the practice of midwifery.' (See also **Scope of practice**.)

Midwife in private practice A person authorised to practise midwifery in their country who works privately and independently of a hospital or health service. See also Independent midwife.

Midwifery caseload practice In midwifery caseload practice, each midwife has a defined number (caseload) of women per year for whom she is the primary or named midwife. She is the first point of contact for each woman and takes responsibility for overseeing her care, and organising consultation and referral as necessary. She provides continuity of carer throughout the antenatal, labour and birth and postnatal periods, with backup from another midwife or small group of midwives who work together.

Midwifery continuity of care Care provided by a small group of midwives whom the woman is able to get to know throughout her pregnancy, labour and birth, and the postnatal period.

Midwifery continuity of carer Care throughout pregnancy, labour and birth, and the postnatal period by a midwife or midwives whom the woman feels she has developed a 'relationship' with and believes she 'knows'.

Midwifery group practice Small groups of midwives (usually four to six) working in a midwifery caseload practice model. Each midwife has her own caseload of women for whom she is the primary midwife and one or more midwives in the midwifery group practice will be identified as backup or second midwife for each woman.

Midwifery models of care Models of maternity services in which midwives are the primary caregivers. These services may include midwife clinics, community midwifery, team midwifery, independent midwifery and birth centres.

Ottawa Charter A charter developed by the World Health Organization in 1986; it recognises that improvement in health requires a secure foundation in a number of basic prerequisites including advocacy, enabling and mediation. Health promotion action was defined as including building healthy public policy, creating supportive environments, strengthening community action, re-orientating health services and developing personal skills.

Postnatal period A period defined by the World Health Organization as extending from 1 hour after the delivery of the placenta until the first 6 weeks after giving birth.

Primary carer The main or first contacted health professional who takes responsibility for coordinating and/or providing all necessary health care required by a woman through pregnancy, labour and birth, and early parenting.

Primary health care An approach to health care that encompasses equity, access, provision of services based on need, community participation, collaboration and community-based care. Primary health care involves using approaches that are affordable, appropriate to local needs and sustainable.

Publicly funded maternity services Maternity services that are funded through a national health system and are available to women at no cost.

Public health An expression used to encapsulate the aims and methods of all whose concern it is to protect and promote the health of all citizens in the interests of both each individual and society as a whole. It includes health promotion activities, disease prevention programs and the treatment of illness as well as care of those who are disabled or disadvantaged. A public health perspective in midwifery is one that explicitly acknowledges the impact of an individual woman's social, economic and psychological life, as well as her personal behaviour, on her health. For midwives this means effective care must focus on the wider context within which each woman's pregnancy occurs, if we are to maintain and improve outcomes for mothers and babies.

Risk management A process of assessing risks and developing strategies to coordinate the prevention and management of those risks.

Scope of practice According to the International Confederation of Midwives (2017), 'the midwife is recognised as a responsible and accountable professional who works in partnership with women to give the necessary support, care and advice during pregnancy, labour and the postpartum period, to conduct births on the midwife's own responsibility and to provide care for the newborn and the infant. Midwifery care includes preventive measures, the promotion of normal birth, the detection of complications in mother and child, the accessing of medical care or other appropriate assistance and the carrying out of emergency measures. The midwife has an important task in health counselling and education, not only for the woman, but also within the family and the community. This work should involve antenatal education and preparation for parenthood and may extend to women's health, sexual or reproductive health and child care. A midwife may practise in any setting including the home, community, hospitals, clinics or health units.'

Team midwifery Care provided by a small team of midwives who are employed in a maternity unit. The midwives in the team share responsibility for providing antenatal, intrapartum and postnatal care for all the women who are allocated to the model of care.

Woman-centred care A concept that implies that midwifery care:

- is focused on the woman's individual unique needs, expectations and aspirations, rather than the needs of the institutions or professions involved
- recognises the woman's right to self determination in terms of choice, control and continuity of care from a known or known caregivers

- encompasses the needs of the baby, the woman's family, her significant others and community, as identified and negotiated by the woman herself
- follows the woman across the interface between institutions and the community, through all phases of pregnancy, birth and the postnatal period, therefore involving collaboration with other health professionals when necessary
- addresses the woman's psychological, spiritual and cultural needs and expectations.

INDEX

Page numbers followed by '*f*' indicate figures, '*t*' indicate tables, '*b*' indicate boxes.